THE Natural Health
GUIDE TO
BEATING THE
SUPERGERMS

This handy book offers a wealth of safe, proven natural methods to help you boost your immunity against the diseases caused by supergerms, and achieve greater overall health.

Did You Know That . . .

- Infectious diseases are the third leading cause of death in the United States

- Antibiotics suppress rather than enhance your ability to fight infections

- Aspirin and acetaminophen can encourage antibiotic resistance in bacteria, leading to more virulent strains

- Yogurt, cheese, sauerkraut, dill pickles, soy sauce, and wine contain good bacteria that help inoculate the digestive tract naturally

- Unlike conventional antibiotics, garlic can kill some viruses, including herpes simplex, parainfluenza (which causes respiratory illness in children), and rhinovirus (which causes the common cold)

- Herbs such as echinacea, goldenseal, barberry root bark, and elderberry can work to boost your immunity

- Selenium, an essential dietary nutrient, can actually prevent some viruses from mutating

- Vitamin C is one of the most inexpensive and effective supplements you can take to achieve optimal health.

THE Natural Health GUIDE TO BEATING THE SUPERGERMS

and Other Infections, Including Colds, Flus, Ear Infections and Even HIV

USE VITAMINS AND NUTRIENTS
TO TURN YOUR BODY
INTO THE ULTIMATE GERM KILLER

Richard P. Huemer, M.D.,

AND

Jack Challem

With the Editors of *Natural Health* Magazine

POCKET BOOKS
New York London Toronto Sydney Tokyo Singapore

The ideas, procedures, and suggestions in this book are intended to supplement, not replace, the medical advice of trained professionals. All matters regarding your health require medical supervision. Consult your physician before adopting the medical suggestions in this book as well as about any condition that may require diagnosis or medical attention.

An *Original* Publication of POCKET BOOKS

POCKET BOOKS, a division of Simon & Schuster Inc.
1230 Avenue of the Americas, New York, NY 10020

Library of Congress Cataloging-in-Publication Data

Huemer, Richard P.
  The natural health guide to beating the supergerms and other
infections, including colds, flus, ear infections and even HIV : use
vitamins and nutrients to turn your body into the ultimate germ
killer / Richard P. Huemer and Jack Challem; with the editors of
Natural health magazine.
    p. cm.
Includes index.
ISBN: 0-671-53764-4
  1. Communicable diseases—Alternative treatment. 2. Drug
resistance in microorganisms. 3. Dietary supplements.
4. Naturopathy. I. Challem, Jack. II. Natural health.
III. Title.
RC112.H78 1997
615.5—dc21   96-29498
                                                        CIP

First Pocket Books trade paperback printing May 1997

10 9 8 7 6 5 4 3 2 1

POCKET and colophon are registered trademarks of
Simon & Schuster Inc.

Cover design by Tai Lam Wong
Text design by Stanley S. Drate/Folio Graphics Co. Inc.

Printed in the U.S.A.

*This book is dedicated
to the health of you,
our readers.*

ACKNOWLEDGMENTS

───────────── ✿ ─────────────

A great many people contributed in small and large ways to this book.

Mark Bittman and Chris Kimball, publisher of *Natural Health* magazine, were instrumental in making this book happen. Claire Zion was astute enough to see the book's potential and helped us simplify many of the technical passages. Danielle Dayen provided many comments that further shaped the book. Shelly Perron's fine copyediting was invaluable, and we are indebted to Amelia Lee Sheldon, an editor whose enthusiasm and effort carried this book through to publication.

Dr. J. P. Kilbourn, director of the Consulting Clinical and Microbiological Laboratory, Portland, Oregon, carefully reviewed and commented on our chapters on microorganisms. Victoria Dolby gracefully accepted the challenge of reading the manuscript and offered valuable comments on each chapter. Other people who contributed in various ways include Alan Bennett, Susan Carlson, Sandi Doughton of the Tacoma *News Tribune,* Charlie Fox, David and Tricia Koon, Dr. Peter Montague of the Environmental Research Foundation, Malcolm Novar, Dr. Lendon Smith, Carrie Swadener of NCAP, and Timothy Triche Jr.

We also must acknowledge the pioneering contributions of Stuart B. Levy, M.D., and Marc Lappé, Ph.D., who were among the first to sound public alarms about the dangers of antibiotic abuse.

Finally, we would, of course, also like to thank our significant others for their patience during the course this project.

CONTENTS

Part III

DEFEND YOURSELF
AGAINST SUPERGERMS

INTRODUCTION

❧

In Seattle, a virulent strain of *E. coli* bacteria at fast-food restaurants kills three children and hospitalizes hundreds of other people. In New York and London, strep-A attacks people by literally eating away at their flesh. In Chicago, tuberculosis is on the rise after once being all but eradicated. In Portland, Oregon, an eerie and deadly strain of meningococcal disease snuffs out the lives of toddlers and teenagers within a day. In Arizona and New Mexico, a previously unknown strain of hantavirus kills dozens of people.

Cholera in Rwanda. Plague in India. Dengue fever in South America. Ebola in Africa. Diphtheria in Russia. Virus mutations in China. A horse virus killing people in Australia. Lyme disease in New England. Parasites in Milwaukee's drinking water. Rabies in Texas. Tuberculosis on airplanes. And, of course, AIDS.

What's happening? Brace yourself for a shock. Bacterial infections, once easily cured with penicillin and other antibiotics, have returned with a vengeance. And the problem isn't just related to bacteria. New strains of viruses, such as those that cause AIDS (acquired immunodeficiency syndrome), cannot be treated with antibiotics—and mutate too quickly for a vaccine to be effective. These *supergerms* are the ultimate moving target, outpacing medicine at almost every step.

Are supergerms hyperbole? A wild idea fanned by newspaper headlines, tabloid TV, and science fiction? We wish that were the case. Supergerms are *very* real. Although we use the term supergerm to describe many life-threatening germs, the idea is based on the medical concept of a *superinfection*—an infection by bacteria impervious to medicine's most powerful antibiotics.

As we approach the twenty-first century, these supergerms are often tougher and more lethal than just about any other microorganism in the history of the world. Even the more common germs, such as those causing colds and flus, pack more of a wallop than they did in the past—and may be next year's supergerms.

Collectively, infectious diseases, including supergerms, have become the fastest growing health menace today. But, you must be wondering, didn't medicine trounce infectious diseases years ago?

Yes. And no.

Worldwide, infectious diseases have always been the number one cause of death. While the leading killers in the United States are heart disease and cancer, infectious diseases are actually one of the leading and fastest growing causes of death. Infections account for one-fourth of all visits to doctors.

How did we get into this predicament? A number of events have led to the emergence of supergerms.

- The excessive use of antibiotics has encouraged the spread of bacteria immune to these powerful drugs. These bacteria are easily spread through day care centers and hospitals.
- The use of antibiotics in livestock has compounded the problem. People often consume antibiotic-resistant bacteria in the food they eat.
- Nutritional deficiencies in people trigger the mutation of at least one virus and likely others. These mutations turn a relatively mild virus into a deadly supergerm, and researchers think new flu germs are created the same way.
- Aggressive deforestation, particularly in tropical rain forests, have brought people into contact with deadly, previously unknown viruses, such as AIDS and Ebola.
- Commercial air travel enables people to spread serious infections around the world in less than a day.

But the questions that kept occurring to us—a physician and a health journalist—as we investigated this issue boiled down to these: why are people suddenly so vulnerable to these supergerms? And what can we do about them?

Unfortunately, physicians and researchers tend to study people who get sick instead of those who stay well. For example, until recently, researchers pretty much ignored long-term AIDS survivors. In doing so, they overlooked important dietary and lifestyle clues that explain why some people stay well instead of get sick.

On your own, you've probably wondered why one person catches a cold, but another does not? Why *E. coli* kill one child who eats tainted meat, but only gives another an upset tummy? Or why 80 percent of the people infected with the Ebola virus die, but 20 percent miraculously live to tell about it?

In a sense, asking those questions puts you a step ahead of many researchers, who have a habit of overanalyzing problems instead of exploring potential solutions. For example, in January 1995 the *Journal of the American Medical Association* joined thirty-five other medical journals in twenty-one countries in simultaneously writing about the growing threat of supergerms and other infectious diseases.

Yet hardly a word was written about the role of people's inborn defenses against germs. That's unfortunate. We believe a big part of the solution is surprisingly simple: *the body's immune system, which guards against infections, works better in some people than in others.*

Why? To some extent, immunity is defined by heredity. If your parents had good immunity, you probably do too.

But there's another important reason: *your immunity can be strengthened or weakened by a variety of lifestyle factors, particularly how and what you eat.*

Does this really seem like such a far-fetched idea? Not at all. Like most people, you probably know that you're more likely to get sick when you're under a lot of stress or don't eat right.

Additional support for the relationship between diet and

immunity comes from researchers, who now see the growing incidence of cancer as a consequence of poor diet and exposure to toxic pollutants. This link is significant because cancer serves as a barometer of immune health, and healthy immune systems attack cancer cells very much the way they attack bacteria. When the incidence of cancer goes up in a group of people, it's a sign that immune competence has gone down. And when immune competence decreases, people become more susceptible to all manner of disease, including infectious diseases.

Over the past fifty years, the same factors that have increased our susceptibility to cancer have also increased our susceptibility to supergerms and other infections. For example, the nutritional quality of the American diet has declined, reducing our consumption of many vitamins and minerals—essential nutritional building blocks of immunity. Excessive consumption of sugary foods compounds the problem because they reduce the ability of white blood cells to fight infections.

In addition, thousands of hazardous chemicals have been added to the food supply and environment over the past five decades, increasing the burden on these weakened immune systems. For example, many of the pesticides sprayed on fruit and vegetables are known to cause cancer, but these same pesticides also impair the immune system's ability to fend off dangerous microorganisms. Perhaps even more disturbing, many common drugs, including antibiotics and pain relievers, also depress the body's ability to fight infections.

So how can you, or anyone else, strengthen your immune system to better your odds against a supergerm—or even a run-of-the-mill germ?

The key is achieving *optimal immunity*. In the pages that follow, we describe the origins and nature of supergerms and propose ways to enhance your immune system—your first line of defense against supergerms and other infections. We explain how to easily avoid antibiotics in meat and immune-depressing pesticides in produce.

Perhaps most importantly, we relate solid scientific research on specific nutrients—including vitamins A and C, selenium, and vitaminlike coenzyme Q_{10}—that can prime your immune system. We explain how garlic and other foods work as natural antibiotics and how fermented foods, such as yogurt and sauerkraut, reinforce your body with armies of "good" bacteria to combat the bad ones.

We also provide guidelines relating to simple hygiene, such as washing your hands, properly handling and cooking foods, and wisely taking prescribed antibiotics. Finally, we provide a list of references, most of which are scientific articles, and a list of resources to help you put all this information into practice. It's our prescription to defend yourself against supergerms and other infections.

JACK CHALLEM
The Nutrition Reporter™
Beaverton, Oregon

RICHARD P. HUEMER, M.D.
Medik Research, Inc.
Vancouver, Washington

Part I

❊

SUPERGERMS:
THE DEADLY
THREAT

❊

The world's airports went on "red alert" when the Ebola epidemic erupted in Kikwit, Zaire, in May 1995. Immigration and customs officials, who typically search for undeclared purchases and illegal drugs, scrutinized passengers for signs of unusual illness. An African passport or itinerary was often enough to justify temporary detention and a medical exam.

But people reading their newspapers and watching television in the comfort of their homes knew that deadly viruses and bacteria could not be identified by baggage checks and X-ray machines, which can so easily spot guns. As distant as that Ebola outbreak was, the average person wondered whether this supergerm would be carried by a passenger on a commercial flight to London, Paris, New York . . . or to their town or city. Luckily, this time, it did not. We were not so lucky in the 1980s, when AIDS emerged from Africa.

The supergerm threat to most Americans, however, is much closer and more immediate than that of Ebola. Supergerms may be in the food you eat, the day care center your child attends, the hospital you trust your life to—and the air you breathe. Sometimes, supergerms erupt as brief but deadly outbreaks, like *E. coli* or the so-called flesh-eating bacteria. Most often, they seem to strike in unpredictable ways.

The threat is very real. And very close to home.

1

MICROBIAL MYSTERIES

❦

January 9, 1993, began as most Saturdays did for Dawn Gould and her husband, Chris Blackwell. But the events of this day, and the following days, would be forever etched in their lives and those of hundreds of other people.

In the course of their usual weekend errands, Dawn and Chris stopped for lunch with their one-and-a-half-year-old daughter, Krystina, at a Jack in the Box restaurant in Puyallup, Washington, a Twin Peaks kind of town near picturesque Mount Rainier. Krystina, excited, insisted on the children's meal. But when the family sat down at a table, Krystina ate only half of the burger.

Some ten miles to the west, two-year-old Michael Nole's father swung by a Jack in the Box in Tacoma to pick up a kid's meal, too. Little Michael loved hamburgers. But he lost much of his appetite when he saw the burger's unfamiliar red center. His family picked at the burger, coaxing Michael to at least eat the cooked edges.

Krystina and Michael's families didn't know it, but that day, thirty miles to the north, two children were admitted to the Children's Hospital and Medical Center in Seattle. They were diagnosed with hemolytic uremic syndrome, a rare disease characterized by the rapid onset of kidney failure, destruction of red

5

blood cells, severe gastrointestinal pain, diarrhea, and brownish-red urine.[1]

Although the cause of hemolytic uremia syndrome is sometimes unclear, doctors do know that it can be triggered by an infection with the *Escherichia coli* 0157:H7 strain, often referred to as simply *E. coli*. Like other food-borne pathogens, or disease-causing bacteria, *E. coli* releases a toxin that irritates the intestine, which in turn tries to expel it with vigorous cramping.

At Children's Hospital, it was pretty much business as usual with a couple of minor exceptions. Ellis Avner, M.D., chief of nephrology, thought it odd to see two cases of hemolytic uremia syndrome in one day. And Phillip Tarr, M.D., one of the hospital's experts in childhood digestive disorders, found himself taking a flurry of calls from area pediatricians. These pediatricians, serving on the front lines of medicine, were getting panicky calls from parents describing children with bloody stools and painful diarrhea.

It wasn't until Tuesday, January 12, that some of the physicians at Children's Hospital happened to compare notes in the hallway. Scott Dowell, M.D., serving a pediatrics residency, talked to Dr. Tarr about whether the problems could be caused by a particularly insidious strain of *E. coli*. Later, Dr. Dowell found the time to scan paperwork from the past couple of days in the emergency room. Out of some two hundred case reports, he found descriptions of a handful of children with bloody diarrhea.

The alarm went out to John M. Kobayashi, Ph.D., Washington state's top epidemiologist. Dr. Kobayashi and his staff started looking for potential causes of food poisoning.

By the end of the week, with help from the Atlanta-based Centers for Disease Control and Prevention (CDC), Dr. Kobayashi and his staff saw a pattern emerging from the hospitalized patients. Most of them, adults as well as children, had eaten hamburgers at Jack in the Box restaurants. With ten children on dialysis machines at Children's Hospital, the scale of the problem was starting to sink in on doctors and health officials. A few days later, doctors removed Michael Nole's colon, ravaged by the toxins secreted by *E. coli* 0157:H7.

Health officials and Jack in the Box managers were scrambling. The same meat, now believed to be contaminated by cow feces, had been shipped from a California slaughterhouse to the chain's restaurants all over Washington state, but people became sick after eating at only a few restaurants. A health official pinpointed the cause, according to reports in the Tacoma *News Tribune* and other newspapers. At some restaurants, the cooking temperature of the burgers barely tickled 140 degrees. That was twenty-five degrees short of state law—and what was needed to kill *E. coli*.

All of the suspect meat was quickly removed from Jack in the Box restaurants after a statewide alert on Monday, January 18. In any event, the epidemic should have been fading anyway. The incubation period for *E. coli* 0157:H7 is twelve to sixty hours. In that time, forty-five people had become sick from *E. coli*.

It was just the beginning.

A couple of days later, Krystina Blackwell started complaining about a tummy ache. When her stools turned bloody, her parents took her to a nearby medical clinic. Not a problem, said the doctor, who attributed her symptoms to the flu.

Meanwhile, state health officials finally confirmed by laboratory analysis what many doctors at Children's Hospital had already believed: the outbreak was cause by *E. coli* 0157:H7 contamination of hamburgers.

On Friday, January 22, a shock wave emanated from Children's Hospital. Michael Nole had died. And *E. coli* infections had sickened another sixty people.

Three days later, Krystina took a turn for the worse. Her parents brought her to Mary Bridge Hospital in Tacoma. Afraid she'd fall into a coma or suffer a seizure, doctors decided not to move her to Children's Hospital.

By Wednesday, January 27, the number of *E. coli* poisonings was up to 250.

One of the Jack in the Box restaurants, publicly cited by

county health officials for *continuing* to undercook its hamburgers at only 137 degrees, sold only six burgers on Friday, January 29.

That night, emergency room doctors at Children's Hospital treated two-year-old Celina Shribbs of Mountlake Terrace, then sent her home. The next day, Celina died from seizures while her parents were driving her back to the hospital.

By this time, Krystina Blackwell, writhing in pain, was moved to Children's Hospital.

Now, Dr. Kobayashi was bracing for a second wave of *E. coli* infections, this time from soiled diapers at day care centers. To head it off, health officials urged day care operators to be especially conscientious about hand washing and sanitizing diaper changing areas. The warning probably helped. Only fifty such secondary infections were noted during the entire *E. coli* outbreak.

But the alarm was too late for sixteen-month-old Riley Detwiler of Bellingham. He contracted *E. coli* from a day care playmate who had eaten a tainted hamburger but whose symptoms had not yet erupted. In desperation, surgeons removed two-thirds of Riley's colon. But by February 20, he became the second child to die from the *E. coli* outbreak.

Krystina Blackwell was one of the luckier children. She recovered slowly but relatively steadily and was released from Children's Hospital after twenty-three days of treatment.

Ten-year-old Sara Brianne Kiner, of Redmond, fell into a forty-two-day coma after eating her burger at Jack in the Box. She remained at Children's Hospital for five months, during which time she suffered a brain-damaging stroke and injury to almost every organ.

On March 5, the *E. coli* epidemic officially ended. It had sickened 540 children and adults. Forty-five of the children had been hospitalized, thirty-eight suffered serious kidney problems, and twenty-one required dialysis during their hospitalization. Three had died.

Within a few weeks, just as people in the Pacific Northwest thought it was safe to return to fast-food restaurants, another massive outbreak of *E. coli* infections was traced to a second restaurant chain, this time to two Sizzlers in Oregon. More than 150 people became ill from what officials suspected was contaminated mayonnaise.

In early August, thirty-seven more cases of *E. coli* sickened people at a Sizzler restaurant in Corvallis, Oregon. The source? Cantaloupe, possibly because someone had sliced it with a meat-contaminated knife.

Inexplicably, this new *E. coli* outbreak followed Sizzler restaurants north along Interstate 5, right back to Seattle. Health officials suspected that lettuce or fruit in the restaurant's salad bar may have come in contact with *E. coli*–tainted meat. The meat was cooked sufficiently, killing the *E. coli*, but most people don't cook their lettuce.

Ultimately, Foodmaker, Inc., the parent corporation of Jack in the Box, settled dozens of lawsuits resulting from the Seattle-Tacoma *E. coli* outbreak. Two years after Sara Kiner's crippling encounter with *E. coli* 0157:H7, almost to the very day, Food-maker agreed to pay her family $15.6 million dollars. All because of a supergerm in undercooked hamburgers.

On June 16, 1995, the *News Tribune* in Tacoma reported that Jack in the Box managers had known about, but chose to ignore, Washington state regulations requiring sufficient cooking of hamburgers. The reason, according to papers filed in U.S. District Court, was that high temperatures made the hamburgers tough, whereas undercooking left them tender. Since the *E. coli* outbreak in 1993, Foodmaker has learned its lesson. Its Jack in the Box restaurants in Washington state have been cooking hamburgers to 180 degrees—far above state requirements.[2]

Emerging and Reemerging Diseases

The emergence of *E. coli* 0157:H7 and the reemergence of other infectious diseases as major health threats means that you no longer have to visit undeveloped nations to contract "Montezuma's revenge"—or much more serious, deadly infections. Many supergerms are already in wide circulation, and *E. coli* 0157:H7 has also been found in salami, yogurt, and apple cider. It was even the cause of infections several years ago among children swimming in a lake near Portland, Oregon. State health investigators thought the cause was undercooked food, but they eventually concluded that the *E. coli* 0157:H7 outbreak began when a swimmer defecated in the water.

E. coli 0157:H7 is related to a more common and usually harmless *E. coli*, a rod-shaped bacterium. Most strains of *E. coli* peacefully coexist in the intestine and even discourage the growth of disease-causing bacteria. (See Chapter 10, Probiotics: Good Bacteria That Fight the Bad.) The virulent *E. coli* 0157:H7 strain was discovered in 1982 by Richard Hebert, M.D., a gastroenterologist in Medford, Oregon. He had admitted patients to the Rogue Valley Medical Center with gastrointestinal pain and diarrhea "unlike anything we had seen before," he told a newspaper reporter.[3] Other physicians were admitting patients with the identical, mysterious symptoms. After some sleuthing, Dr. Hebert discovered that a large number of the patients lived in nearby White City. He alerted local health officials, who called in investigators from the CDC. The new *E. coli* strain was traced back to undercooked hamburgers sold at a McDonald's restaurant in White City.

E. coli are highly adaptable organisms, and the *E. coli* 0157:H7 strain is now a common microorganism in the digestive tracts of cows, where it causes no harm. No one really knows what factors gave rise to *E. coli* 0157:H7, which, according to the U.S. Department of Agriculture, can cause a serious infection with as few as a hundred organisms[4]—a quantity one might expect to find in all but the most well-cooked meat.

❀

SOME DISEASE-CAUSING MICROORGANISMS FOUND IN FOOD

Estimates of food poisoning range from six million to thirty-three million cases and four thousand to nine thousand deaths a year in the United States. These are some of the common ones. They're all very dangerous.[7]

Clostridium botulinum: Known commonly as botulism, this food-borne bacterium releases a powerful toxin that attacks the nervous system, sometimes causing paralysis and death.

Escherichia coli: Several strains of this bacterium cause diarrhea, bloody diarrhea, and other gastrointestinal diseases in people, though most strains are harmless inhabitants of the intestine. The most dangerous strain is *E. coli* 0157:H7, which sickened 540 people in Washington state in 1993.

Campylobacter jejuni: This species of bacteria cause severe abdominal pain and diarrhea. It is one of the most common causes of food poisoning.

Hepatitis: Hepatitis refers to liver inflammation caused by a number of infectious viruses and bacteria. Hepatitis A can be transmitted from feces to food when restaurant workers do not wash their hands.

Listeria monocytogenes: This organism naturally feeds on decaying organic matter in forests and gardens, but it can contaminate food. It is particularly dangerous to infants and people with weakened immune systems.

Salmonella enteritidis, S. typhimurium, S. typhi: These and other forms of salmonella cause a variety of gastrointestinal diseases, ranging from mild to severe. Some strains are carried by pet reptiles, such as snakes and lizards.

Shigella dysenteriae, S. flexneri, S. sonnei: These bacteria cause a broad range of disease, including severe diarrhea, dysentery, and death.

❀

Even worse, *E. coli* 0157:H7 infections are increasing. A recent campaign of vigilant testing in New Jersey found *E. coli* 0157:H7 infections to be ten times higher than previously thought, with many of the cases being sporadic (here and there) rather than indicative of an epidemic emanating from a single source, such as fast-food hamburgers. "The increase in reported cases is believed to reflect both a true increase in incidence and improved laboratory testing and reporting," according to the CDC.[5]

Several other strains of *E. coli* also cause gastrointestinal disease. In 1994, a rare strain identified as *E. coli* 0104:H21 infected eighteen people in Montana. Four of them were hospitalized with bloody diarrhea and fever. This outbreak of *E. coli* 0104:H21, the first to occur in the United States, was traced to a batch of pasteurized milk. CDC officials fear that this strain might become as common and deadly as the *E. coli* 0157:H7 found in hamburgers.[6]

Why don't more people get violently ill? The differences in the intensity of infections often reflect differences in the immune systems among people. Just as some people died and some did not during the Seattle *E. coli* outbreak, many people recover within a day without calling their doctor. Sometimes they don't associate a "blah" day with an infection, or the infection is so slight that it goes unnoticed. Some immune systems are far more effective than others in responding to infections.

Catastrophes in the Making

As serious as the Seattle and Tacoma *E. coli* infections were— and other *E. coli* outbreaks continue to be—they are harbingers of greater catastrophes to come. For thousands of years, infectious diseases, from the bubonic plague to smallpox and typhus, were the scourge of the human race. The discovery of penicillin in 1928, and the widespread use of this and other antibiotics beginning in the 1940s (along with vaccines and improvements in sanitation), gave humankind the upper hand in combatting infectious diseases.

But medicine's "win" in the war against microorganisms may have been temporary at best. The numbers of infectious-disease deaths overseas and at home are nothing short of staggering.

Bacterial, viral, and parasitic infections remain the number one cause of death worldwide. At the top of the list are acute respiratory infections, mostly pneumonia, accounting for 4.3 million deaths a year. Next come diarrheal diseases (3.2 million deaths), tuberculosis (3 million deaths), hepatitis B (1 to 2 million deaths), malaria (1 million deaths), measles (880,000 deaths, though some estimates are as high as several million), and AIDS (600,000 deaths). Around the world, an estimated one million people contract bacterial infections *each day* in hospitals, where most people would think they're safe.[8]

Lest you think infections are primarily a third world problem, pneumonia, influenza, and AIDS are among the top ten causes of death in the United States. The incidence of pneumonia and influenza (lumped together as the sixth most common cause of death in the United States) has jumped 17 percent—from fifty-one thousand to almost sixty thousand annually—since the mid-1980s.[9] AIDS recently tied suicide as the eighth leading cause of death. According to the CDC, fifty-eight thousand Americans die annually because of complications from bacterial infections contracted in hospitals, and nineteen thousand die from antibiotic-resistant infections.

According to the U.S. Department of Agriculture, which oversees much of the food supply, five to seven million people a year become sick from microbially contaminated food, and four thousand of them die. Infections, whether caused by super or not-so-super germs, account for one-fourth of all visits to physicians in the United States, and they have made antibiotics the second most commonly prescribed class of drugs in the country. (The most commonly prescribed drugs act on the central nervous system and include tranquilizers.)[10,11]

But these numbers do not convey the true scale of the problem here at home. In the United States, infectious diseases collectively add up to the *third* leading cause of death, following heart disease and cancer and ahead of strokes, lung diseases, accidents, diabetes, and Alzheimer's disease. Most people, including physicians, do not think about infections in these terms because the numbers are buried in an outdated international classification system for causes of death.

In 1994, for example, infectious diseases officially killed seventy-four thousand Americans.[12] But according to David Satcher, M.D., Ph.D., director of the CDC, pneumonia and influenza deaths are classified separately from other infectious diseases, meningitis is considered a nervous system disease, and cirrhosis a liver disease. Dr. Satcher and his staff contend that "only 17 percent of deaths attributable to infections are actually included in the codes for parasitic and infectious diseases."[13] That means the real number of deaths from infectious diseases may be approximately 435,000—approaching that of cancer. The number of unreported and nonfatal infections can only be guessed at, but it is likely to be in the millions or hundreds of millions.

Even more alarming, the *Journal of the American Medical Association* recently reported that deaths from infectious diseases had increased by 58 percent between the 1980s and 1990s. An aging population susceptible to respiratory infections and AIDS accounted for much of the increase, but even without these two groups, the rate of infectious disease had jumped by 22 to 39 percent![14] Despite the abundance of medicines and medical technologies, people are becoming more vulnerable to infections, not less.

A Combination of Causes

A number of medical and social events have led to the reemergence of infectious diseases and the emergence of supergerms as major public health threats.

First, antibiotics have too often been used cavalierly and

GERMS: WHAT'S THE DIFFERENCE?

Bacteria are single-celled creatures, containing one chromosome, that can be seen with ordinary microscopes.

Viruses, consisting of mere strands of DNA or RNA, are so small that they can be seen only with powerful electron microscopes. Some viruses infect bacteria as well as humans.

Protozoa are much larger than either bacteria or viruses and can be seen with regular microscopes. They are actually considered the smallest animals.

Supergerms are defined by their exceptional ability to cause serious disease and by their resistance to treatment. They include many types of bacteria, viruses, and protozoa.

casually over the past fifty years, a practice that has killed off weak bacteria and allowed virulent, aggressive supergerms to survive and reproduce.[15] These supergerms are actually immune to many antibiotics, and they have triggered new and deadly outbreaks of tuberculosis, pneumonia, sepsis (blood poisoning from bacteria), and many other dangerous infections. As the types of antibiotic-resistant bacteria increase, the odds of getting infected by them also increases. When you do get sick and need antibiotics, the doctor may have to try several before he finds one that works—and in that time you could become even more seriously ill and die.

Second, the extensive use of antibiotics as growth enhancers in livestock has added to the problem of antibiotic-resistant bacteria. When you eat rare or medium-cooked beef, you transport these bacteria right into your gastrointestinal tract. Furthermore, antibiotic-resistant bacteria excreted by livestock—feces are about 75 percent bacteria—become an environmental hazard because the wind can carry the bacteria far away. Even bacteria and viruses exhaled by livestock can travel long distances. Some researchers have documented that gentle winds can carry these germs across the English Channel![16]

Third, day care centers have become a "reservoir" of easily spread infections and antibiotic-resistant bacteria. One recent study found that children in day care centers are thirty-six times more likely to develop serious infections than children who stay at home.[17] Increasingly, these infections are caused by antibiotic-resistant supergerms, which means doctors have difficulty treating them.

Fourth, humankind's encroachment into previously uninhabited areas—the Amazon of South America, the jungles of Africa, and the forests of North America—has exposed people to many new microorganisms, which can be particularly dangerous because people have no inherent or acquired immunity to them. The human immunodeficiency virus (HIV) and Ebola virus are two such supergerms that originated in Africa. In the United States, Lyme disease spread out from the forests of New England and is now found in almost every state. Likewise, a deadly form of hantavirus was discovered in northern Arizona but is now found throughout much of the West.

Fifth, air transportation has made transmissions of all these and other microbes faster and easier than ever before. Each day, more than one million people fly into other countries. Although people and baggage may be scanned and X-rayed to find concealed guns and explosives, potentially dangerous microbes are unnoticed carry-on baggage when their hosts travel from one country to another. When an epidemic of bubonic plague broke out in India in September 1994, health officials monitored U.S. airports to identify possible plague cases among passengers arriving from India.[18] Even greater surveillance was instituted during the Ebola outbreak in Zaire during the spring of 1995. Public health officials had good reason to worry. The entire AIDS epidemic in the United States can be traced to just one promiscuous flight attendant.

Flesh-Eating Bacteria

It hurt like mad, but after all it was *only* a paper cut—one of the professional risks of being an attorney. At first Dan Dudley, of Tucson, Arizona, didn't make a connection between the cut and the rapid onset of his cold and flulike symptoms. But within three days, doctors were trying to stem severe and spreading damage to his hands, legs, lungs, and kidneys from *Streptococcus pyogenes*, the bacterium that also causes strep infections of the throat. To save his life, doctors pumped Dan full of antibiotics. They also had to amputate both of Dan's legs below the knee, his left hand and wrist, and three fingers on his right hand.[19] "I didn't realize that bacterial infections in this day and age are *deadly* infections," he said in an interview.[20]

When outbreaks of *S. pyogenes*, also known as strep-A and the "flesh-eating bacteria," hit the news in 1994, the average person didn't know whom to believe. On one hand, British tabloids fanned fears with headlines such as "Killer Bug Ate My Face," along with photographs of modern-day "scarfaces." On the other hand, American doctors urged calm, insisting there was no new strep-A epidemic.

The flesh-eating infection is more accurately described as necrotizing fasciitis or necrotizing myositis. This especially virulent, or disease-causing, strain of *S. pyogenes* releases a powerful toxin that poisons connective tissue (fasciitis) or muscle tissue (myositis). The alarming "flesh-eating" appellation is based on the observation that strep-A can spread by as much as an inch an hour. While easily treatable in the early stages with antibiotics, such as penicillin or clindamycin, its mild early symptoms do not usually cause alarm. The delay in treatment allows strep-A to kill 30 percent of its victims.

The flesh-eating form of strep-A, however, is more than a simple bacterial infection. It's actually a case of a virus infecting a bacterium, and the bacterium infecting a person with heinous consequences. The virus adapts the bacteria to its own needs—

in this case, producing the toxin—much the way influenza viruses turn human cells into virus-producing factories. Some fifteen thousand people in the United States contract strep-A each year; about 10 percent of the cases evolve into the flesh-eating form of the disease.

Strep-A tends to occur in clusters and, despite official denials, it *has* been increasing in incidence.[21] In an interview, Dan Dudley related that a Tucson man died from a strep-A infection the same week he contracted his—and that nine people in southern Arizona died from it over the course of a year. Dan's doctors suspected that the strep-A infection entered his bloodstream through the paper cut. But it's also likely that far more than nine people were exposed to strep-A—and that a number of factors may have also predisposed Dan to infection. He explained that he had been working very hard, flying weekly between Iowa and Arizona, and feeling very run-down before the infection. The stress and fatigue probably diminished his body's ability to defend against strep-A.[22]

Perhaps the most highly publicized recent outbreak occurred in Stroud, a quaint town located about one hundred miles west of London. At least twelve people contracted strep-A and two died, but the source of the infection was never determined. In February 1994, Les Christie, an engineer and Stroud councilman, may have been exposed to strep-A when he had a routine hernia operation at Stroud General Hospital. A day later, the infection was raging. Christie survived, thanks to an infusion of antibiotics and excision of skin from most of his lower abdomen.[23]

That spring, in Florida, Steve Hillman developed what looked like a pimple on one of his buttocks. A delivery truck driver, Steve didn't think much of it, particularly in the heat and humidity of Florida. The next morning, he had a fever and headache. After one more day, the pimple had grown to the size of a boil, and the pain was agonizing. By that time, Peggy Hillman figured her husband was having a bad reaction to a spider bite. Hillman was nearing multiple systems organ failure as Peggy drove him to the emergency room of Coral Springs Medical Center. Mel Kohan, M.D., diagnosed the boil, now deep purple, as strep-A. A hefty dose of antibiotics brought Steve back from death's doorstep.[24]

Back in Seattle, eleven cases of necrotizing fasciitis were diagnosed and treated at Children's Hospital and Medical Center during 1994 and early 1995. Most occurred between late November and early January. All of the children had chicken pox, and they probably contracted strep-A through open sores. None of the cases was fatal, but Robert Sawin, M.D., a surgeon at the hospital, observed that only one case would normally be diagnosed in a typical year.[25]

If there was cause for alarm, it was sounded by Vincent Fischetti, Ph.D., of Rockefeller University. Epidemics often occur in cycles, and strep-A bacteria caused a large epidemic of scarlet fever and flesh-eating symptoms in the 1880s, then pretty much disappeared except for sporadic cases. Its sudden reemergence could be a presage of a new scarlet fever epidemic, according to Dr. Fischetti.[26]

Fast and Deadly Meningococcal Disease

Sometimes, the factors propelling the spread of a supergerm are obscure at best. And sometimes the supergerm outruns even the best doctors.

That was the case with the Ebola virus, which caused brief but fiery epidemics in Zaire in 1976 and 1995. The contagion caused rapid hemorrhaging—some observers described it as a liquefaction of internal organs—that killed the majority of people infected with the virus. (Ebola is the subject of the best-selling book *The Hot Zone*, as well as the model for the fictional Motaba virus in the 1995 film *Outbreak*.) Ebola spread so quickly that the disease's own virulence helped contain it, because death generally outpaced its victims' ability to travel and infect others.[27]

Another fast-moving and devastating infection recently

gained a foothold in Portland, Oregon, and nearby communities. Like Ebola, an insidious strain of *Neisseria meningitidis*, referred to specifically as Type B Subtype ET-5, often eludes physicians. An estimated 5 to 20 percent of the population harbors this and other strains of *N. meningitidis* without any untoward effects. But some people infected by *N. meningitidis* develop meningococcal disease, a life-threatening inflammation of the meninges, the membranes that surround the brain and spinal cord.

N. meningitidis Type B Subtype ET-5 was identified in Norway in 1974 and caused infections in numerous other European countries and South America before popping up in Oregon. No one knows exactly how it reached the United States. But today, this strain accounts for more than three-fourths of the meningococcal infections in Oregon and southwestern Washington—yet remains extremely rare elsewhere in the United States.[28]

Like many supergerms, *N. meningitidis* strikes with deceivingly mild initial symptoms. In February 1990, it forever changed the life of the Bakamus family of Longview, Washington, just downriver from Portland. Cathy and Bill Bakamus were awakened around midnight on a Saturday night by their thirteen-month-old daughter, Rachel, who had a 103-degree fever and seemed to be developing a flu or ear infection. Cathy spent the night comforting her daughter.

By morning, Rachel's fever disappeared and the toddler was catching up on the sleep she lost during the night. Meanwhile, Bill and Cathy washed the windows of their house. By noon, Rachel remained lethargic and didn't want to drink, but her forehead was cool to the touch. " She just wasn't livening up," Cathy related in an interview.[29]

Cathy and Bill also noticed a tiny but unusual purple spot on Rachel's temple, and called her pediatrician's office. While preparing Rachel for a Sunday afternoon trip to the clinic, Cathy changed her diaper for the first time since midmorning. Rachel had the "worst, most awful-smelling, mucousy diarrhea" her mom had ever seen, and Rachel's body was now covered by "little prickly marks, as if someone had been sticking her with a pin." A second purple spot appeared, this one on Rachel's hand. Cathy, whose father was a physician, had never seen anything quite like this, so she and Bill rushed Rachel to the pediatrician. Reaching the office before the doctor, they reexamined Rachel and began counting the spots: thirty on her front, forty on her backside. "Rachel was in a lot of pain," related Cathy. "The spots were literally popping up as we were sitting there."

By the time the doctor arrived, a few minutes later, the tiny red spots—signs of blood-clotting problems caused by the bacteria's toxin—were coalescing into larger spots and turning purple. The doctor told them to drive right to the emergency room at the local hospital. Once there, the doctors were stymied by another problem: Rachel's blood pressure was now so low that it took them more than an hour to start an intravenous antibiotic. Two hours later, the numerous purple spots had grown completely together, covering large portions of Rachel's body. "The antibiotic is very effective on the meningococcal bacteria," Cathy said, "but now the problem was the bacteria's toxin. It causes irregular blood clotting, and antibiotics have no effect on the toxin."

That night, Rachel was flown by helicopter to the Doernbecker Children's Hospital in Portland. The erratic clotting caused by the meningococcal toxins had already done considerable damage, and over the next few days, scabs formed from Rachel's thighs to her toes. Gangrene developed, and the doctors eventually amputated Rachel's legs below the knees and several of her fingers.

Rachel survived, and with leg prosthetics, acts much like any other child. But while at Doernbecker, Cathy recalled, she asked one of the doctors why only Rachel contracted meningococcal disease, not her older sibling or her parents. About a week before developing meningococcal disease, Rachel had been sick with diarrhea and vomiting. Then she had a perfectly healthy week. The doctor said that Rachel's immune system may have been weakened by the previous illness, making her more susceptible.

How did Rachel contract meningococcal disease? "No one knows," said Cathy. "It could have come from someone who sneezed or picked her up." Such is the unpredictable appearance of supergerms.

Meningococcal disease continues to strike children in the Portland area. For example, Amber Smith's meningococcal symptoms began as nothing more than a headache in the spring of 1995. The seventeen-year-old Portland honor student thought it might be related to a dental retainer her orthodontist inserted the day before. She went to school, then to her part-time job at a grocery store. That afternoon Amber's headache became excruciating and she started to suffer from partial paralysis. Ronald Smith, Amber's father, took her to their family doctor, then rushed her to Providence Medical Center. The paralysis was caused by a swelling of her brain and pressure on the nerves. Amber slipped into a coma, and she died the next day.[30]

In Oregon, the incidence of all meningococcal diseases— dubbed "the fatal flu" by the local news media—had been increasing rapidly. In 1992, sixty-seven cases were reported. In 1993, 106. In 1994, 140. Overall, the incidence in Oregon is five times the national average,[31] and is especially high among those fifteen to nineteen years old.

Not all cases of meningococcal disease are fatal, particularly when it's treated early, but early symptoms are often mild and do not signal alarm. The principal risk factors include crowded living arrangements, gas heat,[32] and another infection (such as the flu and "walking pneumonia") immediately prior to contracting meningococcal disease. Such infections weaken immunity.

In April 1995, the Oregon Health Division published a brief report that noted, in part, that the pattern of meningococcal disease in the Portland metropolitan area was starting to resemble an epidemic rather than a more arbitrary series of outbreaks.

The report read in part that it "is not known if the sustained spread of *N. meningitidis* type B ET-5 reflects increased bacterial virulence, decreased host resistance to a new bacterial strain, changing environmental factors, or some combination of these and other factors."[33]

It's relatively easy for Americans to avoid Zaire, where the most violent Ebola outbreaks have occurred. The country has no attractive resorts or compelling tours. It's much more difficult to guarantee that the food you buy isn't tainted with *E. coli* or your friends and coworkers don't harbor strep or meningococcal bacteria.

The truly sinister aspect of many supergerms is how their infections frequently begin with coldlike or flulike symptoms, which most people simply take in stride. Within hours, however, if a supergerm is the culprit, these small flames can erupt into dangerous fires that consume people's lives.

The answer is not to become a hypochondriac and to overreact to every sniffle. Instead, part of the solution is to minimize risk factors—including suspicious meat, undue stress, and precipitating mild infections—that could leave you vulnerable to a supergerm infection.

2

OLD GERMS, NEW THREATS

⌘

Sometimes old and familiar bacteria, all but vanquished by antibiotics, reappear as modern-day supergerms. Two of the most prominent microorganisms achieving supergerm status in the 1990s are tuberculosis (TB) and bacterial pneumonia caused specifically by *Streptococcus pneumoniae* (formerly known as *Pneumococcus pneumoniae*), a relative of the flesh-eating bacteria.

The resurgence of TB owes itself to several factors: a sense of complacency from the mistaken belief that the disease had been nearly eradicated in the United States, the increased mobility of people (many of whom carry TB), and the spread of AIDS. People with AIDS are especially susceptible to TB.

S. pneumoniae strikes far more people—and in a sense, closer to home—than does TB. It is the microorganism causing most cases of pneumonia, as well as most middle-ear infections in children. *S. pneumoniae* is also increasingly resistant to antibiotics—and these drugs may even encourage repeated ear infections.

The Return of Tuberculosis

A century ago, when it was called consumption, TB was the most common cause of death among adults in the Western world. About all physicians could do was recommend that their patients eat nutritiously, get plenty of rest, and avail themselves of sunlight and fresh air. In the preantibiotic age, and with the stress of six-day work weeks and the thick air pollution of the industrial revolution, it was sound advice for rebuilding the immune system. Unfortunately, such advice was usually too little and too late. As late as 1900, TB killed about 25 percent of Europeans and one-third of Americans.

Establishing sanitariums, which quarantined infected individuals from the general public, improving methods of hygiene and sanitation, and developing vaccines in the 1920s began to bring TB under control. The discovery of streptomycin in 1944, the first antibiotic effective against TB, helped medicine further rein in this wasting disease. In fact, the conquest of TB appeared to be within the grasp of American medicine. Its incidence declined roughly 6 percent annually, from 84,304 cases in 1953, when national statistics on tuberculosis were first compiled, until 1984, when only 22,255 cases were recorded.

Then, in 1985, TB cases started to increase. By 1991, new TB cases were up by 17 percent to 26,000, and by 1993, they had risen by 20 percent to 26,673, with about 2,000 TB-related deaths per year. (In comparison, polio struck roughly 22,000 people a year in the United States until the Salk and Sabin vaccines were developed in the 1950s.) Thanks to renewed eradication efforts, TB cases in the United States declined slightly in 1993 and 1994.[1] Elsewhere, the prognosis isn't very promising. Worldwide, the disease kills three million adults each year, and the World Health Organization (WHO) has estimated that 1.9 billion people—one-third of the world's population—carry *Mycobacterium tuberculosis*, although most do not have symptoms and do not infect others.[2,3]

The reemergence of TB as a major public health threat has been fueled by the spread of AIDS, whose victims are particularly susceptible to opportunistic infection by *M. tuberculosis*. But AIDS cannot take all of the blame for the rise in TB cases. Other factors include the increase in immigration, travel, and tourism. The treatment of TB has become problematic as well, because the misuse of antibiotics—an issue we will discuss in Chapters 3 and 4—has bred strains of TB that shrug off medicine's most powerful antibiotics.

In March 1995, at a press conference in New York City, WHO offered an ominous warning. Hiroshi Nakajima, M.D., WHO's director general, said that without changes in the treatment of TB the death toll would eventually rise to *one new case per second*. He predicted that by the year 2005 far more than two billion people would carry *M. tuberculosis* and four million would die annually from the disease.[4]

You don't have to look to Southeast Asia, where half of all TB cases have so far been diagnosed, to appreciate the gravity of the situation. An estimated fifteen million people in the United States carry dormant tuberculosis infections. In healthy individuals, *M. tuberculosis* shrewdly hides inside macrophages, a type of white blood cell. When the immune system becomes weak, or compromised, *M. tuberculosis* moves to organs, such as the lungs. At this stage, symptoms include fever, weight loss, a deep racking cough, and spitting up blood. The infection is spread through exposure to airborne *M. tuberculosis* from an infected person's coughing, sneezing, singing, or heavy breathing.

The largest U.S. public school outbreak of TB occurred in a middle-class neighborhood near Los Angeles in 1993 and 1994. Almost four hundred students—one-third of the student body—at La Quinta High School in Westminster, California, tested positive for a strain of antibiotic-resistant TB. The contagion was traced to a Vietnamese girl who had contracted TB in her native country before immigrating. The girl's doctor had misdiagnosed her cough as bronchitis in 1990 and let her continue normal activities. Of the students, relatives, and family friends who tested positive for TB, twelve developed active, highly infectious TB. For one student, the infection necessitated the surgical removal of part of a lung.[5]

Commercial aircraft may provide another avenue for the spread of TB and other infectious diseases. Why? Because of air recirculation systems that reuse cabin air instead of exchanging it with fresh air.[6] In 1994, the CDC determined that a flight attendant with TB infected other members of the crew.[7] The following year, the CDC urged that people with active TB not take long flights because of the risk of spreading the infection.[8]

Such infections do happen. In its March 3, 1995, *Morbidity and Mortality Weekly Report*, the CDC related that a woman with active TB had been coughing during an eight-hour flight from Chicago to Honolulu and infected four passengers seated nearby. The woman died several weeks after the flight.[9] In response to airplane-borne infections, some airlines have installed high-efficiency air filters to curb the spread of TB.[10] However, the air is still recirculated rather than refreshed, and the filters won't protect you from the person in the next seat. You might as well be in a crowded elevator for four hours.

As recently as the 1980s, TB was routinely treated with one of two antibiotics, isoniazid and rifampin. They were quite effective, even though the treatment regimen often lasted a year. Recently, several new strains of *M. tuberculosis* resistant to these and other antibiotics have emerged in numerous countries, including the United States, making the infection especially difficult to treat.

Under these circumstances, doctors resort to antibiotic "cocktails" that sometimes work and sometimes don't. Often, treatment becomes a race against time—and doctors lose the race to find a successful combination of antibiotics. Among AIDS patients, the death rate from antibiotic-resistant TB is more than 80 percent. And among patients without AIDS, it's 40 to 60 percent.[11] The size of the problem is frightening. An estimated hundred million people worldwide already carry antibiotic-resistant strains of TB.[12]

Several factors encourage antibiotic resistance, and they are all underscored by the inappropriate use of antibiotics. AIDS patients with dormant TB are often given preventive—but inadequate—doses of antibiotics in a misguided attempt to prevent full-blown disease. A low dose only kills the most susceptible bacteria while enabling stronger ones to survive and reproduce.[13] The consequence is that the patients continue to spread the infection.[14]

Another problem rests not with the physician prescribing the antibiotic but with poor patient compliance—that is, patients who do not or will not consistently take their medication. Taking medication for six to eighteen months, a typical period for treating TB, can be trying for the most committed patients. (How often do you, for instance, skip your medication or vitamins?) Other TB patients stop their medication as soon as the major symptoms subside.

Again, this halfhearted use of an antibiotic encourages antibiotic resistance by wiping out the weaker bacteria and encouraging the survival and reproduction of stronger, antibiotic-resistant strains. For example, one in every million TB germs carries a gene that provides resistance to the antibiotic isoniazid, and one in every hundred million carries a gene that confers resistance to rifampin. Typically, each pocket of TB in a patient's lungs contains ten to a hundred million germs.[15] A lengthy antibiotic regimen creates an inhospitable environment for TB, but abbreviated antibiotic therapy just makes room for the toughest germs.

The problem is far more serious than bacterial resistance to isoniazid and rifampin. One strain of TB is now resistant to as many as seven different types of antibiotics, making treatment especially difficult, costly, and often futile. Resistance to multiple antibiotics is so serious that it's "pushing us back to preantibiotic days," said Louis W. Sullivan, M.D., former secretary of health and human services, at the 1993 World Congress on Tuberculosis in Bethesda, Maryland.[16]

New York City, which saw the incidence of TB rise 125 percent from 1981 to 1991, developed a solution—albeit an expensive one—that has become a model for WHO. Health officials stemmed the increase through "directly observed therapy" in which health-care workers actually wait and watch to ensure that TB patients take their medicine. In addition, homeless shelters, hospitals, and jails were modified to prevent the spread of TB. The total cost was more than $1.6 billion.

Some health officials have naively believed that the increase in TB cases was merely the result of "reactivated" rather than new infections. Two recent studies, however, have found that 30 to 40 percent of TB infections are new. A Stanford University analysis of 473 TB patients reported that about one-third had recently acquired infections. The researchers related that a man infected with AIDS and TB refused to take a prescribed antibiotic and spread TB to twenty-nine others. In another case, a transsexual prostitute infected with AIDS and TB spread the latter infection to twenty-two people.[17,18] In other instances, a homeless man with TB infected forty-one people in a Minneapolis neighborhood bar, and one man spread the disease to four hundred coworkers at a shipyard in Bath, Maine.[19]

The lesson is simple, though sometimes easier said than done: people diagnosed with TB must be treated promptly and effectively, before they have an opportunity to spread the infection. They must also do as the Victorians did, though better: strengthen their inherent immunity to infection.

The Growing Menace of Bacterial Pneumonia

S. pneumoniae, a relatively common germ, is quickly becoming a supergerm. It causes an estimated 500,000, or 80 percent, of the pneumonia cases (infection of the bronchial tubes or lungs) each year in the United States. *S. pneumoniae* is also responsible for six million cases of otitis media (middle-ear infection), fifty-five thousand cases of bacteremia (a type of blood poisoning), six thousand cases of pneumococcal meningitis, and forty thousand deaths a year.[20]

In 1994, a team of researchers described pneumonia as a "silent epidemic" and an "unappreciated killer" in the journal *Annals of Surgery*. They criticized their peers for overlooking pneumonia in the intensive care units (ICUs) of hospitals, where it is the most common major infection to develop after severe trauma, such as automobile accidents or gunshot wounds.

The researchers, from the University of Louisville School of Medicine, Kentucky, made a perceptive observation: though immune suppression was a consequence of physical injury, they could predict the development of pneumonia by carefully tracking patients' immune function. Typically, it takes about five days before pneumonia appears after serious trauma. But by watching for a precipitous drop in immunity, they could identify in two days the trauma patients most likely to develop pneumonia—and begin treatment before the infection became serious.[21]

Penicillin, introduced for broad public use in the 1940s, used to be a highly effective treatment of pneumococcal diseases. Today, penicillin-resistant strains of *S. pneumoniae* are found worldwide, and some strains are resistant to multiple antibiotics, including chloramphenicol, erythromycin, penicillin, tetracycline, and trimethoprim-sulfamethoxazole.[22] One study found that 41 percent of *S. pneumoniae* infections were resistant to antibiotics.[23]

The first reports of antibiotic-resistant *S. pneumoniae* came out of Australia and South Africa in the 1960s and 1970s. These strains of *S. pneumoniae* spread around the world quickly but were not common in the United States until about 1987. To assess the magnitude of the problem, Robert F. Breiman, M.D., and his colleagues at the CDC analyzed pneumococcal strains from twenty-one hospitals in thirteen states.

Dr. Breiman's findings were nothing short of alarming. Among 5,459 bacterial samples obtained in a nine-year period between 1979 and 1987, only one (less than 0.02 percent) was resistant to penicillin. Out of 567 samples obtained in *only* a twelve-month period between 1991 and 1992, seven (about 1.2 percent) were resistant to penicillin—*a sixtyfold increase* in antibiotic resistance. Furthermore, 16.4 percent of the 1991 to 1992 samples were resistant to at least one of the following antibiotics or classes of antibiotics: penicillin, cephalosporins, chloramphenicol, macrolides, and the combination of trimethoprim and sulfamethoxazole.[24] By 1995, according to another researcher, 25 percent of *S. pneumoniae* infections were caused by antibiotic-resistant strains.[25]

Antibiotic-resistant pneumonia is spreading faster and faster, and such infections cannot be treated with the preferred, common antibiotics. Dr. Breiman also found that children were more likely than adults to be infected by antibiotic-resistant bacteria. He wasn't surprised by this finding either. According to his article in the *Journal of the American Medical Association*, children are exposed to a "plethora" of antibiotics early in life, encouraging the growth of resistant bacteria.[26]

Are immunizations a solution? Not likely, at least not soon, because current vaccines do not confer substantial protection to children under age two, who have the highest risk for contracting *S. pneumoniae* ear and blood infections. Dr. Breiman also noted that the elderly, like children, are particularly vulnerable to *S. pneumoniae* infections. Indeed, 40 percent of people over sixty-five years of age who develop pneumococcal bacteremia (when the infection moves to the bloodstream) die from the infection.

Once again, the way we live has contributed to the emergence of *S. pneumoniae* as a supergerm. The transmission of *S. pneumoniae*, including its antibiotic-resistant strains, has been fueled in large part by the rapid increase in the number of day care centers in the United States and other nations. A generation ago, most children were cared for by mothers or grandparents in the home and were not exposed to such a wide range of infectious diseases. Today, one-third of American families pay for day care services, and an estimated ten million American children under age five spend at least part of their week in one of an estimated 250,000 day care centers.[27,28] These centers range from loosely regulated (if at all) home-based services to formal school-like settings. Standards of hygiene and sanitation, and policies regarding sick children, vary dramatically. Some are sterling examples of day care; others leave much to be desired.

Even the best day care centers serve as reservoirs of infectious microorganisms, with transmission as easy as two children playfully touching each other—or each other's toys. Subsequent ear, bronchial, and lung infections, along with quick trips to the pediatrician for antibiotics, become regular and disruptive events.

In a study of several hundred Finnish children, Aino K. Takala, M.D., found that day care outside of a child's own home was the strongest factor affecting risk of pneumococcal infection. But the size of the day care center (and the amount of time the child spent there) were also powerful indicators of risk. Children in large day care centers were thirty-six times more likely than home-reared children to contract pneumococcal infections. Small day care centers (with fewer than six children) posed less risk, but children attending these centers were still almost five times more likely than home-reared children to develop pneumococcal infections.[29]

Dr. Takala urged that children under the age of two in day care centers, as well as those suffering frequent ear infections, be considered a new "high-risk group" for contracting pneumococcal infections—many of which are resistant to common antibiotics. As bad as the situation might be in Finland, it is far worse in the United States, where infants and children under age five were *ten times* more likely than Finnish children to be in day care centers.[30]

Closer to Home: Childhood Ear Infections

A generation ago, faced with a sick infant or child, a mother might have first sought the wise counsel of grandmothers, aunts, or other stay-at-home mothers in her neighborhood. Before the days of health maintenance organizations (HMOs) and prepaid insurance, parents were reluctant to call the doctor unless a child's symptoms failed to improve after a few days. As the extended family shrank down to the nuclear family, and more mothers moved into the workforce, the supportive familial and social fabric has deteriorated and the sense of urgency in medical care has sharpened.

Now, employment pressures on parents result in children being placed in day care centers and often returned to day care centers even when they are still ill. This leads to recurring infections with *S. pneumoniae* and other microorganisms, further quick prescriptions for antibiotics, and then antibiotic resistance builds up in children. All this results in chronically infected children. Pediatricians, especially during the high-infection winter months, oversee what has become, for all practical purposes, a decentralized emergency room. They respond not just to children with symptoms suggestive of infection but to their anxious parents as well.

While most parents are genuinely concerned about their children's health, they are also anxious—and often pressured—to return to work as quickly as possible. They simply do not usually have the time to tend a sick infant or child at home. Pediatricians understand these pressures. They prescribe an antibiotic for the child that, in an odd way, serves as a functional substitute for tranquilizing the parents. It's part of a complex and disastrous medical cycle of infection, antibiotic, and antibiotic resistance, leading to repeated infections.

Unfortunately, pediatricians often find themselves in a no-win situation when it comes to treating "apparent" ear infections, the second most common symptom they see in children after the common cold. Faced with often vague symptoms, they are in the same quandary as veterinarians: they are under pressure to "do something" to help patients often incapable of verbalizing symptoms. In addition to the pressure to deliver a quick fix, they are also discouraged by many insurance companies (particularly HMOs) from ordering laboratory tests that identify the specific infectious microorganism. (Strep tests are the notable exception.) In effect, they are asked to choose a therapy based on an incomplete diagnosis. So, in an age of trigger-fast malpractice suits, they practice defensive medicine, in which antibiotics are routinely prescribed for fear of what *might* happen if they aren't prescribed. (For example, there is a risk of hearing loss from ear infections, but it has been exaggerated. In addition, there is a small risk of a child harboring *Haemophilis influenzae*, which can spread to the brain.)

Some of the best-known pediatricians in the country, among them Lendon H. Smith, M.D., of Portland, Oregon, have long urged their professional colleagues to limit their use of antibiotics and to follow a protocol of "watchful waiting" and perhaps a warm compress to ease pain, for the first forty-eight hours of an apparent ear infection. The reason is that ear infections frequently have a mechanical origin—the shape of the Eustachian tube, which joins the nose-throat cavity with the inner ear, prevents the efficient drainage of fluid. (The position of the ear during breast-feeding, however, does encourage drainage, which may be one of the reasons why breast-fed infants are less prone to ear infections.)

There are other reasons for concern as well, although they are a little more speculative. The use of antibiotics in the earliest stages of an infection may hinder the "programming" of an infant's immature immune system, according to Dr. Smith. Without this programming, the immune system may have continued difficulty identifying and responding to disease-causing bacteria. This could create ongoing susceptibility to the most minor infections and dependence on antibiotics, with the eventual outcome being a serious infection by antibiotic-resistance bacteria. There is even evidence that an overreliance on antibiotics interferes with the immune system's ability to recognize and destroy cancer cells.[31]

One study even found that children taking a lot of antibiotics were more likely to suffer developmental delays than were children given relatively few antibiotics. Investigators reported that children between the ages of one and twelve who had more than twenty antibiotic regimens were more than 50 percent more likely to have impaired learning. In contrast, children taking fewer than three rounds of antibiotics were 50 percent less likely to suffer developmental delays.[32]

In fact, the aggressive use of antibiotics—that is, using them sooner rather than later—in the treatment of middle-ear infections is itself of questionable value for the treatment of infection. The impetus for this common therapy was an apparently well-designed study of several hundred infants and children at Children's Hospital in Pittsburgh, Pennsylvania. The researchers reported in the *New England Journal of Medicine* in 1987 that twice as many ear infections improved after treatment with amoxicillin, a broad-spectrum antibiotic, compared with a placebo.[33]

As Steven Findlay of *U.S. News & World Report* later observed, "Pediatricians seemed to have the proof they had long wanted; antibiotic sales soared."[34] Indeed, one personal friend wryly observed that amoxicillin became the "fifth food group" during his two-year-old daughter's repeated ear infections.

But one member of the Pittsburgh research team vehemently disagreed with his colleagues positive appraisal of amoxicillin. He submitted his own paper to the *New England Journal of Medicine*. Bitter fighting, charges, and countercharges—not rational scientific discourse—ensued, and the journal declined to publish the second paper. Four years later, however, the *Journal of the American Medical Association* published the critical paper. Using the same data, the dissenting doctor calculated that amoxicillin helped only 12.3 percent of the infants and children and, overall, was "not effective." More disturbing, he reported that infants and children treated with amoxicillin were *more likely* to suffer from recurring ear infections than those who took the placebo.[35] The message: if you want your child to suffer from repeated ear infections, give him or her amoxicillin.

While this controversy was still brewing, David M. Jaffe, M.D., of Children's Memorial Hospital in Chicago, and his colleagues in Boston and Philadelphia, chimed in with a separate study of 955 children suffering from fever and infection. Dr. Jaffe stated that without identifying the specific disease-causing microbe, it's very difficult to distinguish a vague bacterial infection from a viral infection in children. It's an important point, because viruses *cannot* be treated with antibiotics.

Dr. Jaffe found that amoxicillin reduced fever and improved the clinical appearance of children with bacterial infections—but, not surprisingly, it provided no benefit to virally infected children. Furthermore, children treated with antibiotics tended to have diarrhea and allergic reactions, whereas untreated children did not. In conclusion, Dr. Jaffe wrote that antibiotics should not be used as a substitute for careful diagnosis. He also reminded his colleagues that it was worthless to prescribe antibiotics unless there was clear evidence of a bacterial infection.[36]

By this time, however, the medical stampede had begun. Many pediatricians were routinely prescribing antibiotics for ear infections, no doubt encouraged by the pharmaceutical companies that manufacture and market these drugs. When children became infected with amoxicillin-resistant bacteria, which became more likely with each prescription, doctors simply switched to other antibiotics, such as broad-spectrum cephalosporins. But the question remained: did an antibiotic help, or did it make the child more susceptible to repeated infections?

A recent "meta," or collective, analysis of twenty-seven well-controlled studies and several thousand children answered part of that question—and it chipped away at the aggressive use of antibiotics to treat ear infection. Robert L. Williams, M.D., of the MetroHealth Clement Center in Cleveland, Ohio, found that only one of every nine children (11 percent) receiving antibiotics for acute middle ear infections improved, and only one of every six children getting an antibiotic for otitis media with effusion (a middle-ear infection in which fluid exerts pressure on the eardrum) improved.[37] Meanwhile, the vast majority of children were needlessly medicated.

There are, in addition, ramifications of excessive antibiotic use that go beyond the health of a single infant or child. Antibiotic-resistant traits can be passed from one species of bacteria to another, and these bacteria can spread easily from one person to another *without* symptoms of infection. When researchers in Houston, Texas, analyzed bacteria from healthy diapered infants in day care centers, they found that 19 percent of the children carried antibiotic-resistant strains of *E. coli*. In a subsequent study, the researchers found that children from day care centers had five times more antibiotic-resistant bacteria than children cared for at home. The researchers proved that day care centers were a major source of antibiotic-resistant *E. coli*.[38]

The problem is not restricted to day care centers and children. The Houston researchers also found that antibiotic-resistant *E. coli* spread from day care children to members of their families. Mothers and siblings are far more likely than fathers to acquire antibiotic-resistant *E. coli* because they spend more time with the child.[39] These *E. coli,* even if harmless themselves, can then share their antibiotic-resistance traits with truly dangerous germs.

Another outcome of recurring childhood ear infections— again encouraged by reckless use of antibiotics—is a referral to an otolaryngologist (ear, nose, and throat specialist) for a tympanostomy ("tubes"). This surgical procedure, which requires a general anesthetic, inserts tiny tubes to siphon off fluid from the middle ear. It is performed on between 700,000 and one million children each year[40] and has become a significant source of revenue among otolaryngologists and hospitals. Neither tubes nor antibiotics address the actual cause of repeated infections and, in our opinion, the tympanostomy is little more than a surgical fad—the tonsillectomy of the 1990s, so to speak.

While these are strong words, our opinion is supported by a major medical study published in the *Journal of the American Medical Association*. Lawrence C. Kleinman, M.D., of Children's Hospital in Boston, reviewed the medical justifications for tympanostomies in 6,611 children under sixteen years of age. Although he made "generous clinical assumptions" in favor of tympanostomies, Dr. Kleinman could justify only 41 percent of the surgeries. Fully one-fourth of the procedures were unjustified and one-third were questionable.[41]

In the meantime, the U.S. Department of Health and Human Services (HHS) Agency for Health Care Policy and Research reviewed published studies and clinical trials and consulted with pediatricians and family physicians. In July 1994, HHS recommended "watchful waiting" for otitis media with effusion because the condition often disappears within three to six months without treatment—and without hearing loss. While antibiotics were considered a treatment option, they weren't the first choice, according to Alfred Berg, M.D., of the University of Washington, Seattle, who served on the HHS review panel. The problem with antibiotics, Berg noted in an interview with the Associated Press, was that they caused side effects and contributed to antibiotic-resistant bacteria capable of causing far more serious disease.[42]

So, what is the real solution for dealing with ear infections in children? Dr. Smith, the author of a dozen popular books on children's health, has long contended that allergy-like sensitivities to foods, such as milk, encourage the retention of fluid in the ear—just as they do in other parts of the body. In the ear, such fluid becomes a breeding ground for infections. At various times, the medical community had downplayed the incidence of food allergies, and it has remained skeptical of such claims.

However, a study published in *Annals of Allergy*, a leading

medical journal, has challenged the conventional view and supported Dr. Smith's contention. Talal M. Nsouli, M.D., and his
colleagues at the International Center for Interdisciplinary Studies of Immunology, Georgetown University, carefully studied
104 children, ages 1.5 to 9 years, with recurrent ear infections.
Dr. Nsouli tested the children for food allergies, then placed them
on diets excluding specific foods for sixteen weeks. Meanwhile,
changes in middle-ear effusion were carefully monitored.

He found that eighty-one (78 percent) of the children had
food allergies, based on skin prick testing, specific IgE tests, and
food challenges. Of the eighty-one children placed on elimina-
tion diets, seventy (86 percent) had a significant reduction in ear
infections. When Dr. Nsouli gave suspected allergenic foods—
principally milk and wheat—to these children, almost all developed ear infections. He commented that food allergy was probably the underlying cause of ear infections and that the resulting
fluid buildup sets the stage for infection. He concluded that
"the present study indicates that food allergy may contribute
significantly to a proportion of cases."[43]

Finally, mothers might prevent many ear infections—and
avoid an incredible medical cascade with risk of subsequent
infection and antibiotic resistance—by exclusively breast-
feeding their infants for at least four months after birth. Burris
Duncan, M.D., a pediatrician at Steel Memorial Children's Research Center, Tucson, tracked more than a thousand infants
during their first year. Infants consuming only breast milk for
four or more months had half the incidence of acute ear infections
as those who were never breast-fed. In addition, the breast-fed
infants had fewer recurrent ear infections.[44]

For all the good antibiotics have done—and there is no question
that they deserve to be called "miracle drugs"—they have been
prescribed and used far too promiscuously in medicine. This is
not by any means strictly an American problem, for many of
the antibiotics sold on prescription in the United States are easily

purchased over the counter in many other countries. In one respect, antibiotics have allowed us to become complacent about addressing the causes of infections and their transmission. In another respect, we have greatly underestimated the ability of bacteria to rapidly evolve and prosper in response to wave after wave of antibiotics.

3

THE MAKING OF
SUPERGERMS

❧

Without a doubt, the discovery of penicillin was one of the most significant events in the history of medicine. It is a profound irony that this and other antibiotics have helped breed supergerms.

For most of human history, the principal cause of death (other than war and old age) was infectious disease. From the bubonic plague, which periodically raced across preindustrial Europe, to the outbreaks of measles, tuberculosis, smallpox, diphtheria, and typhus, epidemics of common infections decimated societies. For the individual, contracting an infection—even from a minor wound—could be a virtual death sentence.

In the nineteenth century, the German bacteriologist Paul Ehrlich began searching for a "magic bullet"—a drug capable of destroying disease-causing bacteria without harming the body. This magic bullet remained out of medicine's grasp until 1928, when Alexander Fleming, at St. Mary's Hospital in London, made a serendipitous discovery. Returning from a brief vacation, Fleming noticed that a staph culture had been destroyed by a common mold, called *Penicillium*, that happened to settle on an unwashed laboratory dish.

Fleming's finding, as well as the discovery of antibacterial sulfa drugs in the 1930s, reignited medical interest in Ehrlich's concept. Sulfa drugs, known more formally as sulfonamides, are bacteriostatic—meaning that they stop the growth of bacteria and give the body's immune system time to mount a stronger defense. The *Penicillium* mold, however, actually destroyed the bacteria. It appeared to work better than the immune system itself.

Research continued on the *Penicillium* mold, and over the next decade a handful of patients were treated with it in England and the United States. In 1940, the Merck Company provided physicians in Boston with a crude form of the drug penicillin to treat *Staphylococcus aureus* ("staph") infections in more than a hundred victims of a fire. Such infections typically killed patients, but penicillin succeeded in curbing the staph infections— and death. Research and development were quickly ramped up, and this rightfully named "miracle drug" saved the lives of thousands of Allied soldiers during World War II.

In retrospect, such stories may sound a bit melodramatic. But for people living in the 1940s and 1950s, the use of penicillin to cure bacterial diseases had the impact that a ten-day cure for cancer or AIDS would have today. Yet among the accolades Fleming and penicillin had received, signs of trouble were already brewing.

Early Signs of Antibiotic-Resistant Supergerms

By the 1940s, physicians knew that penicillin worked against some but not all bacteria. In addition, they started to see signs that some bacterial strains once killed by penicillin had become more resistant to the drug. In 1941, an incident illustrated the looming problem with antibiotic resistance. A policeman in Oxford, England, scratched his face on the thorns of a rosebush, then developed a localized infection around the scratch, and then a more serious systemic infection. He was near death when doctors began giving him injections of penicillin. The policeman improved dramatically, then deteriorated. He died within a couple of weeks, perhaps the first victim of an antibiotic-resistant supergerm.[1]

As it turns out, bacteria evolve and adapt to changes in their environment—including the presence of antibiotics—with incredible speed. While antibiotic treatment often kills all infecting bacteria, a few occasionally survive because they happen to possess a gene that protects them against antibiotics. A small number of bacteria might not seem like much, but some can reproduce in just twenty minutes, creating seventy-two generations and sixteen billion progeny with the same antibiotic-resistant gene in a single day. (It would take your family three thousand years to create seventy-two generations.) The more antibiotics are used, the faster the evolution of antibiotic-resistant bacteria occurs. As rare protective genes become commonplace among bacteria, antibiotics that were once useful become increasingly worthless.

It's the most chilling sort of paradox: the same antibiotics that prevent bacteria from killing people help breed antibiotic-resistant supergerms. Stuart Levy, M.D., of Tufts University, one of the foremost authorities on antibiotic resistance, discussed the details of this contradiction in his book *The Antibiotic Paradox*.[2] In an interview for a *Natural Health* magazine article, he explained, "By taking antibiotics, you are constantly taking out the weaker bacteria and selecting for the stronger ones. This is what creates supergerms."[3]

Penicillin-resistant bacteria were not considered a significant problem in the early 1940s because streptomycin, the second major antibiotic, was discovered in 1944. Streptomycin-resistant bacteria emerged soon after, but again, this was not considered a major problem. The more antibiotics were used, the more common antibiotic-resistant bacteria—supergerms—became.

More than 150 antibiotics have been marketed since the 1940s, and the rapid succession of one antibiotic after another deferred the problem of antibiotic-resistant bacteria for decades. Until relatively recently, few people in medicine thought seriously about the threat posed by bacteria impervious to antibiotics.

But antibiotic-resistant bacteria have become a serious problem today for two reasons. One, there are now many strains of bacteria resistant to many different types of antibiotics. Two, because infectious diseases were mistakenly thought to be "conquered," the big pharmaceutical companies stopped researching new antibiotics in the 1980s. The next new class of antibiotics may not be available until after the year 2000. But even new antibiotics will simply add to the problem of antibiotic resistance rather than provide a long-term solution.

As Bruce R. Levin, Ph.D., an evolutionary biologist from Emory University observed at a recent scientific meeting: "It is reasonable to expect and prudent to plan for the end of the antibiotic era as we have known it. . . . As a consequence of the evolution of resistance, the efficacy of antibiotics for treating bacterial infections has been rapidly waning. 'Natural' selection is almost certainly winning the arms race with the pharmaceutical industry."[4]

HOW BACTERIA SURVIVE

Bacteria have been very adept at defending themselves against the onslaught of antibiotics. Some strains have survived through simple mutations, such as a microorganism with thick, antibiotic-resistant walls. Mutations aren't as common as one might think, though, and most antibiotic-resistant bacteria have persevered because they possess a unique genetic "bag of tricks."

In addition to the genes contained within a bacterium's single chromosome, bacteria also store many accessory traits, including antibiotic resistance, in collections of genes called plasmids. These plasmids function as a genetic toolbox that contains a variety of spare parts. If there's a need, bacteria draw on these genes much the way a handyman might select a particular screwdriver.

Based on the analysis of bacterial samples saved before the advent of antibiotics, it appears that antibiotic-resistant genes always existed, but they just weren't very common. They were presumably an occasional defense against naturally occurring antibiotics, such as the *Penicillium* mold. Widespread antibiotic therapy, however, helped kill off bacteria without these protective genes while encouraging the survival and reproduction of bacteria with them.

The ability of bacteria to adapt against all odds was recently borne out in a series of analogous experiments at the Massachusetts Institute of Technology and the University of Utah. Researchers placed *E. coli* without a chromosomal gene for digesting lactose (milk sugar) into a dish that contained only milk sugar. One would have expected the bacteria to die of starvation. Instead, the lactose ensured the survival of only *E. coli* carrying a spare plasmid gene for digesting lactose. This strain flourished and reproduced faster than anyone had thought possible.[5,6]

This ability to survive would be dramatic in itself. But bacteria also have an uncanny ability to duplicate these plasmids and

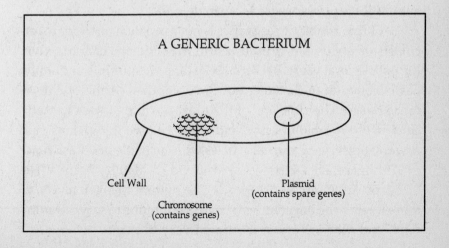

A GENERIC BACTERIUM

Cell Wall

Chromosome
(contains genes)

Plasmid
(contains spare genes)

their genetic contents, kind of like a microbial photocopying machine. So in addition to surviving and passing antibiotic-resistant traits on to their descendants, bacteria can also make hundreds of copies and give them to other bacteria, as if they were people handing out leaflets. They can even transfer these antibiotic-resistant genes to totally unrelated species of bacteria through a process called conjugation. As the name suggests, conjugation is the bacterial equivalent of hot sex. When two bacteria bump into each other—and an estimated ten quadrillion live inside the average person—they pass around these plasmid copies. It's the ultimate in bacterial promiscuity, but *we* suffer the consequences.

INCREASING RESISTANCE TO MULTIPLE ANTIBIOTICS

The ability of bacteria to transfer plasmids from one species to another was identified in 1959 when Japanese researchers found that antibiotic-resistant plasmids from *Shigella,* a type of bacteria that causes severe diarrhea, were also in patients' intestinal *E. coli.* The implications were profound. A generally harmless species of bacteria—*E. coli,* which is common in our intestines—served as a carrier of antibiotic-resistant genes—a bacterial Typhoid Mary, so to speak. But that wasn't half the story. The *Shigella* and *E. coli* had developed resistance to four different antibiotics after exposure to a single one.

Multiple antibiotic resistance is not a problem just with tuberculosis or pneumonia, discussed in the previous chapter. Over the past several years, bacterial resistance to multiple antibiotics has become more the rule, not the exception.[7] Antibiotic resistance has also become one of the most alarming issues in medicine, with normally calm and conservative physicians and researchers writing journal articles with such titles as "Resistance to Antimicrobial Drugs—A Worldwide Calamity"[8] and "The Crisis in Antibiotic Resistance."[9] The bottom line is that you're more likely to be infected with bacteria immune to several antibiotics, and that will make treatment very difficult.

The problem with antibiotic resistance has been amplified by the increasing use of broad-spectrum antibiotics, which theoretically kill a wide range of bacterial species. These antibiotics, including tetracycline and amoxicillin, can select for the survival of many different species of bacteria resistant to many different kinds of antibiotics. The greater the types of antibiotic-resistant bacteria, the less likely it is that antibiotics will be effective.

Today, each one of the hundred major species of disease-causing bacteria has strains (subspecies, so to speak) resistant to at least one antibiotic. Many strains resist three, four, or five antibiotics. Some strains of staph, the cause of many deadly hospital infections, have shown resistance to all antibiotics except vancomycin—and physicians expect to encounter vancomycin-resistant staph at any time. These consequences aren't all that surprising when you consider that more than *forty*

BACTERIA IMMUNE TO ANTIBIOTICS[11]

Some strains of the following disease-causing bacteria are resistant to at least four different antibiotics:

- *Enterobacteria* species, which cause bacteremia (bacteria in the blood), pneumonia, and urinary tract and surgical infections;
- *Haemophilus influenzae,* which cause ear infections, pneumonia, and meningitis;
- *Mycobacteria,* which cause tuberculosis;
- *Neisseria gonorrhoeae,* which cause gonorrhea;
- *Shigella dysenteriae,* which cause dysentery;
- *Pseudomonas aeruginosa,* which cause bacteremia, pneumonia, and urinary tract infections;
- *Staphylococcus aureus,* which cause bacteremia, surgical infections, and pneumonia;
- *Bacteroides,* which cause septicemia (disease-causing bacteria in the blood);
- *Enterococci* species, which cause bacteremia.

million pounds of antibiotics are produced and used annually in the United States.[10]

How did we create such widespread antibiotic resistance among bacteria? Quite simply, through the massive and often uncontrolled use of antibiotics over the past forty-five years. People have unwittingly acted like a combination of God and Charles Darwin to speed the evolution and spread of supergerms.

For years, physicians considered the resulting antibiotic resistance little more than a nuisance. When one failed to work, a doctor could simply switch to another. By the late 1970s and early 1980s, concern about antibiotic resistance was increasingly apparent in medical journals. Dr. Lappé, who has taught medicine at the University of California, Berkeley and the University of Illinois, was the first researcher to go public with a dire warning about the problem in his 1982 book, *Germs That Won't Die*.[12] In a subsequent book, published late in 1994, he described the incredible freewheeling use of antibiotics forty years earlier:

> From the outset, antibiotics were heralded as a panacea for everything from fungus-infected pear orchards to the common cold. Penicillin lozenges were popular as were nostrums such as antibiotic mouthwashes and throat sprays. The unvarnished enthusiasm for using antibiotics was picked up in the ads of the day. Penicillin was touted as a cure-all for bad breath and body odor, and antibiotics were described as the "gold standard" for killing virtually any kind of microbe. Penicillin-containing soaps, mouthwashes, and even drinks were available over the counter. Was it any wonder that when resistant strains emerged, they did so with a vengeance?[13]

Perhaps not surprisingly, some advertisers *still* exploit these antigerm themes. Although they are not marketing antibiotics, these companies reflect and encourage an antigerm mind-set. As recently as 1993, the Clorox Company unearthed one of its preantibiotic themes of the 1930s to prevent food poisoning:

"Start your next meal with Clorox Bleach." Advertising literature for the Lever Brothers Company's Lever 2000 soap asked, "How do you clean up your germiest parts?" The Dial Company became the market leader of antibacterial soaps after leveraging this property of Dial soap. In 1995, Knight's Spray Nine cleaner contained a starburst with the phrase "Kills HIV-1, salmonella,

---

⌘

COMMON CATEGORIES OF ANTIBIOTICS

Penicillins, e.g., phenoxymethylpenicillin, ampicillin, and amoxicillin

Aminoglycosides, e.g., streptomycin, neomycin, and gentamicin

Macrolides, e.g., erythromycin

Lincosamides, e.g., clindamycin

Cephalosporins, e.g., cefaclore, cefazolin, and cefotaxime

Quinolones, e.g., ciprofloxacin

Sulfonamides, e.g., sulfamethizole

Trimethoprim

Beta-lactamase inhibitors, e.g., sulbactam

Thienamycin, e.g., imipenem

Monobactams, e.g., aztreonam

Chloramphenicol

Tetracyclines, e.g., tetracycline and doxycycline

Antituberculosis agents, e.g., isoniazid and rifampin

Urinary antibacterial agents, e.g., methenamine, nitrofurantoin

Various other antibiotics, e.g., vancomycin and bacitracin

⌘

---

staphylococci and pseudomonas in 30 seconds!" Sales of Knight's Spray Nine increased by more than 25 percent after the company added the germ-killing line.

Though these products do not contribute significantly to antibiotic resistance, they encourage the naive view that bacteria can be, and should be, eradicated. As a consequence of this mind-set, antibiotics are often prescribed inappropriately for viral infections (such as the common cold and flu) against which they have no effect, as well as for acne (where the benefits are limited). Patients also contribute to antibiotic resistance by ceasing antibiotic therapy as soon as they feel better, instead of continuing the full course of prescribed treatment. In so many ways, the problem of antibiotic-resistant bacteria grows larger rather than smaller.

Antibiotic Resistance from Your Dentist

In analyzing samples of bacteria, Stuart Levy, M.D., was often troubled by a perplexing finding: antibiotic-resistant bacteria in people who had *not* been taking antibiotics.[14] In the early 1990s, microbiologist Anne O. Summers, Ph.D., of the University of Georgia, Athens, discovered why. Mercury-containing dental fillings, which are toxic to bacteria, select for the survival of mercury-resistant strains—*and* antibiotic-resistant supergerms.

Dr. Summers stumbled across the capacity for this remarkable dual resistance while analyzing the bacteria in fecal samples from 640 hospitalized patients. The feces of more than half these patients contained large numbers of bacteria resistant to mercury and antibiotics, but the patients had not recently taken antibiotics. So in an experiment, Dr. Summers monitored mercury levels and bacteria in six adult monkeys before and after the monkeys were given conventional amalgam fillings.

A couple of weeks after the dental work, the monkeys' mouths and intestines became hosts to significant numbers of mercury-resistant bacteria. The bacteria, which included numerous strep species, were resistant to several antibiotics. When Dr. Summers's team removed the amalgam fillings and replaced them with a nonmercury compound, the numbers of mercury- and antibiotic-resistant bacteria decreased.

What Dr. Summers had discovered was this: the same genes that protected bacteria from the toxic effects of mercury also cross-protected them against antibiotics. Although Dr. Summers couched her hypothesis in conservative medical terms, she contended that the widespread use of dental amalgam was a likely and major contributor to antibiotic-resistant bacteria in people.[15]

Several months later, in a letter to the editor, Brian G. Shearer, Ph.D., of the American Dental Association argued that amalgams could not be the culprit because mercury was "ubiquitous in our environment."[16] In reply, Summers noted that dental amalgams have been the principal source of human exposure to mercury— and that use of mercury amalgams over the past 150 years may have set the genetic stage for widespread antibiotic resistance.[17]

Antibiotic Resistance in the Hospital

Many people believe that hospitals, because of their ready supply of antibiotics, offer supreme protection against supergerms and other infectious microbes. In actuality, the opposite is true. Antibiotic resistance originated in hospitals, beginning in the wards where antibiotics were first administered in the 1940s. And because hospitals use massive amounts of antibiotics, they remain the greatest single source of virulent, antibiotic-resistant supergerms. To use a popular term, hospitals have become "hot zones." If you're hospitalized, you face an unparalleled risk of contracting a deadly infection from supergerms.

This is not an exaggeration. It is serious enough for the existence of a journal, the *Journal of Hospital Infection*, devoted specifically to this problem, and many other medical journals write about the problem as well. Medical jargon often obfuscates this touchy issue—hospital-caused infections are blandly called *nosocomial* infections—but the numbers are simply staggering. More than forty million hospitalizations occur each year in the United States. Two million of these patients develop nosocomial infections, although some estimates go as high as four million.

Upwards of 60 percent—more than 1.2 million—of these people develop antibiotic-resistant infections while hospitalized and treated for other conditions. In some intensive care units (ICUs), patients face a chilling 25 to 70 percent risk of infection. The rates are higher in large hospitals and in teaching hospitals and lower in small hospitals. An estimated sixty to seventy thousand hospital patients die each year from nosocomial infections.[18,19] Those who survive typically have longer and more costly hospital stays. The care of a patient with postoperative fever of an unknown cause adds an average of $9,100 to the bill, and a diagnosed postsurgical infection adds an average of $12,500.[20] According to the CDC, the cost of treating nosocomial infections adds $4.5 billion dollars to the nation's overall health-care budget.

Bacteria are omnipresent in hospitals: in the air, in beds, and on medical equipment. Most nosocomial infections are caused by *S. aureus*, *E. coli*, *Enterococcus faecium*, and *E. faecalis*. In the hospital these microorganisms are more likely to find entry into the body. Each surgical cut in the skin—an attempt at a scientifically controlled knifing—compromises the body's first line of defense against infections. Catheters, which are used to drain urine from the bladder as well as to perform angioplasties on clogged arteries, provide a convenient pathway for bacteria to enter the body. Even though the catheters and many other medical devices are packaged in sterile bags, bacteria immediately settle on them when the seal is broken.

The most vulnerable patients are the sickest, such as those in ICUs, those with immature immune systems, such as infants, and those with weakened immune systems, such as the elderly and patients with cancer and AIDS. But every patient in a hospital is at risk, from the woman with a cesarean section to the man receiving an angioplasty. Indeed, a study at a respectable Canadian hospital found that almost half of the women undergoing cesarean sections developed surgically related infections.[21]

In the mistaken belief that antibiotics can produce a pathogen-free body, antibiotics are frequently dispensed prophylactically before surgery. This has been referred to as the "B-52 approach" to antibiotic use—that is, the saturation bombing of unknown bacteria with broad-spectrum antibiotics. Given the relationship between antibiotic use and the increase in antibiotic-resistant bacteria, this practice aggressively promotes the survival of the toughest antibiotic-resistant bacteria.

Recent trends offer no reason for comfort. By itself sepsis, or blood poisoning caused by infections, strikes 500,000 people annually in the United States, of whom 175,000 die.[22] At one time, E. coli caused the majority of sepsis cases. Soon, if current trends continue, S. aureus will become the leading cause of sepsis.

This is not a good situation because antibiotic-resistant S. aureus is rapidly spreading. Ninety percent of S. aureus strains are resistant to penicillin-family antibiotics,[23] and the numbers of S. aureus strains resistant to methicillin, long the antibiotic of choice, has increased from 8 percent of strains in 1986 to 40 percent in 1992.[24]

Faced with widespread methicillin-resistant S. aureus, physicians increasingly turn to vancomycin, now the antibiotic of last resort. What frightens doctors most is that vancomycin-resistant S. aureus will soon appear, if it hasn't already. Researchers have even figured out how S. aureus will probably gain antibiotic resistance: by swapping genes with a strain of Enterococcus.[25,26] Vancomycin-resistant Enterococcus bacteria are already spreading rapidly across the country, causing death in 60 to 85 percent of people infected with the germ.[27] Infectious disease experts fear that vancomycin-resistant S. aureus could push hospital death rates from infection up to 80 percent, which is where they were half a century ago.

Under these circumstances, antibiotics fit the adage "too

much of a good thing." Calvin M. Kunin, M.D., of Ohio State University, Columbus, has long decried the misuse and overuse of antibiotics by physicians. In a scathing passage in the *Annals of Internal Medicine,* he wrote:

> The pattern of discovery, exuberant use, and predictable obsolescence has been repeated after the introduction of each new antimicrobial drug. No collective memory appears to exist regarding events of the recent past. The prophetic repeated warnings by Maxwell Finland[28] were given lip service and soon forgotten. The opportunity to prolong the effective life of each new antimicrobial drug by more appropriate use was squandered by excessive use.[29]

Antibiotic resistance *can* be slowed by the conservative use of antibiotics. In September 1995, the CDC publicly warned doctors and hospitals to curb their use of vancomycin and the consequential proliferation of vancomycin-resistant bacteria. The CDC recommended that doctors refrain from prescribing antibiotics for viral infections—and that hospitals improve basic sanitation because vancomycin-resistant bacteria can be transmitted via patient charts and telephones.[30,31]

All too often, though, economic forces work against curbing antibiotic abuse. A number of studies have detailed how pharmaceutical company advertising, educational seminars, and expense-paid trips lead to an increase in prescriptions written by physicians.[32,33] In a wry letter to the *Journal of the American Medical Association,* Ronald I. Shorr, M.D., and William L. Greene, Pharm.D., of the Methodist Hospitals of Memphis, Tennessee, described "a food-borne outbreak of expensive antibiotic use."

Drs. Shorr and Greene related an incident in which an intern planned to prescribe a common and inexpensive antibiotic to a patient with a tick bite. The supervising resident ordered the intern to prescribe a "more modern" antibiotic costing $100 per day more. One month earlier, the manufacturer of the "modern" antibiotic hosted an expensive dinner party for the hospital's medical staff. The resident had attended the dinner and was one of many physicians suddenly prescribing the drug. "We do not know if the resident's attendance at the dinner caused his therapeutic choice. . . . However . . . the subsequent changes in hospital-wide prescribing practices should prompt training programs to be wary of such outside sources of medical education," wrote Drs. Shorr and Greene.[34]

A BREAKDOWN IN HOSPITAL CONTROLS

Supergerms are also spread by doctors, nurses, and other hospital workers serving as modern-day Typhoid Marys.[35] Private rooms and simple hand washing between patients or wearing disposable gloves can reduce this problem, but doctors don't consistently wash their hands between patients—or, apparently, at other times. At the 1993 meeting of the Infectious Diseases Society of America in New Orleans, researchers noted that 44 percent of men and 13 percent of women (presumably all physicians) did *not* wash their hands after going to the bathroom.[36]

In June 1995, Duncan W. Clark, M.D., professor emeritus of preventive medicine at the State University of New York, Brooklyn, urged the American Medical Association to remind physicians of the importance of hand washing. In his proposed resolution, Dr. Clark stated that physicians wash their hands only 14 to 50 percent of the time before seeing patients.[37] The AMA passed the resolution without debate.

Several incidents demonstrate how hospital employees can inadvertently promote disease and how sloppy practices can transmit antibiotic-resistant bacteria. In one, CDC researchers investigated an outbreak of twenty postsurgical strep-A infections among patients in a Connecticut hospital. A female technician with a strep infection of the scalp was eventually identified as the source of the infections.[38] She spread the infection directly to patients, often while helping them achieve a more comfortable position in bed.

The spread of a vancomycin-resistant *E. faecium* infection affecting nine patients in a Pennsylvania hospital was traced to the contaminated handles of rectal thermometers. The only controversy erupted after lead investigator Lawrence L. Livornese, M.D., of the Medical College of Pennsylvania, Philadelphia, stated that this was the first time infections were transmitted with electronic rectal thermometers.[39] As if to one-up Dr. Livornese, a nurse from Illinois and a team of doctors from New York wrote letters to the editor pointing out that disease transmission via rectal thermometers had been documented on at least two prior occasions.[40]

These are not rare or isolated incidents either. Recently, researchers tracked the spread of one type of bacteria in a Dutch hospital to the down feathers of pillows.[41] And in a British hospital, investigators traced a salmonella outbreak, which sickened twenty-two patients and seven staff members, to a chef who had been previously disciplined for touching cooked food.[42] Between 1978 and 1987, more than three thousand patients were made ill by 248 separate salmonella outbreaks in England and Wales alone.[43]

Sometimes, microorganisms have the potential to spread as a result of unanticipated consequences of medical technology. Douglas E. Ott, M.D., of Mercer University, Macon, Georgia, has pointed out that the smoke created during laser cauterization can drift more than forty yards, and it has been known to irritate the eyes of surgical teams in separate rooms. Hospitals have air-control systems to remove these ashlike particles, but according to Ott, they are not used consistently. What's a few particles of burned and semiburned tissue? In 1991, researchers at the State University of New York, Syracuse, cultured HIV from the smoke of tissue cauterized with a laser.[44]

A half century ago, antibiotics were heralded as miracle drugs. Although the superlative was well deserved, it encouraged a mind-set that led to the eager and often indiscriminate use of antibiotics. Furthermore, antibiotics had unanticipated consequences that, for too many years, were ignored or avoided. For every million bacteria killed by antibiotics, a few strong ones survived. Today, these antibiotic-resistant bacteria number far more than a few. The situation is compounded by lapses in simple hygiene and sanitation, and home-grown bacteria are emerging as the most serious supergerm threats to Americans.

But medicine cannot shoulder this blame alone. In the next chapter, you'll read how American ranchers and farmers routinely use large quantities of antibiotics to speed the growth of livestock. This profit-driven practice further accelerates the evolution of bacteria and antibiotic-resistant supergerms, including *E. coli* and *Salmonella*. As a consequence, consumers risk encounters with supergerms every time they sit down to eat.

4

DOWN AND DIRTY ON
THE FARM

⌘

Whether physicians prescribe antibiotics wisely or not so wisely, at least they are motivated by a desire to restore the health of their patients. In contrast, the widespread use of antibiotics in animal husbandry is driven by production of and profit from what eventually becomes billions of hamburgers and chicken sandwiches for America's fast-food restaurants.

Ranchers and farmers raising beef cattle, dairy cows, poultry, sheep, and hogs have helped breed large numbers of antibiotic-resistant bacteria. Like people, farm animals develop infections and spread them to other animals, and in this respect, crowded feedlots aren't much different from many day care centers. Ranchers and veterinarians alike view their use of antibiotics as the "humane treatment" of infected animals.

In truth, the rationale behind the use of antibiotics in animal husbandry has less to do with kindness and more to do with maximizing the financial investment in animals and their feed. The most serious abuse of antibiotics in animal husbandry occurs not in the treatment of infections—or even in the dubious practice of preventive treatment. It is in the *subtherapeutic,* or chronic low-dose, administration of antibiotics in feed to stimulate growth. Grain is a business expense—for example, feed accounts for one-half the cost of raising sheep—and relatively small increases in growth and decreases in grain consumption save the livestock industry millions of dollars annually in feed costs.

The problem is exacerbated by a general lack of FDA and veterinary oversight on farms. Unlike antibiotics intended for human consumption, many veterinary antibiotics can be purchased without a prescription at farm-supply stores throughout the country. And the quantities are anything but inconsequential: $500 million worth of antibiotics[1]—half of the forty million pounds produced each year in the United States—are used in animal husbandry. By one estimate, the average farm animal receives thirty times more antibiotics than does the average person.[2]

The health consequences for the consumer are profound. Like antibiotics prescribed for people, antibiotics on the farm speed the evolution of bacteria and select for the survival of drug-resistant supergerms. The average person can be exposed to these antibiotic-resistant bacteria by handling raw meat in the kitchen, eating inadequately cooked meat, and through contact with farmers and ranchers who administer antibiotics. Perhaps most disturbing, the people facing the greatest risk of acquiring a serious antibiotic-resistant infection from food are those who are taking, or have recently taken, antibiotics for medical reasons.[3,4] (We discuss the immune-damaging effects of antibiotics in Chapter 8.)

At this point, you might be anticipating an argument in favor of vegetarianism. We won't argue for or against vegetarianism. Avoiding meat would clearly sidestep this source of antibiotic-resistant bacteria, but it is not the only option available to consumers. In Chapter 9, we will explain how to obtain meats from antibiotic-free livestock. For now, it's the problem of antibiotic-laced meat that concerns us.

Antibiotics As Animal Growth Enhancers

The growth-enhancing property of antibiotics was discovered in the late 1940s by Thomas H. Jukes, Ph.D., then a researcher at Lederle Laboratories and later a professor at the University of California, Berkeley. At first Dr. Jukes thought he had stumbled across a nutritional growth factor related to vitamin B_{12}. This growth factor turned out to be not a vitamin but traces of chlortetracycline, the first of the tetracycline family of antibiotics.

Subsequent experiments revealed that tiny amounts of chlortetracycline—one to five parts per million—dramatically increased the growth and weight gain of chickens. Neither Jukes nor anyone else has ever determined exactly why antibiotics stimulate growth, but some researchers suspect that antibiotics immobilize or kill many bacteria that would otherwise usurp vitamins and other nutrients for their own metabolism. With the bacteria eliminated, these nutrients can be used by the animal. The idea does make sense. Excessive amounts of intestinal bacteria have the opposite effect—they slow an animal's rate of growth.

Chlortetracycline was marketed as a growth stimulant beginning in 1950, with dosages ranging from 2 to 10 milligrams per kilogram (2.2 pounds) of animal weight. Today, virtually every commercially raised chicken is given subtherapeutic levels of antibiotics in its feed, and so are more than half of all cattle, pigs, and sheep.[5] Subtherapeutic doses of these antibiotics, generally one-tenth to one-hundredth that of the therapeutic dose, are ideal for encouraging the survival of antibiotic resistant species because they kill only the most susceptible bacteria and allow those with resistance to survive.

According to *The Stockman's Handbook*, a leading reference book for ranchers, antibiotics increase weight gain in steers, heifers, and calves by 6 percent daily while also reducing feed requirements by 4 percent.[6] Furthermore, antibiotics encourage better marbling of beef than do hormonal growth stimulants, such as "Steer-oid." In other words, antibiotics promote faster weight gain on less food while creating a much more marketable product. The same principles hold true for pigs and sheep. Antibiotics increase the growth rate of young pigs by more than 200 percent! Older pigs being "finished" before slaughter gain weight 10 percent faster on 5 percent less feed when given antibiotics. For sheep, tetracycline increases daily weight gain by an average of 11 percent—and sometimes up to 31 percent.

While *The Stockman's Handbook* provides general guidelines for administering growth-stimulating antibiotics and hormones, in practice it is an imprecise and subjective art. The book notes that the "eye of the expert feeder fattens the cattle"—which translates to a good guess based on experience. Farmers often err on the side of excess, and livestock receive large amounts of antibiotics for all sorts of reasons.

For example, transport is a major stress for farm animals, but ranchers have discovered that antibiotics compensate for the stress and weight loss cattle suffer during shipment. According to the *Merck Veterinary Manual,* a daily dose of antibiotics for two to three weeks after transport significantly lowers the incidence of "shipping fever syndrome," an animal disease of stress, and promotes the rapid regain of weight lost during transport.[7]

ANTIBIOTIC RESISTANCE FROM ANIMALS TO PEOPLE

In an interview published in *Food Insight,* the director of the Food and Drug Administration's Center for Veterinary Medicine downplayed the problems arising from antibiotic use in farm animals. "Many of the microbial resistance issues of concern today, such as tuberculosis, cholera and Streptococcus A, pertain to diseases for which bacteria never occurred in animals," explained Stephen Sundlof, D.M.V., Ph.D. "There are relatively few bacterial organisms that cause diseases in humans."[8]

Although animals and humans do not have many diseases in common, they do share the same antibiotics. Penicillins and tetracyclines are the most common families of antibiotics used in animal husbandry, but cephalosporins, aminoglycosides, chloramphenicol, lincosamides, macrolides, quinolones, and sulfonamides are also used. These antibiotics constitute much of the physician's antibacterial arsenal for treating people.

The real problem, which Dr. Sundlof carefully avoided, is not the types of bacteria infecting farm animals but, instead, the broad use of antibiotics and the ease with which resistance is transferred among bacteria. As in people, the digestive tracts of cattle contain large amounts of E. coli, which serve as a warehouse of antibiotic-resistant genes.

Studies dating back to the 1960s have examined how antibiotic-resistant bacteria, such as E. coli, migrate from farm animals to people. In a remarkable experiment, Stuart Levy, M.D., and his colleagues at Tufts University introduced subtherapeutic levels of tetracycline at a private farm in Sherborn, Massachusetts. The setting was significantly controlled in that no other antibiotics had been used on the farm in at least seven years.

Dr. Levy's team gave about 150 chickens subtherapeutic doses of the antibiotic in feed, as is typically done to speed growth and conserve grain consumption. Another group of chickens received only antibiotic-free feed. The birds were kept in several cages, some inside a barn and some just outside it. At the start of the experiment, only about 10 percent of the E. coli obtained from all the animals' feces showed resistance to tetracycline. Feces obtained from the farmer's family were also low in antibiotic-resistant E. coli. Two days after eating their first meal laced with antibiotics, 60 percent of the E. coli in the chickens' feces were tetracycline resistant, reflecting a dramatic change in the birds' gastrointestinal tract. After two weeks, 90 percent of the chickens were excreting only tetracycline-resistant E. coli.

After four months, 30 percent of the chickens not fed antibiotics also started excreting large numbers of antibiotic-resistant E. coli. About the same time, large numbers of antibiotic-resistant E. coli began appearing in the feces of the farmer's family. All eight family members excreted a large number of antibiotic-resistant *E. coli,* and in three of them 80 percent of the *E. coli* were drug resistant. Even more amazing, the *E. coli* in the chickens and humans were now also resistant to several other antibiotics— including ampicillin and streptomycin—although no other antibiotics had been used.

In another study, Dr. Levy and his team traced the actual spread of resistant *E. coli* on a farm in the absence of any antibiotic. They began with a specific strain of *E. coli* from a cow, genetically tagged it so it could be later identified, and then returned it to the cow. Within four to six weeks, the *E. coli* had spread to mice, pigs, chickens, flies, and even to two farmworkers who took care of the barnyard animals.[9] If the *E. coli* had been a disease-causing strain, the consequences would have been disastrous. Still, the experiment demonstrated the ease with which antibiotic resistance spreads.

In many respects, the agricultural use of antibiotics is more serious than their medical use. Millions of tons of feces containing antibiotic-resistant bacteria are dropped daily—only to be blown long distances by the wind. Cedric A. Mims, Ph.D., a microbiologist at Guy's Hospital Medical School, London, has related that pigs with "foot and mouth" disease excrete 100 million viruses in their breath each day. With favorable humidity, 65 percent of the viruses survive and can be carried from France to England, to infect cows. "Outbreaks of this disease are often explained by studying air trajectories and other meteorological factors," observed Mims.[10]

Agricultural antibiotics—and the consequential antibiotic-resistant bacteria in the environment—pose two serious problems for people, according to Dr. Levy. First, they encourage the swapping of antibiotic resistance among bacteria. Second, antibiotic-resistant bacteria—supergerms—complicate the treatment of infections in people. "The rise in frequency of resistant organisms in our environment is the obvious result of antibiotic usage," wrote Dr. Levy. "The only means to curtail this trend is to control the indiscriminate use of these drugs."[11]

There are, however, few genuine efforts to curb antibiotic

use in animal husbandry. In August 1995, the FDA approved the use of sarafloxacin, one of several types of powerful antibiotics called fluoroquinolones, to treat *E. coli* infections in chickens. The antibiotic does not make chicken safer to eat because the strain of *E. coli* affecting chickens does not cause disease in people. The sarafloxacin is strictly to prevent the loss of chickens—and profits. When sarafloxacin-resistant bacteria appear, as they inevitably will, they will likely be resistant to other fluoroquinolone antibiotics as well. Even *Business Week*, a champion of industry, questioned the FDA's approval of this antibiotic in animal feed: "Given the potential perils . . . is it really so important to save 2¢ on a pound of chicken wings?"[12]

SUPERGERMS FROM ANIMALS AND MEAT

The most immediate risk of infections from farm animals is to the farmers who use antibiotics in animal husbandry and to their families. In October 1992, a thirteen-month-old boy with bloody diarrhea and vomiting was admitted to a hospital in Ontario, Canada. Like the children who ate contaminated meat in Seattle and Tacoma, this boy was diagnosed with an *E. coli* 0157:H7 infection. His five-year-old sister and nine-year-old brother also became sick. The parents raised veal calves in an old dairy barn, and after the farmer broke his ankle, his wife fed the calves and cleaned their pens. She brought along her toddler and, according to a medical journal description, "the mother noted that the boy frequently touched the calves and put his fingers in their mouths and his."[13]

Under the right circumstances, such infections can lead to larger outbreaks. One began at a Connecticut farm on August 16, 1976, when several calves developed diarrhea and one died. The farmer worked closely with the calves and, four days later, developed a mild case of diarrhea. About a week later, his pregnant daughter, who worked on the farm, delivered a full-term boy by cesarean section, but the infant developed a fever and mild diarrhea several days later. Two other newborn infants in the same nursery also developed diarrhea caused by a type of *Salmonella* resistant to several common antibiotics.

An investigation revealed that the first infant contracted the infection in utero from his mother, who had acquired her infection on the farm. In the hospital, the infection was spread by a nurse who cared for all of the infants. In the *Journal of the American Medical Association*, Robert W. Lyons, M.D., of St. Francis Hospital, Hartford, wrote that nurseries seem especially susceptible to these infections, and that the "infecting dose" for an infant may be far less than what's needed to make an adult ill. "There has been concern that the use of antibiotics in animal feed might lead to antibiotic-resistant organisms in animals and that these organisms or their R [resistance] factors could be transferred to human hosts," explained Dr. Lyons. "The present epidemic is consistent with that hypothesis."[14]

In another incident, in 1982, several newborn infants in a Quebec hospital were infected by *Salmonella* resistant to *six* different antibiotics. Again, the outbreak began among dairy cows on a nearby farm and was passed to the mother of one of the infants who regularly drank raw milk from the infected herd.[15] G. S. Bezanson, Ph.D., of Canada's Department of National Health and Welfare, who described the epidemic, pointed the finger at raw milk and urged even more extensive pasteurization of milk.

However, pasteurization failed to prevent the largest *Salmonella* outbreak in the United States and Canada. This epidemic struck in two waves in 1984 and 1985, affecting an estimated 366,000 people in northern Illinois. (More than sixteen thousand of these cases were confirmed by laboratory culture.) The *Salmonella*, resistant to five different antibiotics, was traced to post-pasteurization contamination that persisted for more than ten months in the milk-processing plant. Investigators concluded that the *Salmonella* had originated in dairy cows given antibiotics.

While many people in northern Illinois had low-grade symptom-free infections, those who happened to have taken antibiotics in the month prior to drinking the contaminated milk were *five times* more likely to develop a serious infection. Caroline A. Ryan, M.D., and her fellow investigators at the CDC wrote in the *Journal of the American Medical Association* that the use of antibiotics increased the risk of infection in two ways. First, they destroyed the normal intestinal bacteria, leaving a void that the *Salmonella* quickly filled. Second, the infecting *Salmonella* had the advantage of already being antibiotic resistant.[16]

MEDICAL AND ANIMAL ANTIBIOTICS AS A DANGEROUS COMBINATION

Since the introduction of antibiotics in animal husbandry, the incidence of food-borne salmonellosis has skyrocketed.[17] Using *E. coli* as an indicator of bacterial activity in food, A. H. Linton, Ph.D., and Katherine Howe, Ph.D., of the University of Bristol Medical School, England, traced the transfer of *E. coli* from the farm to the fork. They reported, for example, that rural residents with greater exposure to farm animals were more likely than urban dwellers to carry antibiotic-resistant organisms. The same is true of slaughterhouse workers, because they handle contaminated carcasses.[18] These antibiotic-resistant organisms easily move from the carcass to the kitchen[19] and take up residence in the intestines of people who handle, cook, and eat the meat.[20]

Although *Salmonella* bacteria are common in chickens, few infections are actually caused by chickens. The reason is simple: people almost always cook their poultry thoroughly. This is not always the case with beef, which many people prefer cooked medium or rare—or even eating it raw as steak tartare. And insofar as beef is concerned, hamburger is worse than cuts of beef, such as sirloin or flank steak, because grinding thoroughly mixes bacteria with the meat, and meat on the inside of a patty is less likely to be cooked.

Again, though everyone is susceptible to meat-borne pathogens, people recently taking antibiotics face a much higher risk of infection. In 1983, Scott D. Holmberg, M.D., of the CDC, identified eighteen people in four midwestern states who had been infected by a strain of *Salmonella* resistant to several antibiotics, including tetracycline. Twelve of the patients had been taking penicillin or amoxicillin for a day or two before developing *Salmonella* infections. One of the patients died and the other eleven were hospitalized for an average of eleven days. Each of the patients had eaten ground beef during the week prior to their illness.

Investigators identified the telltale genetic "fingerprints" of the *Salmonella* strain in all of the patients, and Dr. Holmberg traced the source to a slaughterhouse in Minnesota and then to a specific herd in South Dakota. This herd had been fed subtherapeutic amounts of tetracycline as a growth enhancer. Most people eating the meat had asymptomatic infections, but those taking medically prescribed antibiotics were again predisposed to severe salmonella infections. Forty thousand pounds of contaminated meat were distributed from this herd, leading Dr. Holmberg to suspect that many infections probably went unreported.[21]

Another outbreak of antibiotic-resistant salmonella, this one in Los Angeles County, was traced specifically to hamburger from dairy cows. "Dairy cows sent for slaughter, unlike steers raised in feedlots, are older animals that are not in prime condition," observed the CDC's John S. Spika, M.D., who investigated the outbreak. "Acute and chronic illnesses that decrease milk production lead to removal of cows from milking herds. Stressed animals are more likely to shed salmonella in large numbers."[22]

Dr. Spika and his colleagues interviewed 45 of the 298 patients infected by the salmonella, which were resistant to the antibiotic chloramphenicol. Their illnesses were traced to contaminated ground beef, most often eaten in restaurants. But more than half of these patients had also been taking prescribed antibiotics sometime during the month before they contracted the salmonella infection. Once again, the meat was traced to a specific herd of cows fed low levels of tetracycline. The Los

Angeles outbreak was unusual in one other respect. Chloramphenicol cannot be legally used in food production.

In light of such episodes, it's not surprising that numerous countries do not permit the subtherapeutic use of antibiotics in farm animals—or allow the importation of meat from animals whose growth was stimulated by antibiotics.

Mad Cows and Englishmen

In March 1996, a problem that had festered for years on British farms suddenly erupted in headlines and television news reports around the world. A bizarre and deadly infection, dubbed "mad cow disease" had apparently spread to people. The human variant of the disease, called Creutzfeldt-Jakob disease, attacks the brain like a high-speed version of Alzheimer's. Typically, by the time most people are diagnosed with the condition, they have only a couple of months left to live.

Both conditions, mad cow disease and the new strain of Creutzfeldt-Jakob disease, appeared to originate with the practice of feeding sheep offal—parts left over after slaughter—to cows. The emergence of these diseases reflects how seriously the food supply, at least in England, has been compromised by economic greed. There is no reason to use offal as a feed additive for vegetarian animals, except to profit from the waste of slaughterhouses. In the United States, cattle growers have followed the same practice for years, but they have been extremely lucky. There have been no cases of mad cow disease here.

WHAT CAUSES MAD COW DISEASE?

Mad cow disease is technically referred to as bovine spongiform encephalopathy, or BSE. In nonmedical terms, it describes a cow disease that turns the brain into a mass with spongelike holes. The result is a deadly neurological condition—animals shake with palsylike tremors and lose their muscular coordination and ability to stand and walk.

There's no controversy about where BSE came from. Sheep, particularly British sheep, are prone to a similar spongiform encephalopathy called "scrapie," named for the tendency of infected sheep to scrape their legs against each other. BSE was first identified in British cows in 1986, and the use of sheep offal in cow feed was banned two years later. Suddenly aware of the risks, the United States banned the importation of British beef in 1989.

Several events led up to the mad cow panic. Ordinarily, Creutzfeldt-Jakob disease is rare, affecting only people in their 50s or 60s, and then only one person in every million. (It has strong similarities to kuru, a neurological disease that afflicts some cannibalistic natives of Papua, New Guinea.) But British doctors were surprised to recently diagnose ten cases of Creutzfeldt-Jakob disease in a two-year period. Even more striking, the average age of the victims was about twenty-seven. Some were dairy farmers, who obviously worked in proximity to cows, and three were teenagers.

Some scientists and, of course, the general public were getting nervous, and domestic beef sales were slipping. The government kept telling people that British beef was safe—until March 20, 1996, when Health Secretary Stephan Dorrell acknowledged that disease-ridden cows were the most likely cause of the new wave of Creutzfeldt-Jakob disease.[23] An uproar followed. The next day, France banned the import of British beef, and within a few days so did most other European nations. Even though the link to mad cow disease was largely circumstantial, Britain's beef industry was instantly every bit as crippled as a sickened cow. Conversely, sales of organically produced beef—raised the old-fashioned way on grass or grain—increased dramatically.

Scrapie, mad cow disease, kuru, and Creutzfeldt-Jakob disease are not caused by bacteria, viruses, or parasites. The infectious agent—called a prion—is an infectious protein that's smaller than a virus and contains no genetic material.

Not all prions are bad, however. Since the mad cow outbreak, researchers have discovered that normal prions play subtle but important roles in health, helping to manage the circadian rhythm and muscle control. They are best understood as a combination of biology and geometry. Prions behave much like other proteins, in that their function depended in large part on their physical shape. Normal and infectious proteins seem to have the same chemical composition, but they have different shapes. For some reason, as yet unknown, a normal prion can change shape. When it does, the prion seems to trigger a domino effect, and nearby prions also begin to bend in a similar way.

SPEEDING UP AND SLOWING THE DISEASE

What makes a prion go bad? No one knows positively what triggers this transformation, but there's a good chance that it is initiated by dangerous molecules called free radicals. (You'll read more about free radicals in Chapter 6.) In a series of experiments, German researchers may have figured out a big part of the puzzle, with intriguing implications.

Hans A. Kretzschmar, Ph.D., and his colleagues at the University of Göttingen, investigated how prions affected microglia, a type of brain cell that collects metabolic waste products. According to Kretzschmar, microglia release large amounts of free radicals when they are stimulated by prions. Apparently, those free radicals cause the brain damage characteristic of mad cow and Creutzfeldt-Jakob diseases. That means that prions might instigate the deleterious changes, but the actual damage is caused by microglia.

A group of "antioxidant" vitamins and other micronutrients, including vitamin E, are well known for their ability to neutralize free radicals. So in a related experiment, using cultured cells (not animals) Kretzschmar added two antioxidants, vitamin E and N-acetylcysteine. Both prevented prions from triggering the release of free radicals by microglia and, subsequently, brain cell damage.[24] Kretzschmar's findings are significant. Alzheimer's disease, which bears some strong similarities to

Creutzfeldt-Jakob disease, also seems to be aggravated when microglia dump their collected waste products.

This does not mean antioxidant vitamins are a cure for mad cow disease or Creutzfeldt-Jakob disease. These conditions are, in fact, probably irreversible. However, the successful experiments by Kretzschmar strongly suggest there is a way to slow the progression of these diseases. (You'll read much more about antioxidants and free radicals in Parts II and III of this book.)

Antibiotics in Milk

Like other farm animals, dairy cows frequently receive antibiotics to prevent or treat infections. The FDA permits traces of eighty different antibiotics in cow's milk sold to consumers, but milk with significant antibiotic residues is supposed to be dumped. In 1992, however, an analysis by Congress' General Accounting Office discovered that states routinely test for only four antibiotics. When the GAO ran its own tests on milk samples, it found sixty-four antibiotics in amounts "that raise health concerns."[25] The message: milk may not be as well regulated as the average person assumes.

BOVINE GROWTH HORMONE AND ANTIBIOTICS IN MILK

The controversy surrounding the use of antibiotics in dairy cows reached new heights after the FDA's November 1993 approval of Monsanto's recombinant bovine growth hormone (rBGH), also known as recombinant bovine somatotrophin (rBST or rbST). A synthetic hormone, rBGH is injected into dairy cows to increase their milk output by 15 percent. The need for greater milk production has been questioned by a number of consumer groups because milk is generally overproduced, and like tobacco growers, dairy farmers receive generous price supports to bolster their marginal profits. Higher milk production would just seem to add to the glut, narrow profits even more, and increase the need for more federal price supports.

There are serious health considerations with rBGH as well. One is that the hormone increases milk levels of insulin-like growth factor (IGF1), a hormonelike substance linked to breast and colon cancers. Monsanto's rBGH also increases the risk of mastitis, or udder infections, in dairy cows. A higher incidence of mastitis leads to more antibiotic treatment, more antibiotic residues, and more antibiotic-resistant bacteria. The point of contention is not whether rBGH causes more udder infections. It does. The controversy is whether the hormone causes a minor or major increase in mastitis, because the difference influences the amount of antibiotics used to treat the animals. That is what the rBGH issue boils down to.

As you might expect with any argument, the true impact of rBGH is often obfuscated by a careful choice of words and data. According to a report in the November/December 1994 *FDA Veterinarian*, "More than six million injections of Posilac® [Monsanto's brand name for rBGH] have been sold for use in at least 560,000 cows on more than 10,000 farms. In the first six months that rbST was marketed, FDA received 96 reports of adverse reactions in cattle." Left unstated was how many doses of Posilac were actually used in the six-month period—and whether the ninety-six reports were a fraction of a percent or a more significant percentage of the treated cows. Furthermore, while only ninety-six cases were *reported*, more incidents may very well have occurred.

Of the ninety-six reported, twenty-four described mastitis and high numbers of somatic cells (that is, pus-filled white blood cells), twenty-two involved udder swelling or abnormal milk, and twenty-nine described reproductive disorders. Some of the reports refer to more than one condition, including digestive disorders, so there is overlap. Nonetheless, the *FDA Veterinarian* proclaimed, "These reports do not raise new concerns about potential health impacts on consumers."[26]

By February 1995, dairy farmers had filed 806 reports of negative rBGH reactions, including bloody milk, spontaneous abortions, mastitis, retained placentas, and death. Although the FDA's Dr. Stephen Sundlof downplayed the reports, he admitted to the *St. Louis Dispatch* that rBGH complications were probably underreported.

It would, of course, be easy to promote consumer choice in the marketplace by requiring dairies to identify rBGH-containing milk on the label or, conversely, to permit dairies to state that their milk is free of rBGH. Monsanto complained to the FDA about the economic impact when such labeling was proposed by consumer groups. Despite claims of safety, the company may fear that most people would choose rBGH-free milk. In response to Monsanto, the FDA has refused to allow dairies to state on their labels that milk is free of rBGH. Some natural-foods stores and dairies have sidestepped the letter of the law by calling their milk "organic" rather than rBGH free. In addition, some states are now permitting rBGH-free labeling on dairy products.

SCIENTISTS VERSUS BUSINESS INTERESTS

The rBGH controversy overlaps the scientific as well as the regulatory arena. A team of British researchers has charged that Monsanto prevented publication of their highly critical scientific analysis of the company's own rBGH data. Erik Millstone, Ph.D., Eric Brunner, Ph.D., and Ian White, M.Sc., investigated whether rBGH increases the number of somatic cells in the milk of lactating cows. These cells reflect the degree of inflammation in the cow's udder and a large number of the cells indicates mastitis. Since the somatic cells are essentially pus, a large number can alter the taste of the milk. Antibiotics, given prophylactically, can minimize the problem—which is why antibiotics are so closely associated with the use of rBGH.

In a two-page commentary in the journal *Nature*, Dr. Millstone and his colleagues related their difficulties in obtaining all of the rBGH data from Monsanto and getting their preliminary findings published. Based on some of the data, they noted that rBGH increased the number of somatic cells by 19 percent compared with cows not receiving the drug. The increase in somatic cells also raised the number of cows with mastitis, based on European Union standards, from 6 percent to almost 11 percent.[27,28] In an unpublished reappraisal of Monsanto's rBGH data, Dr. Brunner and his colleagues found that the drug increased the risk of mastitis in cows by *39 percent*.[29]

Over the past fifteen years, Monsanto, Eli Lilly, Upjohn, and Cyanamid have spent more than $1 billion on the development of various rBGH products. Like any company, they would like a payoff for their research and development, and it's easy to understand why Monsanto is not fond of Brunner's data. If rBGH were truly safe, Monsanto could quickly quell the controversy by releasing all of its data. We can only speculate about why the company has not yet done so.

Unlike the FDA, the food-regulatory agencies of other nations have so far shown greater skepticism of Monsanto's rBGH data. Neither Monsanto nor the other companies have received approval for rBGH drugs in other countries. Health Canada has refused to allow Canada's dairy industry to use Monsanto's Posilac. Likewise, the European Union has not permitted the use of Posilac or other rBGH drugs.

The administration of low-dose antibiotics in livestock is practically ideal for promoting antibiotic-resistant bacteria. As a consequence, purchasing meat—particularly hamburger—at the supermarket or in a restaurant often risks exposure to dangerous supergerms. The danger can reach a flash point when people taking medically prescribed antibiotics also happen to eat meat tainted with antibiotic-resistant bacteria, such as *Salmonella*. With the body's defenses already weakened by an infection, a new assault by antibiotic-resistant bacteria literally stampedes over the vestiges of immunity.

Similarly, getting milk free of rBGH and antibiotics has become a roll of the dice. Small dairies that refuse to use rBGH may still have their milk pooled with milk from dairies that do use it. Such pooling is a subtle form of arm twisting. Ensuring that the milk ultimately sold to consumers contains rBGH can weaken the will of those who have hesitated using the drug in their herds. And whether the risk of mastitis associated with rBGH is small or great, we believe dairy farmers will inevitably increase their prophylactic and therapeutic use of antibiotics. That action, of course, will promote the selection and survival of more antibiotic-resistant bacteria—and of supergerms. There is, however, a positive sign: large numbers of farmers have stopped using rBGH.[30]

Although antibiotic-resistant bacteria are the types of supergerms Americans are most likely to encounter, other supergerms have emerged for reasons completely independent of antibiotic abuse. With the exception of AIDS, these other supergerms pose a minor threat to Americans. But one outbreak could change that within a matter of days.

5

STRANGERS IN OUR MIDST

———————— ❧ ————————

While the misuse of antibiotics has changed many innocuous or minor bacteria into supergerms, factors completely unrelated to antibiotics have also increased health risks from a variety of bacteria, viruses, and protozoa. Environmental and ecological disruptions, political and social upheavals, unanticipated consequences of common technologies, and simple accidents of twentieth-century life have contributed to the emergence and spread of supergerms.

In its devastating way, AIDS has reawakened the world to just how deadly infectious diseases could be. Since 1981, almost one-half million people in North America have been diagnosed with AIDS, and more than a quarter of a million have died. Worldwide, almost twenty million people have AIDS.

AIDS is not, however, the only "new" germ to emerge and spread in recent years. At least one new, often bizarre microorganism a year now grabs headlines—among them are the Ebola virus, hantavirus, *Borrelia burgdorferi* (which causes Lyme disease), and the Australian horse virus. Just as epidemics of measles and smallpox followed Roman and Asian caravan routes almost two thousand years ago, AIDS and other supergerms often follow our modern travel routes. We encounter them as we explore and develop previously uninhabited regions of the world, and a highly mobile population and commercial air travel enable their rapid globalization.

Most of these microorganisms pass the time harmlessly in their natural hosts, such as rodents or mosquitoes. Human development and deforestation often leads to unfortunate encounters, enabling the microorganisms to infect a new species. Such encounters are dangerous because people have no specific immunity to these germs, and forestry and agricultural workers seem to be at very high risk because they are on the front lines of such situations. Sometimes these infections fester at a low level for years, aided by the poor medical care and haphazard diagnoses in developing nations. At a certain point, the infection reaches a biological flash point, and an epidemic like AIDS or Ebola ensues.

HIV AND AIDS

There is no controversy that the human immunodeficiency virus (HIV), which causes AIDS, evolved from the simian immunodeficiency virus (SIV). This monkey virus is similar in genetic structure to HIV, though not as virulent. What is more controversial is exactly how the virus jumped to people.

Blaine Elswood, an AIDS activist in San Francisco, has proposed an intriguing if unconventional theory: the SIV piggybacked its way to people in a contaminated batch of polio vaccine. Elswood contends that some researchers overlooked SIV while preparing experimental polio vaccines from crushed monkey kidneys in the 1950s. According to Elswood, a suspect batch of polio vaccine was used in 1957 to treat a quarter of a million Africans in what was then the Belgian Congo (now Zaire)—if true, a sizable start for a worldwide infection. It would be easy enough for researchers to analyze stored samples from early batches of polio vaccines, but according to Elswood, the early polio researchers refuse to do so.[1]

The timing is almost too eerie to be mere coincidence. Although doctors reported the first human cases of AIDS in 1981, and identified the virus in 1983, they have since taken a second look at blood samples from people who had earlier died of mysterious AIDS-like diseases. In *Evolutionary Medicine*, Marc Lappé, Ph.D., notes that AIDS has been retrospectively diagnosed from blood samples kept from a number of unusual illnesses during the 1960s and 1970s.[2]

Like influenza, HIV is a highly adaptable, rapidly mutating virus. Researchers at Oxford University have suggested that the exceptionally fast mutation rate and other characteristics of HIV might make a protective vaccine impossible.[3] According to Lappé, HIV remains relatively quiescent unless the immune system is stimulated by another infection. In Africa, malaria might serve as the primary stimulus. Elsewhere, just about any infection might suffice.

A contrarian view of AIDS has been espoused by virologist Peter H. Duesberg, Ph.D. He has pointed out that HIV fails to fulfill Koch's postulates, a set of rules that links a germ to a specific disease, and thus cannot be the cause of AIDS. Dr. Duesberg and his colleague Bryan J. Ellison, Ph.D., argue against an infectious origin of AIDS altogether, favoring instead an explanation based on exposure to immune-suppressing drugs such as narcotics. Whatever the actual cause, AIDS is characterized by profound immune suppression with concomitant malnutrition and opportunistic infections.[4]

We have addressed only a few key points about HIV and AIDS here, mainly because so much has been written about them. In later chapters, we will discuss various nutrients that can bolster the immune system, improve the well-being, and extend the life span of people with this deadly infection.

EBOLA HEMORRHAGIC FEVER

In the spring of 1995, a brief but major outbreak of Ebola hemorrhagic fever erupted in Kikwit, Zaire. By the time it was declared over—several months after it was first reported by the Associated Press—244 of the 315 infected people had died, including six Roman Catholic nuns and at least three Red Cross volunteers. The first major Ebola outbreak, in Zaire nineteen years before, had killed 274 of the 300 people infected with it. A second outbreak occurred in Sudan in 1979, and a number of isolated, nonepidemic cases have also been reported over the years.

Ebola's initial symptoms—fever, diarrhea, and weakness—resemble many other infections and are not terribly alarming. Its later symptoms, however, are grisly: blood from leaky vessels pours through the mouth, nose, eyes, and ears—and sometimes it is expelled projectilely—making humane care for the sick difficult and risky. Although "the red diarrhea," the local name for Ebola, is not spread by casual contact, extensive bleeding encourages transmission. Blood can infect a caretaker or family member through a minor cut in the skin. There is no cure and no vaccine.

The 1995 Ebola outbreak began with a forestry worker who made charcoal from trees—or someone he had been near. His work may have placed him in proximity to a rodent or insect that is the natural host of the Ebola virus. (The natural host of Ebola, for now, is unknown.) The forestry worker died in January, and other members of his household succumbed in the following weeks. At the time, no one had suspected Ebola as the cause of their deaths.

The epicenter for the actual epidemic was a 350-bed hospital in Kikwit, a city of 600,000. The reuse of unsterilized syringes and a lack of surgical gloves hastened the infection's spread from a surgical patient to doctors and nurses in mid-March. When they realized the infection was Ebola, doctors and nurses fled the hospital in panic, likely infecting other people. News reporters who arrived a week later found the hospital virtually deserted.

In response, the government quarantined Kikwit. Angola, to the south, sealed its borders to prevent the infection from spreading. By mid-May, immigration officials at airports around the world were wary about travelers from Zaire. CDC quarantine personnel, which works at seven major U.S. airports, screened some overseas passengers as many as three times. On May 17, a man arrived at Toronto's Pearson International Airport via a circuitous route from Zaire, where his mother had died. Quarantined, the man was released ten days later when it was obvious he was not infected. In France, all passengers arriving from Zaire had to undergo a medical checkup before leaving the airport.

Meanwhile, in Kikwit, traditional funereal rites, which involve washing the corpse, spread body fluids and fueled the epidemic. In response, the Red Cross distributed fifty thousand brochures urging people to avoid the blood of Ebola victims, to wear gloves when handling the clothing belonging to the sick, to boil the clothes before washing, and to break tradition and not wash bodies before burial.

Toward the end of May, the movement of bright orange trucks carrying bodies was a sign that the epidemic would soon end. People were forgoing traditional burial practices and permitting the government to place all the bodies in a mass grave.

After two decades, researchers have still failed to identify the Ebola virus's natural host. They may have also overlooked an important clue: the two largest Ebola outbreaks occurred in the nation where the HIV epidemic originated and remains concentrated. For reasons that will be discussed in Chapter 14, the population itself may suffer from seriously compromised immune systems.

To underscore the potential risks of Ebola to Americans and to the doctors and nurses who would treat them, the CDC and the *Journal of the American Medical Association* published a list of guidelines for handling patients with hemorrhagic infections. Among the protective measures recommended were face shields, rooms with negative air pressure (to prevent the escape of an airborne virus), cautious use of needles and scalpels, limited medical tests, the sealing of waste in leak-proof bags, and the prompt cremation of corpses.[5,6]

DENGUE FEVER AND DENGUE HEMORRHAGIC FEVER

Dengue fevers have existed for at least two hundred years. The most common type causes a high fever and pain in the bones. Though not usually deadly, it does feel considerably worse than a very bad flu. Dengue *hemorrhagic* fever is more serious, though not as deadly as Ebola. As the name suggests, this variation of dengue fever causes spontaneous bleeding.

All dengue fevers are spread by the Asian tiger mosquito *(Aedes aegypti)*, but extensive mosquito-control programs had confined it to southeast Asia. During the 1970s, dengue fevers spread to the Philippines and South America. In 1981, it infected more than a quarter of a million Cubans, more than one-third of whom required hospitalization.

In 1995, more than one-half million cases of dengue fever were reported in Central America and Mexico, with a number of cases occurring near the Texas border. What accounts for the spread? Paul Epstein, M.D., of Harvard University believes that the mosquitoes' spread has been aided by rising global temperatures over the past several decades. The mosquito can now be found at elevations of about five thousand feet in Colombian mountains—a cooler setting than its original jungle home. That also means the mosquito can live farther north and south.[7]

Thanks to a shipment of old tires from Southeast Asia, Asian tiger mosquito larvae containing the dengue fever virus entered Florida in 1985. The mosquito is now spreading through the South, but the virus itself seems to be moving much more slowly. That may be because Americans have a history of diligently destroying mosquitoes and many of their breeding grounds.

HANTAVIRUS

The death of a young, otherwise healthy Navajo Indian with flulike symptoms puzzled doctors in March 1993, but it wasn't until May that a pattern emerged. By that time eleven people had died and nine others had become seriously ill on or near the Navajo reservation in northern New Mexico and Arizona. During the summer, the CDC identified the cause as a type of hantavirus. The largest previous hantavirus outbreak caused hemorrhaging and kidney damage in thousands of United Nations soldiers during the Korean War, although the virus itself was not identified until the late 1970s. (The name hantavirus was derived from the Hantaan River in Korea.)

Unlike its predecessor, the newly discovered hantavirus caused respiratory symptoms—hence, its flulike nature—and a 67 percent fatality rate among confirmed cases. The hantavirus is spread by deer mice, which do not exhibit any ill effects, to people who inhale or touch virus-containing particles of deer mice feces. Since 1993, the CDC has confirmed almost fifty deaths in fourteen western states from this hantavirus, now named the *Sin Nombre* virus. One fatality occurred as far north as Edmonton, Canada, in a man who had caught and handled a wild deer mouse. The virus has also been identified in Louisiana, where researchers suspect a different rodent to be the carrier.

What accounted for the hantavirus outbreak in the Southwest? Researchers now suspect that the *Sin Nombre* virus may have gone unnoticed for hundreds of years. In 1993, heavy rainfall led to an abundance of flora and seeds, which produced an expansion in the deer mouse population.

This particular type of hantavirus is one of four strains; the others cause kidney diseases. A study in the Netherlands suggests hantavirus may be more common than originally thought. Researchers found that 6 percent of animal trappers and 4 percent of forestry workers carried hantavirus antibodies, a sign of exposure to the virus, but most had no symptoms. That suggests many people might suffer only mild symptoms.[8]

SABIÁ VIRUS

In 1990, a twenty-five-year-old agricultural engineer in São Paulo, Brazil, was hospitalized after suffering from fever, headache, vomiting, and weakness for twelve days. Until this time, she had been unremarkably healthy and had not traveled out of the São Paulo province for two months. Four days after being hospitalized, the woman died.

A laboratory technician analyzing the woman's contaminated blood in Belém, Brazil, apparently accidentally breathed in some of the virus from the sample and became infected. Although seriously ill for fifteen days, he recovered.

The infections were caused by a previously unknown arenavirus related to the one that causes Lassa fever in South America and Africa.[9] Rodents are the natural reservoir for arenaviruses, and researchers suspect that the agricultural engineer contracted what became known as Sabiá virus in the course of her work.

In August 1994, a virologist diagnosed himself with malaria and entered the Tropical Medicine Clinic at the Yale-New Haven Hospital. Laboratory tests failed to confirm malaria, so the man was queried for possible exposure to the Sabiá virus. While working on an experiment, the virologist was exposed to a small amount of the Sabiá virus. Although the laboratory was outfitted with negative air pressure (to keep viruses inside) and a high-efficiency air-filtration system, and the virologist was wearing a surgical mask, he apparently breathed in sufficient numbers of the virus to cause an infection. He was treated with ribavirin, a drug effective against other arenaviruses, and recovered.[10]

The origins of Sabiá in equatorial South America parallel those of Ebola in Africa. However, it is not clear how widespread of a threat Sabiá poses.

LYME DISEASE

Identified in the 1970s, Lyme disease is caused by the *Borrelia burgdorferi* parasite, which ticks transmit from deer to cats, dogs, and humans. Aside from an initial tick bite, the symptoms of Lyme disease are varied and may be slow to appear. If the infection is not quickly treated with antibiotics, the parasite attacks the central nervous system and causes neurological and arthritis-like symptoms, depression, seizures, and memory loss.

In 1994, Lyme disease cases rose to 13,083, a 58 percent increase over the previous year. The jump was due to improved reporting by physicians *and* a genuine increase in cases, according to the CDC.[11]

Why has Lyme disease become a problem relatively recently—after all, Americans have lived near forests for hundreds of years? And why did this disease originate in New England? The reasons are not entirely clear. One possible explanation is that the carriers of the tick, deer and rodents, increased in numbers because they lost natural controls, such as wolves and cougars. It may have taken years for a "critical mass" of infected animals to form and quickly spread the disease.

In 1991, doctors identified a bacterial disease transmitted by the same tick that carries Lyme disease. This germ causes human granulocytic ehrlichiosis (HGE), which is more difficult than Lyme disease to diagnose. HGE causes sudden fever, chills, and muscle aches. By 1995, more than sixty people in the United States—mostly in the upper Midwest and Northeast—had been diagnosed with HGE. More than a dozen cases have been identified in the suburbs of New York City.[12]

AUSTRALIAN HORSE VIRUS

In September 1994, a previously unknown virus killed thirteen of twenty-one infected horses, as well as one of two people who had worked with the horses near Brisbane. In just twelve days, Australian researchers pinpointed the cause as a new type of morbillivirus, later named the equine morbillivirus. Other types of morbilliviruses cause distemper in dogs, plague in sea mammals, and measles in humans. The equine morbillivirus was the first virus of this type to affect people since measles was identified a thousand years ago. It was also the first morbillivirus to cross species.

Although the equine morbillivirus outbreak was brief, it was particularly virulent, killing two-thirds of the horses infected with it. The virus causes cells in blood vessel walls to clump, which creates holes and allows blood to leak into the lungs.

With amazing speed, Australian researchers also developed a test for the equine morbillivirus, which they subsequently administered to 1,600 horses and ninety people in proximity to the outbreak. No other infections were detected. However, analysis of the morbillivirus indicated that it was not caused by a recent mutation. Instead, it appears to have hopped from its natural host, an Australian fruit-eating bat, to horses and to people.[13]

DIPHTHERIA IN RUSSIA

Before the collapse of the Soviet Union in 1991, immunization programs were carried out with almost military precision and citizens required permits to travel far from home. In just a few years, the public health system has eroded and a highly mobile population has helped spread a diphtheria epidemic infecting more than eighty thousand people and killing two thousand.

It began in 1990 when a few soldiers returned to Moscow from southern Russia with infections of *Corynebacterium diphtheriae*. In southern Russia, this bacterium causes only a mild skin disease, but it apparently becomes more virulent in populations exposed to it for the first time. Initial flulike symptoms can lead to heart and brain damage, which kill 13 percent of patients. The epidemic spread to all fifteen republics of the former Soviet Union, and cases were identified in Poland, Finland, Norway, and Germany. Americans are potentially at risk, also. Two Russian-born Americans visited their homeland, only to return with *C. diphtheriae* infections. Once diagnosed, their infections were successfully treated.

Back in Russia, the government began mounting a new immunization campaign, but as John Maurice wryly noted in *Science*, Russian officials "are understandably anxious to get the diphtheria epidemic out of the way so they can get on with the other problems of daily life, such as cholera, dysentery, tuberculosis, AIDS, and even malaria."[14]

CHOLERA IN MEXICO

Cholera, a life-threatening diarrheal disease, has reached epidemic proportions in Mexico. The incidence is highest in the southern state of Chiapas and the northern state of Nuevo León, although cases are regularly being reported in Mexico City, Monterrey, and other large cities. The disease is caused by *Vibrio cholerae*, a bacterium that lives in human feces and easily contaminates food and water. Mexican officials said the brunt of the epidemic occurred in Nuevo León, located just 150 miles south of the Texas border.[15,16]

PARASITES IN MILWAUKEE WATER

In March and April 1993, protozoa from the *Cryptosporidium* genus contaminated the water-treatment plant serving Milwaukee, Wisconsin. The microorganism caused cryptosporidiosis, a severe type of diarrhea, in an estimated 403,000 residents. One hundred people died. The most common symptom was severe watery diarrhea, followed by abdominal cramps, fever, and vomiting. Infections lasted an average of nine days, although they ranged from one to fifty-five days. The average maximum number of bowel movements was twelve per day, though they ranged from one to ninety per day—a testament to the seriousness of the disease.

People rushed to the store to purchase bottled water, or boiled tap water before drinking it. In a scene reminiscent of small towns in Europe and South America, many Milwaukee residents lined up to fill bottles and jugs with uncontaminated spring water bubbling up at the Pryor Avenue Iron Well, a nineteenth-century public pump. The suspected cause of the cryptosporidiosis outbreak was agricultural runoff into Lake Michigan, the source of Milwaukee's drinking water. *Cryptosporidia* are commonly found in the digestive tracts and excreta of animals.

As it turns out, *Cryptosporidia* may be very common in drinking water. In June 1995, a study by the National Resources Defense Council reported that the protozoa were found in raw and treated water from a hundred public utility systems affecting forty-five million people.[17] The CDC recommended that all people with AIDS, cancer, and organ transplants boil their water before drinking or use filtered or bottled water.[18]

BIOLOGICAL TERRORISM

While the specter of biological warfare has been present for decades, no country has actually unleashed infectious microorganisms on another country. (One reason is the unpredictable release pattern of microorganisms.) That doesn't mean someone might not try. In a disturbing event in May 1995, a self-described white supremacist in Columbus, Ohio, ordered $300 worth of freeze-dried *Yersinia pestis*, the bacterium that causes the bubonic plague. The bacteria could have easily been reconstituted with warm water.

The man worked for a food-testing laboratory and represented himself as a microbiologist, although he was legally certified only to test drinking water for bacteria. When he ordered the plague bacteria from American Type Culture Collection in Rockville, Maryland, and asked that the bacteria be sent via Federal Express, the employee who took his order thought it sounded suspicious and called the police. Different species of bacteria have different legal shipping requirements, and *Yersinia pestis* is not shipped by Federal Express.[19]

Several hundred disease-causing viruses have been identified in people and animals, and about a hundred species of bacteria account for the majority of bacterial infections in people. With the exception of HIV, most Americans face far greater risks close to home with antibiotic-resistant bacteria than they do from viruses emerging out of Africa, South America, or Asia.

Still, it is troublesome that many serious and deadly infections begin with similar, common symptoms—fever, diarrhea, and flulike respiratory problems. That makes an early and accurate diagnosis difficult—and often delays appropriate treatment.

Obviously, none of us can go through life living in a microbe-free bubble. Nor is it realistic to assume that medicine will develop antibiotics or immunizations effective against all of these microorganisms. So, how can you protect yourself when you have no idea when or where you're going to be accosted by a supergerm?

We believe that a person's first line of defense is his or her own immune system. A strong immune system is like a large number of watchful sentries and a powerful army positioned to counterattack bacteria, viruses, and parasites. With optimal immunity, you may still become infected—but the symptoms will probably be less severe and recovery much faster. The following chapters describe how immunity works, what dietary and environmental factors reduce immunity, and which nutrients optimize it.

Part II

❖

IMMUNE STRENGTHS AND WEAKNESSES

❖

We are awash in a sea of germs—some causing disease, others promoting health, and still others acting as little more than innocuous bystanders. They live in the food we eat, the air we breathe, the hands we shake. They take up residence in our intestine, on our skin, and elsewhere in the body. Most of the time, however, these germs do not bother us. The real question is: why does one infected person become very sick, and not another?

The emergence of antibiotic-resistant bacteria and encounters with previously unknown species of deadly viruses form only part of the equation affecting your susceptibility to infectious disease. Germs, in a sense, are the external pressure bearing down on you. The other half of the equation is internal and consists of your immune system. A well-tuned immune system, with vigilant molecular eyes, defends against the majority of pathogenic bacteria, viruses, and protozoa. And if you can resist or weather infections without antibiotics, you will reduce the numbers of antibiotic-resistant bacteria.

But something has gone dreadfully wrong as we approach the twenty-first century. Our ability to resist disease—and not just infectious disease—has been severely compromised. The rates of cancer, Alzheimer's disease, diabetes, multiple sclerosis, and many types of heart disease have been increasing steadily.

The decline of our health—and, specifically, our immunity—is due in large part to a decrease in the quality of our food supply and what most people put on their plate. Malnourished, in a manner of speaking, on full stomachs, our health suffers, and we become more vulnerable to a broad range of degenerative diseases—and to supergerms.

On the positive side, most of us *can* control what we eat, and we *can* make dietary changes that bolster our inborn defenses against diseases, including infections by supergerms. But before we work to strengthen our immune systems, let's take a closer look at the fundamental role of diet in health and immunity.

6

DIETARY DEFENSES
AGAINST DISEASE

⌘

Could something as simple as a good diet and vitamin supplements really protect you against supergerms? Although you might initially be skeptical, the answer is *yes*—for many of the same reasons that a good diet reduces your risk of heart disease, cancer, diabetes, and other serious diseases. Vitamins and many other nutrients are essential for overall health and, specifically, for the health of the immune system.

So why haven't more doctors put down their prescription pads and just recommended vitamins to their patients? Nutrition, in many respects, has been the missing link in medicine—overlooked and ignored. After years of being all but dismissed as worthless, vitamins and other nutrients are currently gaining newfound respect. Understanding why requires a brief glimpse of an amazing transformation—one that's still in progress—in medicine.

Over the past century, most medical advances were driven by the idea that diseases could be conquered, given the right combination of drugs, surgery, and other therapies. This feeling was reinforced by a series of dramatic victories. In the 1940s, antibiotics vanquished some of the biggest bacterial killers, including staph and tuberculosis. In the 1950s, vaccinations eliminated the fear of polio, a terrifying crippler of children. In the 1960s, doctors succeeded in doing what they once thought impossible: open-heart surgery. By most measures, modern medicine had forced disease into retreat—and everyone was promised long, productive lives.

In retrospect, medicine had become a bit too arrogant and overly self-confident. The fact of the matter is that in recent years people have been getting sicker, not healthier, and medicine has lost as many battles as it has won. The highly publicized "war on cancer," declared by President Richard Nixon a quarter of a century ago and financed with billions of dollars, has had no clear victor—and some people have described it as a medical Vietnam. The incidence of cancer continues to increase, and survival today is generally no better than it was thirty years ago. A similar well-funded assault on AIDS has failed to produce a cure, although safer sexual practices (which are essentially nonmedical) have slowed the spread of this disease in the United States.

The only modest success has occurred with coronary heart disease, which has declined in incidence steadily since the 1960s. But this remarkable improvement has less to do with drugs or surgery than it does with the fact that large numbers of people have reduced their consumption of dietary fat and stopped smoking. Still, it's a dubious victory. Even with this improvement, cardiovascular diseases remain the number one cause of death in the United States and kill almost twice as many people as does cancer.

Why have major medical advances stalled?

Part of the reason is that much of medicine remains committed to an outdated approach to treating people. At the cornerstone of this approach is the belief that diseases have well-defined causes that respond to well-defined treatments. This paradigm has an inherent fault. Because diseases are more easily defined (diagnosed) in their late stages, doctors' emphasis has naturally been on treatment rather than on identifying causes or preventing the progression of diseases.

For example, in treating a tumor with surgery or chemotherapy, doctors do not address the cause of the abnormal growth, which often recurs. In hypertension, drug treatments lower blood pressure but they do not deal with the cause of the disorder. If you take away the drug, the hypertension returns and is often even worse. Emphasizing treatment over prevention in this way is a little like repeatedly applying Band-Aids® to wounds instead of asking why people keep cutting themselves.

The causes of most chronic diseases are actually biochemical, and while biochemistry is exceedingly complex, its origins are not. The raw materials for our bodies' biochemicals are nutrients, and the quality and quantity of these biochemicals are based on the quality and quantity of their nutritional raw materials. If you think about it, what we are as people—our hands, our hearts, our ability to think—comes from our diet. The machinery that processes these raw materials is based on genetics, but the materials themselves are dietary. We are most definitely what we eat.

Do Diet and Vitamins Fight Disease?

Faced with a declining return on a massive investment of time and money, medicine has slowly but surely begun to correct its focus. Researchers and physicians are returning to biochemical basics and reexamining the role of vitamins and other nutrients—the raw materials on which our health is based.

Foods are extraordinarily complex collections of chemicals— a small garlic clove yields more than two hundred different chemicals. Without food, we die. Without good quality food, our biochemistry is shortchanged and health impaired. We all know that calcium (such as from milk) is needed for bones and vitamin A (such as from liver) is needed for good vision. When essential nutrients are lacking, health disasters usually follow.

One dramatic illustration occurs when a pregnant woman is deficient in a single B vitamin, folic acid, which is required in minuscule amounts: her baby is born with a life-threatening deformity called spina bifida.

Throughout life, when the nutritional raw materials of our biochemistry are good—like well-made parts for a car—the end result is of high quality. When these raw materials are of poor quality, the result is comparable to a car made with inferior parts. It's always back in the shop, the mechanic's equivalent of the doctor's office. Cars, however, are typically in the shop for routine maintenance (checkups) or to replace minor parts long before they require a major overhaul. The same is true of you and your health. Osteoporosis, heart disease, cancer, and other diseases do not appear in a single day. They develop slowly over many years. The many gradations between health and serious disease mean there are ample opportunities to treat the early signs of diseases and their causes.

For years, a relatively small number of physicians have used vitamins and other nutrients to do just this—that is, to treat minor conditions before they develop into far more serious diseases. These doctors published their experiences in obscure and often unread medical journals, and for the most part, they were shunned—or even castigated by the medical establishment. This situation started to change in the 1950s when cholesterol was recognized as a cause of coronary heart disease, and low-cholesterol diets have since been recommended to prevent coronary heart disease.

Nobel laureate Linus Pauling, Ph.D., was a catalyst for the further rehabilitation of nutrition as an influence on health. In 1968, he published an article suggesting that nutrient intake be manipulated to achieve optimal health.[1] Two years later, he published *Vitamin C and the Common Cold*.[2] Although criticized, the book stimulated (sometimes begrudgingly) a wave of scientific research. Pauling followed this book with one on vitamin C and cancer,[3] generating still more controversy—and research.

By the late 1970s and early 1980s, the clock could not be turned back. Nutrition research was clearly becoming more prominent in mainstream medical journals, and several events further raised the medical establishment's consciousness about nutrition and health. In 1982, the University of Arizona, Tucson, sponsored an international medical conference on the role of vitamins in cancer prevention and treatment. Scientists from fourteen nations gathered to describe research showing that vitamins boosted the body's immune system against cancer.

Later that year, the U.S. National Academy of Sciences published *Diet, Nutrition and Cancer.*[4] This report recommended a diet low in fat, red meat, and smoked foods and high in vegetables (particularly those containing beta-carotene) to prevent heart disease and cancer. The following year, in a landmark article in the journal *Science*, Bruce N. Ames, Ph.D., a preeminent researcher at the University of California, Berkeley, described the importance of vitamins and minerals in preventing cancer.[5]

Although medicine continues to be wed to drugs, surgery, and high-tech (and high-priced) treatments, it would not be an exaggeration to say that most doctors now believe that the majority of degenerative diseases are preventable through dietary and lifestyle changes. But like the adage you can bring a horse to water but you cannot make him drink, the difficulty now, as you might surmise, is putting this belief into practice.

GROWING MOMENTUM OF NUTRITION IN MEDICINE

Several factors have given nutrition and nutritional therapy additional momentum. One is the growing recognition that free radicals are probably a fundamental cause of aging and disease. When Denham Harman, M.D., Ph.D., conceived the free radical theory of aging in 1954, the words "free radical" and "antioxidant" were used only by chemists, and very few at that. Thanks in part to vitamin advertising, "free radicals" and "antioxidants" have practically become household words.

Free radicals are molecules with an unpaired electron. In the process of acquiring an electron to make a pair, free radicals "oxidize" nearby molecules or atoms.[6] Oxidation is what makes butter rancid or turns iron to rust—it ages them. Essentially the same process occurs in our bodies, with free radicals aging cells and causing or aggravating diseases. Free radicals also oxidize cholesterol, leading to coronary heart disease, and genetic mutations, which leads to cancer cells.

*Anti*oxidants quench these free radicals and prevent oxidation. Some of the most effective antioxidants are nutrients: vitamins C and E and beta-carotene. As medicine has increasingly embraced the free-radical theory of aging, it has had to acknowledge the disease-preventing roles of vitamins and other nutrients. One cannot accept the role of one without the other.[7]

Studies comparing the health of people living in different countries and eating different diets have also convinced many physicians of the value of diet. For example, researchers have found that Japanese and Eskimos eating diets high in fish oils suffer fewer strokes from blood clots than those who eat little or no fish.[8] Similarly, researchers have suggested that Japanese men have a low incidence of prostate cancer because they eat large quantities of nutrient-rich soy. In contrast, Finnish men eat little soy and have a high incidence of prostate cancer.[9] Another example shows that Japanese women have a low incidence of breast cancer compared with American women—until the Japanese women began eating Western foods either in Japan or after moving to the United States.[10,11]

Thousands of medical studies like these have now made nutrition an irresistible force in maintaining health. This body of evidence, now easily accessible via the Medline database, is too large to ignore. In general, the findings boil down to two key points:

• a low intake of vitamins and other nutrients is associated with disease, and
• a high intake of the same nutrients is associated with health and well-being.

In other words, the *cure* for many diseases is not a miraculous new drug or a high-tech panacea. It is prevention through good nutrition.

NUTRITION IN HEALTH AND DISEASE

Because our focus is on enhancing immunity against supergerms, we won't attempt to present a comprehensive discussion of the role of nutrients in disease. But at this point, we will convey the flavor of the research on this topic and some recent discoveries. (Some additional discussion on the role of nutrients in heart disease will be included in the subsequent chapters on individual nutrients, and sources for additional information on vitamins and health will be noted in the Appendix.)

Heart disease and vitamin E. Harvard University researchers have found that vitamin E supplements decrease the risk of coronary heart disease by 54 percent in men and 26 percent in women.[12,13] In 1996, a British study found that vitamin E reduced the incidence of heart attacks by 77 percent.

Blood pressure and calcium. More than a hundred studies have found that high dietary levels of calcium or supplements reduce blood pressure.[14]

Blood pressure, cancer, and fish oil. Patients taking several fish oil capsules daily had significant reductions in blood pressure.[15] Fish oils also suppress the spread of cancer.[16]

Bladder cancer and vitamins. A simple "one a day"–type vitamin supplement slightly reduces the recurrence of bladder cancer, and a high-potency vitamin supplement reduces the recurrence rate by 40 percent.[17]

Cancer survival and vitamins. Cancer patients taking high doses of vitamin supplements live up to twenty times longer than patients who do not take supplements.[18]

Osteoarthritis and B vitamins. Supplemental vitamin B_{12} and folic acid reduce pain and increase flexibility in patients suffering from osteoarthritis.[19]

Osteoporosis and calcium. Numerous studies have reported

⌘

**KEY PRINCIPLES TO DEFEND YOURSELF
AGAINST SUPERGERMS**

1. A low intake of vitamins and other nutrients is associated with most diseases.
2. A high intake of vitamins and other nutrients is associated with health and well-being.
3. Nutritional deficiencies can interfere with the immune response to infections.
4. Infections increase the body's requirements for many nutrients and can induce deficiencies.
5. Dietary improvements and large doses of some micronutrients can bolster weak immune systems.

⌘

---

that high dietary intake of calcium (and sometimes vitamin D) slows the loss of bone in postmenopausal women.[20,21,22]

Cataracts and antioxidants. A high intake of vitamin C, glutathione, and other antioxidant nutrients protects against cataracts.[23]

Just as vitamins and other nutrients build a healthy body and protect against cancer, heart disease, and other conditions, they also boost your immunity and defend against supergerms.

Vitamins and Diet Essential for Immunity

In medical journals, physicians and researchers frequently refer to the crucial role of "host defenses"—the immune system—in fighting infections. Like other aspects of health, the foundation of a person's immunity ultimately depends on a large number of biochemical building blocks essential for all aspects of health, growth, and healing. The raw materials for these biochemicals originate in the diet and include such macronutrients as proteins, carbohydrates, and fats and such micronutrients as vitamins and minerals.

This is hardly a revolutionary concept: the general relationship between diet and resistance to infection has been recognized for thousands of years. The ancient scriptures of India noted the association between food and health in 5000 B.C., and medieval church records from England acknowledged the relationship between crop failures and famine and subsequent epidemics.[24] Furthermore, the modern medical literature has documented the role and precise mechanisms of these nutrients in immunity for years.[25]

DIET AS THE MISSING LINK IN IMMUNITY

Most physicians, however, have routinely assumed diet is clinically unimportant unless they see signs of severe protein-calorie malnutrition or gross immune depression. When something does go awry with immunity, it's generally interpreted as a call for pharmaceutical intervention, rather than to check whether the immune system's nutritional building blocks are present.

Even in AIDS, now the most commonly recognized type of immune suppression, nutritional deficiencies are frequently thought to be clinically irrelevant. This is a serious oversight because deficiencies of beta-carotene and vitamins A, C, and E are common among AIDS patients,[26] and each of these nutrients plays an important role in immunity.

The consequences of a good or bad diet cannot be understated. HIV-positive men with a high intake of vitamins do not develop full-blown AIDS as quickly as do men with low intake of vitamins.[27] Furthermore, patients with AIDS require large doses of micronutrients to achieve and maintain what would be normal levels of these nutrients in a healthy person.[28,29]

Some people might argue that HIV and AIDS are extreme examples of immune dysfunction, even in the context of supergerms. While HIV may pose the greatest microbial challenge to the immune system, every infection poses challenges to the immune system, and every infection disturbs nutrient levels in the body.[30] If physicians fail to recognize the important role of nutrition in the most serious infectious assault on the immune system, how likely are they to view the role of nutrition in other infections?

An effective immune system response to an infection, or even to an immunization, depends largely on the quality and quantity of a person's nutritional intake. Variations in the diet result in ups and downs in immunity. For now, keep in mind two key points that we will discuss in more detail in the following chapters:

- nutritional deficiencies and toxic chemicals can interfere with the immune response, and
- dietary improvements and large doses (so-called megadoses) of some micronutrients can bolster weak immune systems.

The role of nutrition is so basic that it's hard to believe it is often ignored or assumed to have little influence on immunity. As one researcher observed, "The nutritional status of an individual has a profound effect on both host susceptibility to specific infectious diseases and on their outcome."[31] Other infectious disease experts have noted that vitamin and mineral deficiencies interfere with immune responses, antibiotic treatment, and vaccines, impairing the body's ability to recover from infection.[32]

How the Immune System Works

Just what *is* the immune system?

When you were in school, you learned that white blood cells fought infections, whereas red blood cells delivered nutrients and oxygen to tissues. Such a description was a necessary oversimplification of the immune system, which is an extraordinarily complex set of biological defenses.

Immunity is essentially the body's ability to identify and attack foreign or "nonself" molecules, be they microorganisms

KEY COMPONENTS OF THE IMMUNE SYSTEM

Phagocyte: A general name for white blood cells, which eat bacteria or virus-infected cells.

Macrophage: One specific type of white blood cell.

Polymorphonuclear leukocytes: Another type of white blood cell.

Neutrophil: The most common type of polymorphonuclear leukocyte.

Interferon: An immune stimulant released by macrophages.

Lymphocyte: Either a B cell or a T cell.

B cell: The cell that produces antibodies, which fight infections.

Antibody: A chemical tag that helps the body identify some types of infecting germs.

T cell: The "brains" of the immune system.

T4 (or CD4) cell: One of the most sophisticated T cells that fights infections.

T8 (or CD8) cell: This cell turns off T4 cells to prevent them from overreacting.

Natural-killer cell: An immune cell that destroys virus-infected and cancer cells.

or toxins. Under ideal conditions, a series of immune system trip wires automatically activate a cascade of biological and chemical responses to the invaders. These defenses are analogous to a well-coordinated police department and diversified military force fighting individual criminals or an invading army. In some of us, these biological police officers and soldiers are physically fit and well equipped to do their jobs; in others, they are not.

FIRST LINES OF DEFENSE

The first lines of defense against infection actually consist of physical barriers, not parts of the immune system. They are the skin and other epithelial tissues (covering the surface of organs) and mucous membranes. Like the ancient Great Wall of China, the skin and epithelial cells serve as major obstacles to invaders.

When bacteria or viruses breach the skin, such as through a cut, they can access the innermost parts of the body via the bloodstream or the lymphatic system (which maintains fluid levels in the body). Similarly, when microbes penetrate weak portions of membranes, they can attack the lungs and other organs. In a very real sense, these microbial invaders threaten the heartland of the body.

But invading bacteria or viruses do not go unnoticed or unchecked. Almost immediately, alert lookouts spot these microbes and prepare for battle. To cause an infection, or death, bacteria or viruses must run the gauntlet of many powerful and coordinated immune system defenses.

WHITE BLOOD CELLS

The infantry of the immune system consists of white blood cells called *phagocytes.* They provide a generic defense against a broad range of infectious microbes and, as the immune system's front-line troops, may be the most important part of the body's defense against microorganisms.

The body produces two principal kinds of phagocytes in bone marrow. *Polymorphonuclear leukocytes* (sometimes called *granulocytes*) are one type. The body actually relies on several different kinds of polymorphonuclear leukocytes, but the most common are *neutrophils.* These white blood cells circulate through the blood, patrolling their territory, and respond very quickly to infection.

Macrophages are the second type of phagocyte. Some of them circulate through the body, but other macrophages remain on reserve duty in tissues, ready to be called into action. Wherever they happen to be, macrophages act as sentries monitoring the blood for circulating microorganisms. They respond to infections slower than leukocytes, but they are much more adaptable when it comes to outwitting bacteria. In addition, macrophages produce their own antibiotics, such as *interferon,* which also stimulate the immune system.

Both leukocytes and macrophages kill bacteria by eating and digesting them, a process called *phagocytosis*. The details of how white blood cells kill bacteria surprises many people, because it depends on free radicals, those dangerous molecules that cause aging, cancer, and heart disease. Phagocytes generate enormous quantities of free radicals to fight infections. Unless the excess free radicals are mopped up by antioxidant nutrients, such as vitamins C and E, they can damage healthy cells, increase the risk of heart disease and cancer, and even impair immunity.[33,34,35] (We'll explain more about good and bad free radicals, and the relationship between infection and heart disease in Chapter 12.)

As you might expect, many bacteria and viruses have developed defenses against phagocytes. Some microbes actually destroy phagocytes, and others camouflage themselves to evade white blood cells. Bacteria and viruses can also hide within healthy cells of the body. When faced with this type of microbial attack, the body's immune system quickly falls back on a number of sophisticated countermeasures to fight infections.

B CELLS AND T CELLS

Lymphocytes, which include *B cells* and *T cells*, are types of white blood cells produced by the thymus gland. They are called lymphocytes because they travel primarily through the lymphatic system, though they also move through the bloodstream. B cells and T cells are among the most sophisticated components of the immune system and counter invaders that make it past ordinary white blood cells.

B cells can produce more than one million types of *antibodies* in response to invading microorganisms (or other nonself substances, such as pollens and donated blood cells). If you have been treated for allergies, you might recognize the name of one of these antibodies, immunoglobulin E, or IgE. Antibodies attach to bacteria, viruses, and parasites either damaging the microorganisms or tagging them so they can be recognized and destroyed by macrophages.

If the immune system is an army, the B cells are its special forces. During their first encounter with a microbial threat, they require several days to mount an effective antibody response. Perhaps most remarkable is that B cells possess a memory, a molecular "wanted poster" of sorts. They learn to recognize specific disease-causing microorganisms after a single encounter and subsequently mop them up quickly and efficiently. That's why a person gains lifelong immunity after the first exposure to many infectious diseases (such as measles).

Over the past twenty years, many researchers have come to believe that T cells provide the actual intelligence that guides the immune system. There are many types of T cells. *Natural-killer cells* roam through the body seeking out and destroying virus-infected cells. T4 cells are particularly adept at fighting bacteria and viruses, even when these germs seek cover inside the body's own cells. The T4 cells identify and destroy the virus and the cell it has taken hostage. To prevent T4 cells from over-reacting and attacking normal cells, T8 "suppressor" cells eventually intercede and turn off the T4 cells.

In HIV, however, the virus strikes at the brains of the immune system by infecting and destroying T4 cells. Immunity is hampered further by a relatively large number of T8 cells, which proceed to turn off many of the remaining T4 cells. AIDS is diagnosed when large numbers of T4 cells have been killed by HIV. At this point, immunity is virtually nonexistent, and the body becomes defenseless against infection. That's why even a simple infection can kill a person with AIDS.

The immune system is one of the most complex biological systems found in nature. Immunologists continue to probe its depths to learn more about how immunity works. In sum, it provides both a generic defense against a broad range of known and unknown bacterial intruders and, through antibodies, learns to recognize and attack specific viruses. But to accomplish these remarkable feats, the immune system depends on the biochemical building blocks found in foods.

A SIMPLIFIED VIEW OF THE IMMUNE SYSTEM
AND SOME OF THE NUTRIENTS IT DEPENDS ON

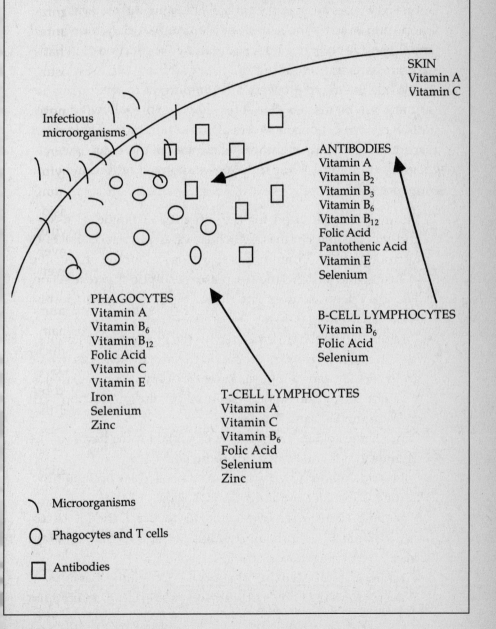

SKIN
Vitamin A
Vitamin C

Infectious
microorganisms

ANTIBODIES
Vitamin A
Vitamin B_2
Vitamin B_3
Vitamin B_6
Vitamin B_{12}
Folic Acid
Pantothenic Acid
Vitamin E
Selenium

PHAGOCYTES
Vitamin A
Vitamin B_6
Vitamin B_{12}
Folic Acid
Vitamin C
Vitamin E
Iron
Selenium
Zinc

B-CELL LYMPHOCYTES
Vitamin B_6
Folic Acid
Selenium

T-CELL LYMPHOCYTES
Vitamin A
Vitamin C
Vitamin B_6
Folic Acid
Selenium
Zinc

Microorganisms

Phagocytes and T cells

Antibodies

MICRONUTRIENTS AND IMMUNITY

The first details of the link between vitamins and immunity were described in 1921, when researchers noted how deficiencies in B vitamins affected the lymph glands and decreased immunity. Sixty years later, in the early 1980s, a pivotal medical workshop sponsored by the American Medical Association reviewed the expansive body of evidence detailing the function of individual nutrients in immunity.[36]

While the micronutrients most important to optimizing immunity will be discussed in later chapters, the following nutrients have basic, noncontroversial roles in immunity and other aspects of health. Even minor deficiencies of these nutrients can degrade immunity, while supplementation can restore and often enhance it.[37,38]

- Vitamin A is required for the integrity of epithelial tissues and mucous membranes, which serve as physical barriers to microorganisms. Vitamin A is also essential for the production of T cells, and its deficiency increases susceptibility to infection. The best food sources are liver, eggs, fish, and vitamin A–fortified milk.
- Vitamin B_2 (riboflavin) is needed for the production of antibodies. All of the B vitamins are found in liver, meats, eggs, whole grain cereals, and to a lesser extent in leafy green vegetables.
- Vitamin B_6 (pyridoxine) is essential for the production of B cells, antibodies, and T cells.
- Pantothenic acid, a B vitamin, is essential for the health of the thymus gland and antibody production.
- Folic acid, another B vitamin, is also needed for optimal functioning of B cells, antibodies, and T cells.
- Vitamin B_{12} is required by phagocytes to attack and kill bacteria. Vitamin B_{12} is difficult, though not impossible, to obtain from strictly vegetarian sources.
- Vitamin C is needed by phagocytes for killing bacteria. It also promotes the body's production of interferon, an immune

stimulant. Vitamin C is found in fruit and vegetables—with higher levels in fresh rather than cooked foods.

- Vitamin E is needed to ensure normal phagocyte and antibody activity. It's found in whole wheat grains and natural vegetable oils sold at health food stores.
- Selenium enhances the production of antibodies and lymphocytes. It is also a key component of glutathione peroxidase, an antioxidant that detoxifies bacterial toxins and other hazardous chemicals. This essential mineral is found in broccoli, fish and shellfish, cereal grains, and meats.
- Zinc is "mitogenic" for T cells, meaning that it helps the body produce more of them. High-protein diets, containing meat and cereal grains, provide this mineral.[39]

Deficiencies of any of these and many other nutrients interfere with an effective response to infections. As a consequence, people are sometimes more susceptible to common infections, such as the common cold or influenza.

Some years ago, Dr. Derrick Lonsdale treated a number of children suffering from recurrent fevers and enlarged lymph glands but whose symptoms of infection had not responded to antibiotics (even after taking them for years). Typically, blood tests showed inadequate vitamin B_1 or abnormalities that interfered with B_1 levels, and symptoms would disappear after B_1 supplementation. In one case, a five-year-old boy's response was so dramatic that his mother resisted Dr. Lonsdale's suggestion that they briefly stop B_1 supplementation to see what would happen. When she finally consented and supplementation was withheld, her son's symptoms of infection returned—only to disappear again when the B_1 was resumed.[40]

Some nutritional deficiencies can also prompt common viruses to mutate into much more dangerous strains. In many regions of China, peasants commonly suffer from cardiomyopathy, a form of heart failure. A few years ago, researchers discovered that these peasants were deficient in either vitamin E, selenium, or both nutrients. But the disease seemed to be worse in some years than in others. So the researchers looked for an associated infectious microorganism, which turned out to be the Coxsackie virus.

The Coxsackie virus is a common germ and generally causes nothing worse than the common cold or sore throat. But researchers discovered what no one had ever expected: when the virus infected people deficient in vitamin E or selenium, it mutated into a much more dangerous form that attacks the heart.[41] The implications are chilling, and researchers are now investigating whether nutritional deficiencies might also cause mutations in the flu, HIV, and Ebola.[42] This research will be discussed in greater detail in Chapter 14.

Severe, lengthy, or frequent infections and fever take their toll on the body and can induce deficiencies of protein and many vitamins and minerals. William R. Beisel, M.D., of Johns Hopkins University, has described how normal immune responses to infection can lead to life-threatening malnutrition, particularly among infants, children, the elderly, and people who are already seriously ill.[43] Replenishing these nutrients becomes critical to prevent the "darker side" of immunity from being unleashed. That dark side impairs recovery and increases the risk of subsequent infection. Malnutrition caused by the stress of infection is also very different from malnutrition caused by inadequate diet or starvation—and, in many respects, is much more dangerous.[44]

Some of the doctors exploring nutritional therapy seem to go out of their way to describe vitamins as "drugs," or to say that they are using "pharmacological" rather than nutritional doses. Doctors choose such words because they don't want to look unprofessional in the eyes of their more conservative colleagues. Would eating two steaks be a pharmacological dose of meat? Would eating more fruit to prevent cancer make the fruit a drug? It's very doubtful—and downright silly. We tend to favor what our friend and associate Linus Pauling once said when asked about this very issue: a vitamin is a vitamin regardless of its dosage.

The evidence is overwhelming that an optimal intake of vitamins, minerals, and other nutrients protects against heart disease, cancer, and most other diseases. Conversely, a low intake of these nutrients increases the risk of disease. The lesson is simple: just as nutrients guard against degenerative diseases, they also protect us against infectious diseases, including supergerms.

Fighting an infection, whether the common cold or the flesh-eating bacteria, when you're missing some of these nutrients is a little like baking a cake without flour. The immune system simply is not going to work as well as it could. Unfortunately, that is the situation in which we find ourselves. In the next chapter, we discuss specifically how the quality of the American diet has declined—and how the average person's immunity is now very much like a cake without flour. The consequences leave us extremely vulnerable to all types of diseases, but especially supergerms.

7

THE DECLINE OF THE
AMERICAN DIET

❦

Despite official pronouncements that Americans enjoy the best food supply in the world and that malnutrition is rare in the United States, our food has undergone massive changes since 1900, and the pace of these changes has accelerated over the past fifty years. Though food production is at record highs, and food-distribution channels have never been better, the nutritional quality of our food has declined measurably. Sheer quantity, often in the form of carbohydrates, has been substituted for quality—at the expense of key vitamins and minerals.

These changes mean the adequacy of your diet should not be taken for granted. Our thesis is simple: if the nutritional building blocks of our immune system are of poorer quality than in the past, it is inevitable that our immune defenses will be less effective in protecting us against infections, particularly when confronted by germs stronger than ever before.

The Manufacturing of Food

Most people think of food as something that has been grown (grains, fruit, and vegetables) or raised (beef cattle and chickens).

While food is still *initially* grown or raised, it is also manufactured, and its nutritional content is substantially altered from its original form.

REFINED FLOUR AND BREAD

The first major change in food processing occurred with the milling of wheat and refining of flour. Until about a hundred years ago, virtually all bread was made from whole wheat or rye grain rich in vitamin E, the B vitamins, and minerals. In the late nineteenth century, new milling technology enabled the easy separation of the wheat "germ," which contains most of the nutrients, from the kernel's endosperm. The endosperm yielded a flour and bread lighter in weight and color, and this refined white bread quickly became popular with the public.

Bread made from this white flour, however, was nutritionally void except for starch. Because experiments showed that it could not sustain the lives of laboratory animals, the federal government eventually required that a handful of essential vitamins be restored to partially compensate for the twenty-some nutrients that had been removed during processing. Despite this partial reenrichment with vitamins, white bread has remained more of a marketing than nutritional wonder. A century after its popularization, it's still a highly refined and nutritionally lacking food product.

REFINED AND MANUFACTURED FOOD OILS

Another profound dietary change has been the increased consumption of polyunsaturated fatty acids (PUFAs)—that is, oils derived from corn, soy, safflower, and other vegetables. After the oils are extracted, they are refined even further. For example, the vitamin E in the oil is distilled for use in supplements.

PUFAs are used to fry foods, such as french fries and chicken, and in baked goods, salad dressings, margarine, and hundreds of other processed and packaged products. In the 1970s and 1980s, health authorities urged people to help prevent coronary heart disease by reducing their intake of saturated fats from beef and increase their consumption of PUFAs from vegetable oils. The rationale was that saturated fats raised blood levels of cholesterol, whereas PUFAs lowered cholesterol levels. In response, consumption of PUFAs rose dramatically, though this was also because PUFAs were added to many processed foods. By some estimates, the average American now eats twice as much margarine as butter and fifteen times more vegetable oil than lard.[1]

Our health is not better and may be worse as a result. Over the last few years, researchers have noted a sharply increased risk of coronary heart disease among margarine users—the very product they were urged to eat to prevent heart disease.[2] Margarine contains a particular class of PUFAs called trans-fatty acids, which have a chemical structure not found in naturally occurring PUFAs.

Although Americans have reduced their consumption of beef (and the associated saturated fat) and increased their intake of chicken, much of the chicken is breaded and fried in PUFAs of one type or another. Heating PUFAs speeds their oxidation and the generation of damaging free radicals, which set the stage for heart disease and cancer. Most of the vitamin E naturally associated with PUFAs, which would protect against this free radical oxidation, is removed during the refining of the oil. So while PUFAs technically do not contain cholesterol, refined PUFAs still increase the risk of coronary heart disease and cancer. Not surprisingly, a number of studies have noted that a person's vitamin E requirements increase with higher consumption of PUFAs.[3,4]

Equally disturbing, PUFAs play havoc with the immune system. Large amounts of PUFAs, such as from corn oil, may stimulate the growth of breast cancers.[5] Researchers have also discovered that PUFAs impair immunity by interfering with the ability of white blood cells to fight infections.[6] In fact, PUFAs dampen the immune response so appreciably, one team of researchers found them useful in preventing organ rejection among kidney-transplant patients.[7]

MANUFACTURED FOODS

Still another dramatic change affecting our food supply has been the emergence of a large number of highly processed manufactured food products. These common, heavily advertised brand-name foods include highly refined and sugar-drenched cereals (which sometimes contain more sugar than cereal), candy bars sold as breakfast meals, imitation whipped cream, reconstituted potatoes pressed into chips, reconstituted meats, dehydrated soups, sandwich spreads, salad dressings, and soft drinks sweetened with sucrose or high-fructose corn syrup. Even highly touted "fat-free" foods require extensive processing to remove the fat, and fat phobia sometimes leads to deficiencies of fats necessary for health.

Designed largely for taste, convenience, and marketplace appeal, these foods tend to be high in simple sugars and nonnutritive additives (artificial colors, preservatives) and low in vitamins, minerals, fiber, and protein. A century ago, few of these foods existed, but today these foods dominate supermarket shelves and freezers, and most people assume they are the norm.

The latest assault on the diet is Procter & Gamble's olestra, a synthetic fat that is not absorbed and thus provides no calories. If it were simply neutral, it might have a place in a nation in which one-third of the population is overweight. But olestra is not a passive dietary constituent. Fat-soluble nutrients, such as vitamins A, D, and E, and beta-carotene dissolve in olestra and are excreted by the body. When the nutritional health of many people is already questionable, an oil that removes vitamins from the body is the last thing anyone should have.[8]

NUTRIENT LOSSES FROM THE FARM TO THE FORK

Fifty to a hundred years ago, most of the food people consumed was locally grown, minimally processed, and fresh. Thanks to a combination of rail, interstate highways, shipping, and air traffic, Americans now enjoy oranges from either coast and grapes and tomatoes from South America. It seems like a great improvement. In many respects it is, but the complexity of modern food distribution and preparation can also degrade the nutritional quality of food.

Each of the many steps in food processing "from the farm to the fork"—harvest, shipping, refining, precooking or freezing (or both), storage, shipping again, sitting on the shelf in supermarkets and at home, defrosting, cooking again, refrigerating, and reheating—leads to measurable and significant losses in nutrient values, particularly for water-soluble vitamins, which include vitamin C and the B complex. Many of these nutrient losses have been described by Emanuel Cheraskin, M.D., D.M.D., professor emeritus of the University of Alabama School of Dentistry in *Diet and Disease*[9] and *The Vitamin C Connection*.[10] Although Dr. Cheraskin focused on vitamin C, what happens to this vitamin likely reflects what happens to other vitamins.

The vanishing act with nutrient levels often begins on the farm with poor soil quality. Soils lacking minerals or natural fertilizers cannot yield healthy plants, and unhealthy plants are not good vitamin producers. In one study cited by Cheraskin, produce from "underdeveloped" Mexico had higher levels of vitamins than food grown in the United States. Although the finding was puzzling, it may very well be explained by American farmers' dependence on chemical fertilizers. In experiments, Sharon B. Hornick, Ph.D., of the USDA's Agricultural Research Service, found that conventional nitrogen fertilizer reduces vitamin C levels in chard, green beans, and kale by as much as one-third.[11]

Even when the soil is rich in nutrients and the food crop is off to a good start, the time of harvesting significantly influences nutritional values. Consider that vitamin C levels in tomatoes peak just as the fruit starts to ripen. Left to overripen, vitamin C levels in tomatoes start to diminish.[12] Unfortunately, farmers tend to pick produce at the time optimal for shipping, not for vitamin C levels or human consumption.

The longer food is stored, the more its vitamin content decreases as a result of oxidation. Refrigeration slows this deterioration, but it still takes place. While you may not store large quantities of produce for long periods in root cellars, you do store foods in cans on the shelf or in bags in your freezer. These nutritional losses accelerate during food preparation. Defrosting frozen foods, washing, and cutting lower vitamin levels still more. One team of researchers found that the vitamin C levels in spinach and amaranth leaves decreased by as much as 65 percent with typical household refrigeration and cooking.[13]

More than anything else, however, cooking (i.e., heat) is the true enemy of vitamins. L. J. Prochaska, Ph.D., of Wright State University, Dayton, Ohio, has reported that vitamin C levels decrease by 20 percent when vegetables are fried and by 50 percent when they are boiled. Processed and packaged foods are often cooked and recooked several times—at the cannery, on the stove, and in the microwave oven—before being completely eaten. The repetition of cooking, chilling, and reheating takes an even greater toll on vitamin levels.[14] Similar nutrient losses occur when other foods, such as meat and milk, are heated.[15,16]

How Common Are Nutritional Deficiencies?

Under such circumstances, it comes as no surprise that large numbers of Americans experience deficiencies—often undiagnosed by their physicians—in one or more micronutrients. These deficiencies, of course, result from poor food choices as well as from a questionable food supply. In a major analysis of eating habits, researchers at the University of California, Berkeley, found that on a given day almost half the people surveyed did not eat fruit or drink juice, and almost one-quarter did not eat any vegetables. Only a meager 9 percent of the people questioned ate the five daily servings of fruit and vegetables recommended by U.S. Health and Human Services Department, and their vegetables lacked variety and nutritional diversity.[17]

Investigations of nutrient intake in the United States have determined that one-half of the population consumes substantially less than 50 percent of the Recommended Dietary Allowance (RDA) for vitamins C, A, E, and other micronutrients. Although many of these studies are based on questionnaires, and therefore may not be a precise reflection of dietary intake, one group of researchers came across a highly disturbing finding while analyzing blood levels of nutrients. They reported that 15 to 30 percent of men had vitamin C levels reflecting consumption of just 16 percent of the RDA daily over a month![18]

ARE THE RDAS VALID?

Many experts believe that the RDAs have been set on the higher side as insurance against nutritional deficiencies. But if they have been set too low, the findings of these dietary studies are all the worse.

The RDAs were conceived in 1941 as a "guide for the planning and procuring of food supplies for national defense"—basically to keep Americans at home and at the front nourished. At that time, severe nutritional deficiency diseases, such as scurvy (vitamin C), rickets (vitamin D), pellagra (vitamin B_3), pernicious anemia (vitamin B_{12}), and beriberi (vitamin B_1) were still relatively common and perceived as the first sign of deficiency. Viewed fifty years later, these gross nutritional deficiencies are clearly acute symptoms of nutritional deficiencies, which are preceded by more subtle signs. For example, gums that bleed during tooth brushing suggest inadequate vitamin C intake and deep fissures on the tongue indicate B-vitamin deficiencies. (Take a moment to look in the mirror.)

After World War II, it seemed rational to use the RDAs as the basis of the United States' peacetime public nutrition policy. Today, the RDAs of vitamin and minerals are listed on everything from packages of hot dogs to cartons of orange juice, and they're used as nutrition guidelines for federally funded school lunches. They have become the default setting for peoples' nutritional requirements, and most people don't question them.

There are dangers in relying too much on RDAs or similar

guidelines for large numbers of people. Despite their authorita-
tive ring, the RDAs remain a conservative and often erratic
standard. Consider the case of vitamin E. Discovered in 1922, it
was not declared essential to health until 1968. Selenium, another
essential nutrient, was long considered toxic because high levels
were known to poison livestock. In 1978, in an about-face, the
Food and Nutrition Board of the National Academy of Sciences
acknowledged that "selenium must be essential for man . . ."[19]
In 1989, the RDA for folic acid was cut in half because researchers
thought it was unimportant. Now, prominant researchers are
urging that it be raised to prevent birth defects and heart disease.
Many other important nutrients, such as the carotenes, flavonoids, and coenzyme Q_{10} warrant RDAs, but they are unlikely
to be blessed with RDA status for years.

What if the rationale behind the RDAs is entirely wrong?
What if the RDAs are an overly conservative and antiquated
dietary standard? Paul Lachance, Ph.D., and Lillian Langseth,
Dr. Ph., who are far from being nutritional firebrands, are among
those who have eloquently made this very argument.

These two researchers have pointed out that the RDAs originated as safeguards against now-rare gross deficiency diseases,
not as targets for *optimal* nutritional intake or for the prevention
of heart disease or cancer. To wit: the latest edition of *Recommended Dietary Allowances* describes the RDAs as appropriate
for "practically all healthy persons."[20] But, as Drs. Lachance
and Langseth have observed, "A large proportion of the general
population cannot truly be described as 'healthy.' About 30 percent of Americans smoke, and many drink to excess. Others
have diabetes, elevated cholesterol levels, or high blood pressure. After age forty-five, most people are not 'healthy' in the
strict sense of the word and relatively few qualify as having no
chronic or acute problem."[21]

Changes to the RDAs have become bogged down in arguments between nutritional conservatives and liberals—those
who want to keep RDAs low and those who want to raise them.

Drs. Lachance and Langseth have suggested a reasonable two-tiered approach, one addressing basic requirements and the other focusing on more optimal levels of nutritional intake.

NUTRITIONAL INDIVIDUALITY

The very concept of a population-wide nutritional standard can also be questioned. Forty years ago, Roger Williams, Ph.D., discoverer of the B vitamin pantothenic acid, developed the concept of biochemical individuality in which he argued that people need the same nutrients—but in very different quantities. These differences are the result of wide individual variations in biochemistry and physiology. As Dr. Williams pointed out, our nutritional needs are as unique as our fingerprints.[22] Today, doctors are reexamining how our *genetic* individuality affects our nutritional requirements.

Put into practice, biochemical (or nutritional) individuality means that 100 milligrams (mg) of vitamin C might be sufficient for one person, whereas another might require 3,000 milligrams—thirty times more. The late Nobel laureate Linus Pauling, Ph.D., helped shape the concept of biochemical individuality into one that emphasized optimal nutrition, and he routinely recommended that people take anywhere from one hundred to three hundred times the RDA level of vitamin C for *optimal* health.[23] In this context, the concept of RDAs becomes increasingly irrelevant.

When you consider how people respond to higher levels of vitamins, the idea of optimal requirements far above RDA levels makes sense. For the moment, two examples should suffice. In analyzing twenty-one studies on vitamin C and the common cold, Harri Hemilä, Ph.D., of the University of Helsinki, noted that 2,000 to 6,000 milligrams daily—thirty-three to a hundred times the RDA—was the optimal dose for reducing symptoms.[24] Similarly, Meir Stampfer, M.D., of Harvard University, has reported that 400 IU of vitamin E—forty times the RDA—greatly reduces the risk of coronary heart disease.[25,26] (IU is an abbreviation for international unit, a measurement standard for some vitamins.) These and other nutrients will be discussed in greater detail in Part 3 of this book.

Still another problem occurs when RDAs are set too low: nutrient-poor foods look more nutritious than they are. Consider how advertising touts many highly refined, sugar-rich cereals as containing 100 percent of the RDA for vitamin C and other vitamins. One hundred percent sounds nutritionally complete. But if the RDA was set at higher, more optimal levels—let's say 500 to 1,000 mg for vitamin C—today's cereals would look nutritionally inadequate. Thousands of such foods and RDA claims populate the shelves of supermarkets, but in reality they may be woefully inadequate to maintain health and immunity.

A SIGN OF WIDESPREAD DEFICIENCIES

Although nutritional deficiencies impair the immune system, one of the best documented signs of widespread deficiency may actually be related to coronary heart disease. In a sense, this is the stage where a mediocre RDA falls apart in the face of optimal requirements.

Based on accumulating research over the past quarter century, a substance called *homocysteine* has become recognized as a major risk factor in coronary heart disease, stroke, and other cardiovascular diseases. In some respects, homocysteine is the "new" cholesterol, but it is not found in food. It is actually a by-product of the breakdown of protein, and it normally exists only briefly in the body. Levels of homocysteine in the blood build up only when people inherit a peculiar genetic defect *or* when they do not consume adequate amounts of the B vitamins, including B_6, B_{12}, folic acid, and choline.

The association between high homocysteine and low folic acid intake is so strong that researchers and physicians have come to accept homocysteine as an indicator of folic acid deficiency—and as a risk factor for coronary heart disease and stroke. So how common are deficiencies of folic acid and the other

B vitamins, which also happen to be essential for immunity? Numerous studies have found that about one-third of elderly men and women have elevated homocysteine levels and that half of those who are middle-aged and elderly are deficient in folic acid and other B vitamins.[27,28] Even people with normal blood levels of vitamins, reflecting RDA intake, benefited greatly when the researchers gave them vitamins.[29]

The situation becomes more grave wherever institutional diets are served, such as in hospitals, schools, nursing homes, and prisons. The emphasis in these environments is more on the logistics of serving food to large numbers of people, and processed and packaged foods are easier than fresh foods to prepare and serve in mass quantities. Nutrition gets the short shrift. The consequence? Malnutrition by RDA standards increases the risk of infection by five times among hospitalized patients.[30] By higher standards, the risk of infection would be greater.

It's clearly time to stop thinking about malnutrition strictly as a problem of third world nations and to take a good hard look at our own shopping carts. At the very least, ignoring the nutritional health of Americans leaves us vulnerable to criticism as well as to disease. Not long ago, José Ignacio Santos, M.D., an infectious disease specialist at the Hospital Infantil de Mexico Frederico Gomez Hospital in Mexico City, gently offered such criticism. Experienced in the problems of malnutrition in his own country, Dr. Santos wrote, "Physicians in affluent countries are becoming aware of the association between malnutrition (deficiencies or excesses) and various conditions, including sepsis, multiple trauma, cancer, AIDS, renal disease, hepatic failure, cystic fibrosis, prematurity, and aging. An acute or chronic condition can be compounded by associated nutritional deficiencies, placing the sufferers at increased risk of severe, often fatal, opportunistic infections."[31]

Sugar—An Antinutrient That Impairs Immunity

Unfortunately, it's not just nutritional deficiencies that impair immunity. Some nutritional excesses, such as the high consumption of sugary foods, diminish immune function.

At the beginning of the twentieth century, the average per capita consumption of refined sugar was an estimated five pounds per year. Sugar was expensive and a special treat. Then, as with wheat and bread, new manufacturing technology allowed the efficient and relatively inexpensive production of sugar from beets and cane. Without the previous constraints of manufacture and cost, the nation's sweet tooth grew. Today, the combined annual consumption of sucrose, high-fructose corn syrup, and other caloric sweeteners averages 150 pounds per capita. As with any average, some people eat more and others less—and for each person who limits his sugar intake, someone else eats 300 to 400 pounds per year.

Much of this sugar is added to soft drinks and hundreds of other processed and packaged foods, including some brands of salt, before it reaches your kitchen table. Although manufacturers of sucrose and high-fructose corn syrup attribute many superlatives to their products, these sugars provide nothing except carbohydrate calories—no vitamins, no minerals, no protein. In a nation with at least one-third of its population overweight, such calories are completely unnecessary from a dietary standpoint. But sugar is not simply a dietary bystander. It functions as an *anti*nutrient because it displaces nutrient-dense foods and drains B vitamins to metabolize it. Sugar also reduces your body's ability to fight infections.

In the 1970s, John Yudkin, M.D., Ph.D., a professor at Queen Elizabeth College, London, moved the discussion of sugar from medical journals to a public forum with the publication of his book *Sweet and Dangerous*. Yudkin, a conservative and methodical scientist, had carefully documented the relationship between sugar and heart disease.[32] In an interview, he commented that if sugar were reintroduced as a "drug," it would probably not be permitted on the market because of its health hazards. Yudkin documented that sugar—in this case sucrose—raised blood levels of cholesterol and triglyceride, fats associated with increased risk of heart disease. It also increases platelet aggregation, setting the stage for blood clots.[33]

The relationship between sugar and infection goes back to 1908, when researchers noted that diabetics, who characteristically have high blood sugar levels, were more susceptible than nondiabetics to infection.[34] In 1942, researchers determined the reason was that diabetics' white blood cells were unusually sluggish.[35]

One of the most significant studies on sugar and white blood cell activity was conducted by three dentists at the Loma Linda University School of Dentistry in Loma Linda, California, and published in 1964.[36] Ernest Kijak, D.D.S., George Foust, D.D.S., and Ralph R. Steinman, D.D.S., investigated how different levels of blood sugar (glucose) influenced the performance of white blood cells in blood drawn from diabetics and nondiabetics. Dr. Kijak and his colleagues fed their human subjects different concentrations of glucose, then drew blood samples from them.

Next, Dr. Kijak and his colleagues measured blood sugar levels and added *Staphylococcus* bacteria to the blood. They then incubated the blood for thirty minutes, during which time the white blood cells engulfed the bacteria. Then they measured the "phagocytic index"—that is, the effectiveness of white blood cells in capturing bacteria. They quite literally counted the average number of bacteria a group of a hundred white blood cells captured and digested. The more bacteria captured, the higher the index; the fewer, the lower the index.

Among both diabetics and nondiabetics, the higher the sugar consumption and the more blood sugar levels rose, the lower their phagocytic indexes dropped. More sugar meant white blood cells that were less efficient. White blood cells from people who consumed the equivalent of a candy bar and a soft drink captured only one-tenth the bacteria of people who ate half a candy bar. These changes did not take long to occur—only forty-five minutes.[37]

Several years later, Albert Sanchez, Ph.D., of Loma Linda University looked at how other sugars and starch affect the phagocytic index. Dr. Sanchez and his colleagues gave human volunteers 100 grams of a variety of individual sugars, including glucose, fructose, sucrose, or simple starch. All of the sugars lowered phagocytosis by 50 percent, but the starch had little effect. The highest phagocytic index was noted right before the subjects were fed the sugars, and it reached its lowest point two hours after the sugars were eaten. Furthermore, the depression in phagocytic activity lasted for more than five hours. The implications? Regular sugar eaters have a perpetually depressed response to infecting microorganisms.[38] If you're one of the many people who eat a donut for breakfast, drink a soft drink with lunch, and relish a dessert after dinner, your white blood cells are chronically groggy defenders of your body.

Around the same time, researchers at Utah State University, Logan, examined how increases in dietary sugar lower the body's production of antibodies. Using laboratory rats as a model for the human immune system, they increased dietary sucrose levels in 10 percent increments while decreasing vitamin, mineral, and protein levels by comparable percentages. The rats were exposed to Salmonella, and levels of antibodies were measured after each change to the diet. As little as a 10 percent decrease in the nutritional quality of the diet—10 percent more sugar, 10 percent fewer vitamins, minerals, and protein—resulted in a 50 percent decrease in antibodies. When the diet was 75 percent sugar, antibody production was down by 90 percent.[39]

After conducting their own study on how sugar affected white blood cells, William M. Ringsdorf, D.M.D., and Emanuel Cheraskin, M.D., D.M.D., of the University of Alabama, Birmingham, observed that major drops in phagocytosis—resulting from sugar-rich institutional foods—would increase the likelihood of

TEST YOUR NUTRITIONAL HEALTH

It's easy to lose sight of your nutritional health. This brief questionnaire will help you assess your nutritional status. If the statement on the left is true, add the number at the right. Check your total score at the bottom.

1. I often skip breakfast, or just eat a breakfast bar.   3

2. I often skip lunch because I don't have the time.   3

3. I eat in restaurants at least once a day.   2

4. I eat in fast-food restaurants at least three times a week.   2

5. I don't like fruits or vegetables, so I don't eat the five recommended servings per day.   3

6. When I eat at home, I tend to heat frozen meals.   2

7. I buy most of my food at the supermarket rather than at natural foods stores.   1

8. I have two or more beers, glasses of wine, or hard liquor drinks each day.   2

9. I enjoy snacking on chocolate, candies, cookies, or cake and have some every day.   2

10. I have a medical condition that has made me change the type or amount of food I eat.   2

11. Without trying, I've lost or gained ten or more pounds over the past few months.   2

YOUR TOTAL SCORE   _____

If your score is

  0–4. Your diet is good.
  5–8. You need to pay more attention to your diet.
  9–12. Your diet is marginal, but if you change it, you can probably avoid some health problems.
  13–17. You are not eating a sound diet, and you're at risk for serious health problems.
  18–24. Your diet is severely lacking, placing you at risk of coronary heart disease, cancer, and infection.

infection after surgery. "Is there any group who needs optimal phagocytosis any more than the hospitalized?" they asked.[40] As recently as 1994, researchers were still trying to impress upon the medical community that sugar consumption and blood sugar levels have a direct effect on resistance to infection.[41] It's not clear, however, how many people have been listening.

There's one final, important note about sugar consumption. Over the past twenty-five years, much of the sucrose used in foods has been replaced with high-fructose corn syrup, which sounds like a natural sweetener. It isn't—it's as refined a product as sucrose. The makers of sugar and high-fructose corn syrup compete fiercely with each other—there are differences in taste—but from a chemical standpoint their products are almost identical. Although no studies have been conducted on high-fructose corn syrup and phagocytosis, the chemical similarity to sugar would suggest an identical effect. No refined sugar would seem to enhance immunity. In contrast, the bulk of fruits prevents people from consuming large quantities of natural sugars.

Too often, people take the contents of their shopping carts for granted and assume they buy and eat nutritionally worthwhile foods when they do not. A large number of foods are marketed simply for reasons of taste, novelty, and profit—not for their nutritional value. Even with good foods, such as produce, grains, and meat, fragile vitamins and other nutrients deteriorate during processing, packaging, refrigeration, and cooking. The effect of these nutrient losses is compounded by poor food choices, such as skipping a salad to save room for dessert.

According to major surveys, half of Americans do not obtain RDA levels of at least several nutrients. These nutritional deficiencies may actually be far worse because the RDAs are increasingly viewed as a conservative standard of nutritional intake. Whatever your standard, though, large numbers of people simply do not obtain adequate amounts of the nutrients necessary for a strong immune system. Their resistance to infectious disease has been further compromised by the consumption of poly-unsaturated fats and sugars. If you have come to see nutrition as the foundation of health, you can only conclude that it has become seriously weakened.

8

IMMUNE SYSTEM ATTACKERS

❡

A poor or unbalanced diet is not the only factor that can degrade your resistance to infectious diseases. Numerous non-nutritional substances can also harm your immunity as well.

For example, few physicians and researchers realize that some antibiotics and common pain-relieving drugs can also interfere with normal immune function. Antibiotic use often leads to infections with *Candida albicans* yeast, which further compromises immunity. Still other immune system attackers include pesticides, alcohol, stress, and overexercise. Together, they leave you less able to defend yourself against the surrounding sea of bacteria and viruses.

All this might strike you as a bit overwhelming. How do you cope? How do you change those things that can leave you susceptible to disease? There's actually a lot you can do, and most of it is relatively easy. We will begin discussing how you can achieve optimal immunity in the next chapter. For now, though, you have to recognize that there are a few more immune "enemies" that require caution on your part.

Antibiotics and the Erosion of Immunity

Physicians know that some antibiotics are toxic and must be used judiciously. For example, tetracyclines interfere with calcium and magnesium absorption and therefore the growth of bone and teeth, and chloramphenicol occasionally causes aplastic anemia long after antibiotic therapy has ceased. As we described in Chapter 4, antibiotics can predispose people to infection by destroying the normal intestinal bacteria that compete with disease-causing bacteria.

Back in 1950, a team of researchers noticed that an antibiotic reduced phagocytosis, that is, the ability of white blood cells to capture and destroy bacteria.[1] Because other scientists could not confirm this finding, it was dismissed as a fluke.[2] Then, in 1972, researchers at the Baylor School of Medicine, Houston, rediscovered that a number of antibiotics, sometimes in very low concentrations, interfered with the ability of white blood cells to move toward and kill bacteria.[3,4] A small number of researchers have continued to investigate this paradoxical effect of antibiotics, but most physicians remain unaware of the research.

The almost heretical discovery that some antibiotics depressed immunity stimulated other research along the same lines in this country and in Europe.[5] Scientists subsequently determined that common tetracycline-class antibiotics were among the worst offenders.[6,7,8,9,10] Other common antibiotics, such as erythromycin and chloramphenicol, significantly decreased T cell numbers, but plain old penicillin did not seem to affect them or other immune cells.[11]

These are disturbing findings for people raised to believe in the miracle of antibiotics, and more recent evidence backs them up. In 1987, F. C. Sheng, M.D., of the University of California School of Medicine, Los Angeles, investigated the effect of clindamycin and netilmicin in rabbits with peritonitis, a type of abdominal infection. In people, this infection is often life threatening. Dr. Sheng found that the antibiotics dramatically decreased the activity of white blood cells and phagocytosis and concluded that "antibiotics, while vitally important in fighting infections, may in and of themselves be agents of immunosuppression at the cellular level."[12]

Over the past several years, Gerhard Pulverer, M.D., and his colleagues at the Institute for Medicine, Microbiology and Hygiene at the University of Cologne have been among the most steadfast investigators of these undesirable antibiotic side effects. They have carefully documented that various antibiotics, including the penicillin-class mezlocillin, suppress the activity of macrophages and T cells.[13]

The Cologne researchers have also discovered one of the reasons why antibiotics hurt immunity. Some species of intestinal bacterial (such as *Bacteroides*, *Clostridium*, *Lactobacillus*, and *Propionibacterium*) produce peptides that enhance and even appear essential for the immunity of their animal and human hosts.[14,15] These peptides, like amino acids, are constituents of protein. In experiments, Dr. Pulverer and his colleagues used antibiotics to destroy the intestinal bacteria of laboratory animals and, consequently, to stop their production of peptides. As a consequence, T cells (considered the brains of the immune system) failed to mature, proliferate, or activate. Restoring the peptides returned the T cells to normal.[16] Such findings support the idea that intestinal bacteria and their hosts share a true symbiotic relationship. (You'll read more about beneficial bacteria in Chapter 10.)

Antibiotic therapy disrupts this symbiotic relationship and the general health of the gastrointestinal bacteria,[17] and regular antibiotic use prevents their recovery. But whether an antibiotic destroys a person's natural colony of intestinal bacteria—which weigh a couple of pounds or so in a healthy adult—depends partly on other factors: the type of antibiotic and how well it is absorbed.

Unfortunately, nearly every oral antibiotic disrupts intestinal bacteria to some extent. The most damaging oral antibiotics are ampicillin, piperacillin, third-generation cephalosporins (e.g., cefixime), cefoxitin, erythromycin, clindamycin, and tetracyclines. Antibiotics also alter the bacterial balance in other parts of the body. For example, during antibiotic therapy traces of clindamycin, erythromycin, and tetracyclines appear in the saliva and change the microbial environment of the mouth, teeth, and nose.[18]

Disturbances in the normal intestinal bacteria also create a "microbiological vacuum" that *Candida albicans* and some disease-causing bacteria quickly fill, causing diarrhea, colitis, or infections of the blood. These disease-causing bacteria are often resistant to antibiotics. Even normal intestinal bacteria, such as *Enterobacteria* and *Pseudomonas* species, can flourish under such circumstances and cause life-threatening infections. Some antibiotics, such as the third-generation cephalosporins and tetracyclines, disrupt the intestinal bacteria so much that patients risk secondary antibiotic-resistant "superinfections."[19,20] As Judy Belsheim, M.D., a pioneering researcher in antibiotic side effects, once observed, impaired white blood cells "cannot be advantageous to the patient."[21]

All this does not mean you should always refuse antibiotic therapy, for such drugs may save your life. They just need to be used judiciously. Like any medication, antibiotics can be good or bad, creating both desirable changes and unwanted side effects. In light of these findings, it might be best to remember that antibiotics assist, but do not replace, a healthy immune system.

Such a view, in fact, was stated in 1944, during the early days of penicillin's medical use. Sir Howard W. Florey, Ph.D., who was instrumental in developing penicillin as a commercial drug, observed that penicillin's antibacterial activity gave the body the extra time it sometimes needed to mount its own effective attack on pathogens.[22] Antibiotic suppression of immunity is one more reason to use these drugs conservatively—and to build up one's natural defenses against infection.

Pain-Relieving Drugs
and Supergerm Susceptibility

In December 1994, the Canadian politician Lucien Bouchard thought he had accidentally pulled a leg muscle. To relieve the pain, he did what many other people do in similar circumstances: he took common nonsteroidal anti-inflammatory drugs (NSAIDs), which include such common pain relievers as aspirin, ibuprofen, and acetaminophen. Within days, Bouchard found himself in a life-or-death struggle with the so-called flesh-eating bacteria, a strain of strep-A. To stop the rapidly spreading infection and save his life, doctors amputated the leg.

As it turns out, the association between NSAIDs and succumbing to the flesh-eating bacteria may be more than mere coincidence. The occurrence of life-threatening strep-A infections following the use of NSAIDs was first noted in 1985, and the evidence linking the two has continued to mount. For example, flesh-eating bacteria infections sometimes occur after a child has had the chicken pox. But a sharp increase in flesh-eating bacteria infections in children occurred after ibuprofen was marketed for pediatric use.[23]

Obviously, not everyone who takes NSAIDs develops an infection with flesh-eating bacteria, known formally as necrotizing fasciitis or necrotizing myositis. The virulent form of strep-A must be present, and other factors, such as fatigue and poor diet, no doubt make a person more susceptible.

Dennis L. Stevens, M.D., an infectious diseases specialist at the Veterans Affairs Medical Center in Boise, Idaho, recently theorized what happens. NSAIDs work by reducing inflammation, which is why they reduce arthritic symptoms. However, NSAIDs suppress white blood cells' ability to move toward, capture, and kill bacteria. In other words, NSAIDs force white blood cells to largely ignore bacteria, giving them the opportunity to reproduce and grow into dangerous infections. Furthermore, NSAIDs alter the immune response in other ways, leading to shock and organ failure.[24]

Bouchard probably had strep germs on his skin or in his blood, and the stress of constant political campaigning may have weakened his immunity. Even though Bouchard's immune system was stressed, he might have successfully fought the infection—had the NSAIDs not stymied the activity of his white blood cells.

But NSAIDs open the door to not only strep germs. According to Dr. Stevens, NSAIDs could conceivably play a role in toxic shock syndrome, a sometimes deadly staph infection associated with tampon use. Many women take NSAIDs to relieve pain during menstruation. A combination of superefficient tampons that change normal vaginal bacteria, the presence of an infecting organism, and NSAIDs could also set the stage for a dangerous infection.[25]

Although Dr. Stevens addressed the possible role of NSAIDs in only strep and staph infections, the same immune-suppressing mechanisms would affect the body's response to any infection. NSAIDs are very common drugs sold without a prescription and are effective at relieving pain. But it may be prudent to use them more conservatively because of their ability to disable the body's response to infection.

There's one more reason to be concerned about NSAIDs. Some of them may encourage antibiotic resistance in bacteria, leading to more virulent strains. In one experiment, Stuart B. Levy, M.D., and his colleagues at Tufts University found that *E. coli* exposed to aspirin and acetaminophen developed resistance to not just one but multiple antibiotics. Although the experiment was conducted in a test tube, not a living animal, the implications are chilling.[26]

Fungal Infections and Immunity

Symptoms of oral and vaginal thrush, caused by *Candida albicans*, were described more than two thousand years ago by Hippocrates. But this type of infection did not become common until antibiotics were widely used.

Candida albicans, often referred to simply as *Candida* or "yeast," is normally present in the body but usually controlled by the immune system and by competing microorganisms. It emerges as an opportunistic fungal infection when antibiotics destroy large numbers of intestinal bacteria. C. Orian Truss, M.D., one of the leading experts in *Candida* infections, observed, "The first broad-spectrum antibiotic, aureomycin, became available in 1947. The next thirteen years saw a proliferation of articles in medical journals detailing the rapid increase of intestinal and vaginal yeast infections as these drugs attained wide usage."[27] Today, the large number of prescription and over-the-counter antifungal drugs suggest that *Candida* has reached epidemic proportions.

Physicians sometimes prescribe nystatin, a safe antifungal drug, to treat vaginal or systemic infections caused by *Candida*. Systemic, or bodywide, yeast infections are generally considered rare, and their diagnosis often raises eyebrows among conservative physicians and the insurers who often pay for drugs. But such *Candida* infections may be fairly common, according to Dr. Truss, chief of allergy and clinical immunology at St. Vincent's Hospital, Birmingham, Alabama. A methodical scientist, he approached the issue of *Candida* infections skeptically and collected data for sixteen years before publishing his first paper on the subject. Dr. Truss became convinced that *Candida* can easily migrate from the skin, mucous membranes, or gastrointestinal tract to the bloodstream, where it can then cause systemic infections.

These *Candida* infections can often be unusual in that they provoke a diverse number of apparently inexplicable symptoms, including abdominal bloating, nausea, diarrhea, constipation, menstrual problems, memory and concentration difficulties, depression, rhinitis, and wheezing.[28] William Crook, M.D., of Jackson, Tennessee, another expert in *Candida*, has pointed out that the yeast can cause fatigue, headache, muscle pain, premenstrual syndrome, and endometriosis.[29]

By disrupting the intestinal bacteria, *Candida* also depresses immunity, increases susceptibility to subsequent bacterial infections, and weakens defenses against infection.[30] The first direct link between *Candida* and immune disturbances was established in the late 1960s by Kazuo Iwata, Ph.D., of the University of Tokyo. Dr. Iwata noted that the number of T cells decreased during *Candida* infections.[31] He and other researchers subsequently determined that *Candida* produces a substance that prevents the activation of both T cells and white blood cells.[32,33,34] Furthermore, aminoglycoside-class antibiotics (which include streptomycin and gentamicin) directly interfere with the ability of white blood cells to capture and digest the fungus.[35]

All of this leads to a near ideal environment for *Candida*, since in most people the immune system has already been weakened by a primary infection and possibly by an antibiotic. It is conceivable that the immune effects of *Candida* reverberate biochemically and contribute to the wide range of symptoms observed by Drs. Truss and Crook.

The situation has been further aggravated by the spread of HIV and its concomitant immune suppression. *Candida* infections have reached epidemic proportions among AIDS patients, but they are not the only ones at risk. People taking immune-suppressive drugs following organ transplant surgery or as part of cancer therapy also risk serious *Candida* infections.[36] It's worthwhile remembering that, aside from AIDS, most infectious diseases and immune suppression occur in various degrees of severity. It's very likely that low-grade *Candida* infections increase susceptibility to milder bacterial and viral infections and slow recovery from them.

The Pesticide Assault on Immunity

Until the late 1940s, nicotine, kerosene, and turpentine were the most common pesticides—administered occasionally to control insect pests. Farmers did not expect to entirely eradicate insect pests and, like consumers, resigned themselves (however painfully) to periodic blights and blemished produce. The development and commercialization of DDT and other modern pesticides, used regularly to blanket fields, rapidly altered both farmers' and consumers' expectations of food crops—and, more slowly, their health. Since the introduction of pesticides, researchers have progressively investigated their effects on the nervous, reproductive, and endocrine systems, and now on the immune system.

Developed during World War II to protect Allied soldiers against lice and malaria-carrying mosquitoes, DDT was the first of many pesticides in a new class of chemicals called organochlorines. It was a remarkable chemical achievement. Both carbon (which is what *organo* refers to) and chlorine occur naturally, but until that time, they rarely existed as a compound. Looking for new markets after the war, the chemical industry aggressively marketed DDT and other pesticides to farmers, much the way pharmaceutical companies marketed antibiotics to physicians. By the 1950s, expectations among farmers and consumers changed. Farmers started believing they could vanquish insect pests, and consumers thought that anything less than a perfect, spotless vegetable was unworthy of purchase.

People are exposed to pesticides in a number of ways, most often through the food they eat and by spraying around the home or office. An estimated eight hundred million pounds of pesticides are used each year in American agriculture—roughly three pounds for every man, woman, and child.[37] Pesticides permeate the food on which they are sprayed and, because they are oil based, do not wash off with rinsing. Although the amount of pesticides ingested in individual foods is generally very low, it is a chronic and cumulative exposure. Pesticides are stored with fat—in the breasts, torso, and buttocks.

People are also exposed to pesticides during the routine spraying of offices and schools, and the hazards are amplified by sloppy handling of these chemicals. "In a representative incident," reads a recent Oregon Health Division report, "an office was commercially treated with chlorpyrifos after work hours. The building was not properly ventilated before workers returned. The next day, sixteen employees complained of symptoms such as headache, dizziness, throat irritation, and nausea, most of which resolved upon leaving the treated area."[38] Farmworkers may receive larger and more frequent exposures to pesticides, from simple spills and their proximity to sprays, but many of these incidents go unreported.

For the average person, pesticides in the house or yard, whether applied by the home owner or a commercial pest-control company, dwarf the amount of pesticides found in food, according to Sheldon L. Wagner, M.D., professor of clinical toxicology at Oregon State University and lead investigator for the Environmental Protection Agency's National Pesticide Medical Monitoring Program.[39] A number of studies support Dr. Wagner's view. An analysis of the habits of 239 Missouri families, which may be representative, found that 98 percent of them used pesticides in the home or yard at least once a year and 64 percent used these chemicals more than five times a year. Twenty-eight percent of the families used pesticide-containing flea collars on their pets.[40]

It's easy for even well-meaning people to overdo—and overdose—with pesticides. In 1994, Dr. Wagner reported the case of a twelve-week-old infant who developed muscle paralysis. After several months, investigators discovered that her home had received an "excessive application" of Diazinon five weeks before her symptoms appeared. Months after the Diazinon was applied, levels on the floor, in the air, and in the infant's urine remained high. The infant recovered completely only after she was removed from the house.[41] In another case, a woman sprayed her house intermittently over three weeks with two cans of a commercial ant spray. Her seventy-five-year-old husband, who suffered from a number of physical problems, couldn't leave the house. After several weeks, when his condition worsened, he was hospitalized, and laboratory tests show pesticide poisoning. He was discharged after sixteen days, and died nine days later.[42]

THE THREAT OF ORGANOCHLORINE PESTICIDES

Research on the immune effects of pesticides over the past fifty years has accumulated slowly but steadily. "The worldwide use of pesticides makes it urgent to know as much as possible about the effects of pesticides and their degradation productions on humans and animals," observed Walter B. Dandliker, Ph.D., of the Scripps Clinic and Research Foundation, La Jolla, California. "Immediate toxic effects are relatively readily assessed, but slow or delayed effects are more difficult to detect and may be the more important—possibly leading to altered susceptibility to disease, damage in utero, accelerated aging, etc."[43]

Not surprisingly, pesticides have selected for the survival of resistant insects much the same way antibiotics have selected for resistant bacteria. As with antibiotics, the chemical industry has "solved" the problem by recommending stronger concentrations and developing a steady stream of new pesticides. But organochlorines have turned out to be resilient, long-lived chemicals. While they can have a dramatic and rapid effect—death—on susceptible insects, their effects on the more complex physiology of mammals are more subtle.

The first signs of trouble—reproductive disorders in animals—were described by Rachel Carson in her 1962 book, *Silent Spring*. Carson suggested that people view animals in the wild as analogous to the canaries miners carried deep underground to detect poisonous methane gas: a sick or dead bird was a sign of imminent danger. Carson's book prompted a reassessment of DDT and other pesticides, and a bitter fight ensued with the chemical industry and farmers on one side and environmentalists and regulatory agencies on the other. It took ten years, but DDT was banned as an environmental pollutant and carcinogen in the United States. However, many other organochlorine pesticides are still used in this country. In addition DDE, a breakdown product of DDT, is still commonly found in land, water, and the food supply. It is not only a legacy of the past. DDT is still used in Central and South America and finds its way back into our food supply and environment through imported produce.

Nonpesticide organochlorines have become common as well—about eleven thousand different ones are manufactured as products or by-products of industry. These chemicals are found in polychlorinated biphenyls (PCBs), used in the manufacture of electronics; in many of the plastics used in baby bottles, water jugs, and food can linings; and in chlorine compounds, such as dioxin, used to bleach paper. Dioxin is particularly well documented as a toxin to the immune system, even at very low doses. It alters the behavior of T cells and suppresses the body's production of antibodies.[44,45] Dioxin also increases susceptibility to *Salmonella* infections,[46] and just recently researchers reported that dioxin speeds the replication of HIV.[47]

For the most part, people concerned with the effects of pesticides were dismissed by industry as environmental extremists or, pejoratively, as health food nuts. Organochlorines aroused only minor concerns until several years ago, when researchers stumbled across something really big: many organochlorines, including pesticides, mimicked the female hormone estrogen in animals and humans. These estrogen mimickers are not limited to pesticide contaminants of foods. Butylated hydroxyanisole (BHA), a widely used food preservative, and butyl benzyl phthalate (BBP), used in paper and cardboard packaging for foods, are also potent estrogen mimickers—and food contaminants.[48]

Estrogen, the "feminizing" hormone, serves an essential role in reproduction. But it also proliferates breast and uterine tissue, increasing the risk of endometriosis and breast and uterine cancers. Chemicals that mimic estrogen could conceivably increase a woman's estrogen load by hundreds of times. With that insight, the increasing human incidence of reproductive disorders and cancer started to make a little more sense to researchers.

Devra Lee Davis, Ph.D., M.PH., and other researchers have started to document the link between synthetic estrogens in the environment and breast cancer, hinting that these chemicals affect both the reproductive and immune systems.[49] Mary Wolff, Ph.D., of the Mt. Sinai School of Medicine in New York City, has established a clear link between blood levels of DDT and a woman's subsequent risk of developing breast cancer. By analyzing blood samples from fourteen thousand women, Dr. Wolff found that women with high blood levels of DDE, a by-product of DDT, had four times the risk of developing breast cancer compared with women who had low levels of the chemical.[50]

Cancer is arguably different from susceptibility to infection, though both conditions share elements of immune dysfunction. (It's generally believed that cancer cells form on a regular basis, but that a healthy immune system destroys them.) Recently, Albert D. M. E. Osterhaus, Ph.D., a virologist at Erasmus University, Rotterdam, unequivocally demonstrated that mammals exposed to organochlorine pesticides and other pollutants become more susceptible to both cancers and viral infections.

For two years, Dr. Osterhaus and his colleagues fed seal pups herring from either the relatively pollution-free North Atlantic or the industrially polluted Baltic Sea. The Baltic fish contained ten times the quantity of organochlorines as the North Atlantic fish. Immediately after the start of the experiment, levels of vitamin A, natural-killer cells, T cells, and antibody-producing B cells dropped in the seals eating the contaminated Baltic fish. These seals also began producing elevated levels of white blood cells, a sign of chronic infection.[51] The implications in terms of human susceptibility to infection are profound.

The body also seems to use the estrogen mimickers a little

differently than normal estrogen. Peter Montague, Ph.D., who directs the Environmental Research Foundation in Annapolis, Maryland, explained the difference: "Natural hormones do their work as messengers (or as stimulants of a cascade of other effects), and then the body disassembles them and removes them from the bloodstream. In contrast, when industrial chemicals and pesticides mimic hormones, they do not disappear quickly. They tend to remain in the body for very long periods, doing the work of hormones at times, and in ways, that are inappropriate and destructive."[52]

Furthermore, the body's metabolism of DDT, DDE, and atrazine (currently the most widely used pesticide in the United States) leads to a highly potent form of estrogen capable of damaging DNA.[53] Damaged DNA generates large numbers of free radicals, and both the damaged DNA and free radicals increase the likelihood of cell mutations and cancers.

PESTICIDES, IMMUNITY, AND THE DIET

Whatever the exact mechanism, pesticides *do* have established, deleterious effects on immunity. In the early days of pesticides, researchers assumed their effects were limited to the nervous system, because this is the organ system these chemicals attack in insects. Of course, the body's organs are not isolated entities. The same blood that flows through the nervous system also flows through the endocrine and immune systems. In time, researchers documented that pesticides affected the hormone-producing endocrine system, which includes the thymus gland, the source of T cells. By the late 1960s, these findings helped create the new field of immunotoxicology. Much of the research has been conducted on animals, since exposing people to hazardous chemicals in a laboratory (but not at the farm or grocery store) is considered unethical.

As one might expect, different pesticides have different effects on the immune system. The animal evidence is disturbing, if not always consistent: these man-made chemicals reduce immunity and increase susceptibility to infectious disease. After concluding a study on how some pesticides affected the immunity of hamsters, Dr. Dandliker observed that "a single dose of orally administered pesticide may exert large, long-lasting effects on the immune response. . . . the depression of the immune response . . . could lower resistance to a variety of infectious diseases."[54] In many cases, however, the real "canaries" are people, not birds. A study of eighty-five workers found that white blood cell impairments and upper respiratory tract infections correlated with how long the workers were occupationally exposed to pesticides.[55]

Organochlorine pesticides also alter how the body uses vitamins C and A, which are essential for immunity. This has been well documented with two pesticides, aldrin and lindane. These pesticides disrupt thymus function and lower vitamin C levels in the adrenal glands, which produce defensive "fight or flight" hormones.[56] In turn, a vitamin C deficiency makes it more difficult for animals to break down DDT, dieldrin, and lindane—resulting in greater tissue accumulation of the pesticides.[57] Of these pesticides, aldrin and dieldrin were banned in 1974. Lindane is still used in the treatment of lice, and the FDA received eighty-eight reports of severe neurotoxicity—six of them resulting in death—from lindane prescriptions between 1972 and 1995.[58] It's likely that many reactions, especially milder ones, go unreported.

A small but significant study at the University of Wisconsin, Madison, looked at the interplay between malnutrition, environmental chemicals, and susceptibility to infection. William P. Porter, Ph.D., and colleagues exposed "laboratory" white mice and "wild" deer mice to a number of chemicals, including PCBs, immune suppressants, and viruses. As long as the mice were well nourished, they generally resisted the effects of the chemicals and viral infections. When both the white and wild mice species were malnourished and exposed to the chemicals, they both gave birth to offspring with low birth weights and shorter life spans.

"Our results suggest the possibility of added danger to humans and animals if they are malnourished and exposed to a combination of infectious agents and environmental chemicals," Dr. Porter wrote.[59] He suggested that well-fed white mice, which are usually used in toxicology studies, might not accurately indicate a chemical's true effect. The reason is that wild animals—like most people—don't always eat an ideal, balanced

---

✼

SOME PESTICIDES AND THEIR EFFECTS ON IMMUNITY[62]

Atrazine: Decreases T cells in blood

Benzene hexachloride: Inhibits immune response to *Salmonella typhimurium*

Captan: Lowers T-cell count and reduces weight of the thymus gland, which produces T cells

Carbofuran: Reduces resistance to *Salmonella* and likely other germs

Chlordane: Suppresses T-cell activity

DDT: Causes thymus atrophy

Dieldrin: Inhibits response to *Salmonella* and increases susceptibility to viral infection

Dinoseb: Depresses white blood cells and antibodies

Malathion: Suppresses T cells

Methylparathion: Causes thymus atrophy and decreases resistance to *Salmonella* infection

Mirex: Decreases antibody levels

Parathion: Depresses white blood cells and antibodies

Pentachlorophenol: Reduces resistance to cancer-causing viruses

Tributyltin oxide: Suppresses antibody responses

Triphenyltin hydroxide: Decreases T cells in blood

✼

laboratory diet. As a consequence, wild animals (and not-so-wild people) may be more prone to infection. "Interactions of certain 'harmless' chemicals at low levels may prove more deleterious than higher doses of 'dangerous' toxicants acting alone," added Dr. Porter.[60]

As with antibiotics, the end of the line for pesticides is within sight. Though the chemical industry claims pesticides are better than ever, and most farmers fear what might happen if they stop using them, pesticides simply don't work as well as they once did. In the journal *Science,* Constance Holdren summed up the situation by writing, "Efforts to control crop damage solely with pesticides have by and large failed and, in developing countries, insect-borne diseases remain as serious a threat as ever."[61]

A PROBLEM THAT WON'T GO AWAY

Problems with pesticides continue, largely because of a lack of firm regulatory oversight, and deregulation will make the situation worse, not better. Once sprayed on fruit, vegetable, and grain crops, pesticides migrate throughout the environment. They are found in meat and fish—and in our drinking water. In 1994, the Environmental Working Group, based in Washington, D.C., warned that 14.1 million people in 121 midwestern communities consumed the pesticides atrazine, cyanazine, alachlor, metolachlor, and simazine through their drinking water. The pesticides are sprayed routinely on corn and soybeans in the Midwest,[63] and the summer growing season levels exceed federal standards.[64]

In February 1995, the Environmental Working Group charged that the Food and Drug Administration routinely ignored the illegal use of sixty-six pesticides on forty-two species of fruits and vegetables. Some of the pesticides had been banned, and others were used on crops for which they were not legally intended.[65] While the FDA downplayed the dangers, the charges were reminiscent of the largest single outbreak of acute pesticide poisoning, which had occurred ten years before. In that incident,

⌘

FOODS WITH LARGE AMOUNTS OF PESTICIDE RESIDUES

Peanuts	Bologna
Raisins	Salami
Fast-food Hamburgers	Ground Beef

**FOODS WITH MODERATE TO HIGH AMOUNTS
OF PESTICIDE RESIDUES**

Apples	Lettuce
Apricots	Peaches
Broccoli	Spinach
Cantaloupe	Rye, White, and Whole Wheat
Cherries	Bread
Cranberries	Beef Round Steak
Eggplant	Ham
Grapes	Pork Chops
Green Bell Peppers	

FOODS WITH FEW OR NO PESTICIDE RESIDUES

Alfalfa sprouts	Hawaiian Pineapples
Asparagus	Cornflakes
Avocadoes	Granola
Cauliflower	Game Meats
Peas	Turkey
Tangerines	

Adapted from *Diet for a Poisoned Planet,* by David Steinman (Ballantine Books, 1990).

⌘

264 people in Oregon were sickened by California watermelons contaminated by aldicarb, a pesticide legal for cotton crops but not for watermelon. Investigators believed the aldicarb was either misapplied or that the pesticide persisted in the soil from previous seasons.[66]

In 1995 as well, researchers reported that pesticides used more than fifteen years earlier had contaminated wells in fifty towns and cities—including Fresno, Lodi, and Modesto—in California's farming communities. The principal contaminant, dibromochloropropane (DBCP), was originally pumped into the ground to kill root-eating worms. DBCP was banned because it causes sterility in people and is a suspected carcinogen.[67]

To the north, rapid population growth has forced officials in the Portland, Oregon, metropolitan area to contemplate new sources of drinking water. They are focusing on the Willamette River, but stretches of that river contain parasites and toxic chemicals in sufficient quantities to cause deformities in fish, a bad sign. State environmental quality experts concluded that the water-quality problems have not been caused by the dumping of sewage or leaking landfills. Rather, they are the result of agricultural runoff, including pesticides and untreated animal waste, from Oregon's Willamette Valley farm belt.[68] The conclusion is unmistakable: humans are the only adult animals that soil their own nest.

Other Immune System Attackers

Numerous other factors can diminish the performance of the immune system, including alcohol and drug abuse, stress and fatigue, and overexercise. Any combination of these factors, especially in association with a poor diet, can weaken immunity and interfere with your ability to effectively fight infections.

ALCOHOL, DRUG ABUSE, AND TOBACCO

Low or moderate alcohol consumption seems to stimulate immune functions in a positive way.[69] However, the immunotoxic effects of excessive alcohol consumption have been documented for more than a century. Alcohol reduces the activity of white blood cells and the body's antibody responses, and heavy alcohol consumption has been associated with pneumonia, tuberculosis, and other infections.[70]

Similarly, drug abuse has been recognized as a cause of immune dysfunction since 1907. Heroin, morphine, and cocaine cause a variety of immune-system abnormalities. Some of the chemical components of marijuana, including tetrahydrocannabinol and cannibinoids, exert a powerful immunosuppressive effect, reducing the body's production of T cells, natural-killer cells, and interferon. The use of alcohol and drugs increases the susceptibility to AIDS[71] and, likely, other infections.

Tobacco, tobacco smoke, and the chemicals they contain are recognized for their roles in causing cancer. Tobacco smoke contains many free radicals, which lead to mutations, and the body generates more free radicals in trying to detoxify it. It's not enough not to smoke—chewing tobacco and breathing in secondhand tobacco smoke are just as bad.

STRESS AND FATIGUE

In Japan, *karoshi* refers to the growing problem of death from overwork. Americans may not be dying from overwork, but they do seem more stressed than ever. Much of this stress comes from the pressures of work, trying to do too much, and not getting sufficient rest.

The downsizing of businesses has resulted in more and more people being asked to simply do the job of 1.3 people with no additional benefits and less vacation time. Furthermore, many people are connected to work twenty-four hours a day via cellular phones, pagers, and modems. Overtime now averages 4.7 hours per week, an all-time high, but the figure is a little misleading because many people work sixty to seventy hours per week and face many additional everyday stresses, including the demands of commuting and parenthood.[72] Emotional and physical stresses alter the bacterial population of the intestine, decreasing numbers of beneficial *Lactobacilli* and increasing numbers of neutral or dangerous *E. coli* strains.[73]

Fatigue is the most common complaint physicians hear from their patients, and one-fourth of patients say their fatigue has lasted longer than two weeks. While some of the immune consequences are direct, others are the result of a complex cascade of events involving the brain and the endocrine and immune systems.[74] Interest in how the brain and hormonal fluctuations affect immunity has led to a new medical discipline, psychoneuroimmunology.[75] The end point, however, is the same: stress and fatigue weaken the body and affect the immune system's ability to resist infectious diseases and cancer.

In one study, physicians used a questionnaire to assess the stress levels of 394 healthy volunteers, then infected them with respiratory viruses. Although everyone received viruses nasally, not everyone became sick. The rates of respiratory infections and symptomatic colds were related directly to the level of psychological stress of the subjects.[76] Other researchers have reported that reducing stress levels, increased socializing, and positive thinking can increase the activity of T cells and natural-killer cells and dramatically extend the life of cancer patients.[77] Studies by Lee S. Berk, D.H.Sc., M.PH., of the Loma Linda University School of Medicine, have found that laughter significantly increases the activity of T cells and other markers of healthy immune function.[78]

OVEREXERCISE

Moderate exercise stimulates and enhances all cellular activity.[79] More, however, is not necessarily better. The negative effects of overexercise have been documented by researchers.[80] Overexercise stresses the immune system and can increase the risk of upper respiratory infections, particularly during marathon training and races.[81] Such strenuous exercises depress the activities of T cells and natural-killer cells.[82]

Kenneth H. Cooper, M.D., who defined the term "aerobics" and has written numerous books advocating high-intensity exercise, moderated his recommendations in his 1994 book, *Antioxidant Revolution*.[83]

Dr. Cooper was perplexed after a number of exercising and physically fit friends developed cancer. On investigating possible causes, he realized that exercise generates large numbers of free radicals, which can damage DNA. In his book, Dr. Cooper recommends that people take antioxidant nutrients, such as vitamins C and E and beta-carotene, to minimize the numbers of these free radicals. He also suggested that running ten miles a week is sufficient for cardiovascular fitness but that there is no reason for anyone to run a hundred or more miles per week.

The health of the immune system is shaped by the interplay of both internal and external influences. The internal factors are nutritional, particularly vitamins and minerals, which provide the essential biochemical building blocks for optimal health. When intake of even one of these nutrients is inadequate or marginal, resistance to infectious disease declines.

In addition, a variety of external factors create an unnecessary burden on the immune system, and the effect is amplified when the diet has been compromised. The use of antibiotics and NSAIDs, exposure to pesticides, and stress constitute serious immune system stresses.

The number of deleterious dietary changes and immune-damaging chemicals may seem a bit overwhelming to you, odds that are insurmountable. But the fact is there's a lot you can do—and, surprisingly, with relatively little effort and few major changes to your diet. In the remainder of the book, we focus on ways that you, as an individual, can rectify this situation and optimize your immunity.

Part III

❧

DEFEND YOURSELF AGAINST SUPERGERMS

❧

Try as we might, there is no escaping supergerms and other disease-causing microorganisms. Worse, the misuse of antibiotics has greatly accelerated the evolution of supergerms, creating new strains of bacteria resistant to the very drugs designed to eradicate them. We have also, inadvertently, devised highly efficient means of spreading supergerms via hospitals, day care centers, airplanes, and the very foods we mass produce and consume.

With new strains of supergerms constantly bearing down on us, many doctors have fallen back on the concept that "the best defense is a strong offense"—that the aggressive use of broad-spectrum antibiotics will keep supergerms at bay. Not only has this approach failed, but it has also aggravated the underlying problem of antibiotic-resistant bacteria and supergerms. Overall, the situation is so bad that microbiologists and other researchers at a major scientific meeting in 1995 urged their colleagues to prepare for life in the *post*-antibiotic era.

If the external forces shaping supergerms have grown stronger, peoples' internal defenses against them have clearly weakened as well, doubling the problem. Immunity has been impaired by a declining diet, exposure to pesticides and other chemicals, and in some cases, the deleterious effects of antibiotics and other drugs.

What's the solution? We believe that the best offense is actually *a strong defense*—what we call optimal immunity.

By optimizing your immune system, similar to how you might optimize the performance of a computer or a car, you can enhance your body's inherent defenses against supergerms and other disease-causing microorganisms. This does not mean you will never get sick or never need antibiotics. Rather, with optimal immunity, your body's natural defenses will respond more effectively to these challenges, and you will resist and recover from most infections better than you would otherwise.

So how does a person strengthen immunity and minimize the risk of infectious disease?

In the chapters that follow, you will learn about specific dietary changes and nutrients that provide the building blocks of optimal immunity. By improving the nutritional foundation of immunity, you will

- maintain the immune system's vigilance against microorganisms,
- promote an effective response to infection,
- reduce the duration and severity of infections,
- prevent the mutation of some supergerms, and
- provide the added benefit of protection against cancer, heart disease, and other degenerative diseases.

We make recommendations with the knowledge that most people dislike making major dietary or other lifestyle changes. For this reason, our suggestions add up to relatively minor changes in how and what you eat. We group our recommendations into three tiers. First, we suggest a baseline diet that points you toward nutrient-rich foods that provide nutritional building blocks for immunity. Second, we recommend several specific supplements that form a powerful first line of defense against infections. These supplements can also be used to jump-start a weak immune system. Third, we describe a number of foods and additional supplements that you can use to tweak your immune system a little more.

As you read about the benefits of vitamin and mineral supplements in optimizing immunity, keep a couple of important points in mind. One, the nutrients that enhance the immune system's response to common infections, such as colds and flus, also enhance the body's defenses against much more serious supergerms. Two, the nutrients that bolster the immune system against AIDS also help the body fight less serious infections. The difference is in dose—the immune system generally needs larger amounts of micronutrients to fight more serious infections.

In the last chapter, we address a number of basic issues, including the value and limitations of immunizations, the appropriate use of antibiotics, the critical importance of hygiene, and the need for proper food handling and preparation. We also suggest some dosage ranges for supplements.

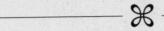

9

ORGANICS: THE WAY FOOD USED TO BE

❡

People *know* that much of the food supply has become tainted by pesticides and many other chemicals. Concerned about the long-term health effects of these food additives, most people would prefer eating organic foods.

This is not merely our opinion. Two opinion polls have demonstrated the extent of these feelings about organic foods. In a Louis Harris Poll conducted for *Organic Gardening* magazine, 84.2 percent of the people questioned said they would opt for organic foods if price was not an issue—and 49 percent would even pay more for organics. Similar feelings were echoed in a poll conducted by The Gallup Organization for *Newsweek*. Seventy-three percent of people queried stated that the food industry should use fewer pesticides and chemicals, even if it meant higher food prices. Forty-five percent bought organic foods either regularly or occasionally.[1]

Some people might quibble about the meaning of the term "organic," which to chemists means any compound containing a carbon molecule. In this book, however, organic refers to a method used to produce food. Organic farming avoids the use of synthetic chemicals while emphasizing "sustainable" agricultural practices, including the use of natural fertilizers to enhance soil quality and biological controls to control insect pests. In some states, the term organic is a legal definition of these foods. Conversely, we use the term "conventional" to describe the large-scale production of nonorganic crops and meat, which are routinely treated with nitrogen and other types of commercial fertilizers, pesticides, herbicides, fungicides, and other chemicals.

One of the obvious beauties of organics is their absence of immune-toxic pesticides. Missing as well are harsh fertilizers, fumigants, waxes, and colorings—additives that improve crop yield, shipping, appearance, and shelf life, but contribute nothing to a food's nutritional value. But the full value of organics is not just in what they *don't* contain, but in what they *do* contain.

Higher Nutrient Levels in Organics

Two recent studies reported that organically grown produce contains substantially higher levels of vitamins and minerals than does conventional produce. While the studies were small and could be criticized from a scientific standpoint, they strongly suggest the nutritional superiority of organics.

In the first study, researchers at the Campden Food and Drink Research Association, Great Britain, compared the nutrient levels of organic produce from health food stores with conventional produce from supermarkets. To avoid one or two very good or bad samples skewing the results, researchers determined the average nutrient levels based on thirty samples of each fruit or vegetable. Some foods, such as cabbage and carrots, had virtually identical vitamin levels, regardless of whether they were grown conventionally or organically. Others showed dramatic differences in vitamin and mineral levels.

The vitamin C level of organic apples was 12 percent higher than that of conventional apples. Organic tomatoes contained 21 percent more vitamin C and 33 percent more carotenes than did the conventional varieties—percentages that were virtually unchanged after the samples were dehydrated and measured by dry weight. Organic carrots, while relatively equal to conventional carrots in vitamin levels, contained 24 percent more potassium. Mineral levels in organic potatoes were lower, but after adjusting for their higher water content, researchers discovered that they contained 21 percent more iron, 13 percent more calcium, and 37 percent more zinc than conventional potatoes.[2]

Such findings did not reflect well on conventional, processed foods or on the purveyors of large-scale agricultural production—on whose behalf the Campden Food and Drink Research Association generally serves. Written in 1990, the Campden report was originally marked "confidential" and restricted to food-industry distribution. For four years it was virtually ignored. A request by the researchers to fund further research on organic foods was denied, and a single copy of the report was tucked away in the library of Britain's Ministry of Agriculture, Fisheries and Food. In May 1994, *Living Earth and the Food Magazine* described the findings of the Campden report and charged that it had been intentionally suppressed.[3]

Another study, focusing strictly on mineral levels, was conducted by Bob L. Smith, former president of Doctor's Data, Inc., a licensed analytical laboratory in West Chicago, Illinois. Over a two-year period, Smith collected and analyzed comparable varieties of apples, pears, potatoes, sweet corn, and whole wheat from area health food stores and conventional supermarkets. His motivation was simple. Smith, who eats organic foods but has no ties to the organic foods industry, explained in an interview that he grew tired of people saying there was no nutritional difference between organic and conventional foods.[4]

Using the mineral levels of conventionally grown produce as his baseline, Smith determined that organic produce contained an average of *90 percent* more nutritional minerals, including calcium, chromium, magnesium, manganese, potassium, selenium, and zinc. Sometimes, the amounts were nothing short

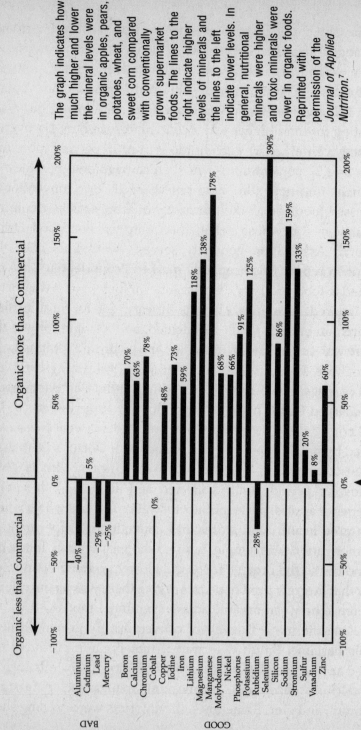

AVERAGE: ORGANIC VS. COMMERCIAL

Organic less than Commercial

Organic more than Commercial

Organic = Commercial

The graph indicates how much higher and lower the mineral levels were in organic apples, pears, potatoes, wheat, and sweet corn compared with conventionally grown supermarket foods. The lines to the right indicate higher levels of minerals and the lines to the left indicate lower levels. In general, nutritional minerals were higher and toxic minerals were lower in organic foods. Reprinted with permission of the *Journal of Applied Nutrition*.[7]

BAD

GOOD

Aluminum −40%
Cadmium 5%
Lead −29%
Mercury −25%

Boron 70%
Calcium 63%
Chromium 78%
Cobalt 0%
Copper 48%
Iodine 73%
Iron 59%
Lithium 118%
Magnesium 138%
Manganese 178%
Molybdenum 68%
Nickel 66%
Phosphorus 91%
Potassium 125%
Rubidium −28%
Selenium 390%
Silicon 86%
Sodium 159%
Strontium 133%
Sulfur 20%
Vanadium 8%
Zinc 60%

of astounding. For example, organic wheat contained 1300 percent more selenium, and sweet corn contained 1800 percent more calcium and 2200 percent more iodine. Conversely, organics generally contained substantially lower amounts of toxic metals, such as aluminum, cadmium, lead, and mercury.[5] "When there's a difference [between organic and nonorganic], it's usually a substantial difference," Smith said.[6]

Many advocates of organics claim that these foods taste better than conventionally grown foods. Because such a view has never been confirmed in scientifically controlled taste tests, it's easy to dismiss it as nothing more than opinion. However, several factors might account for the better taste of organics.

One factor is that organic fruits and vegetables tend to be vine ripened, whereas conventional foods are routinely picked and shipped while green. As any home gardener will attest, vine-ripened fruit tastes better. Vine ripening has nothing to do with the absence of pesticides, but it is a hallmark of the exceptional care that organic farmers generally exercise.

In addition, organics are not waxed or sprayed with fungicides, so they have a shorter shelf life. That means time to market is critical—and food fresh from the farm also tastes better than food that has been stored or shipped long distances.

Yet another reason may be the broad variety of plant species and the increasing use of heirloom, or older and genetically diverse, seeds by organic farmers. According to the United Nation's Food and Agricultural Organization, 75 percent of the genetic diversity of agricultural crops has been lost since 1900, largely because a handful of seed companies dominate the market.[8] Growing interest in heirloom seeds, however, has preserved a broad genetic heritage of plant species, many of which yield sturdier and tastier food crops than the more common conventional varieties.[9]

Better Soil Quality Enhances Organics

While food safety and nutritional value are the primary issues attracting consumers to organics, organic farmers consistently emphasize the importance of sustainable agriculture. The term "sustainable agriculture," which forms the philosophical under-pinning of organic farming, refers to farming methods that consistently build up rather than tear down soil quality. Over the past twenty years, soil microbiologists have given sustainable agriculture a solid scientific foundation and documented that soil is more than just dirt. It consists of a rich, complex microenvironment that forms the foundation of the entire food chain.

In any ecological system, higher levels of life depend on lower ones. The microorganisms that inhabit soil and the plants that grow in it share a delicate interdependence. A single gram of healthy agricultural soil—about the weight of a paper clip—is home to from ten to a hundred million bacteria that digest, recycle, and synthesize soil nutrients. In arid regions, soil typically contains fewer than one million bacteria per gram.[10] Without such bacteria, the soil cannot retain nutrients, and higher forms of life, including plants, cannot prosper. When organic farmers or home gardeners build up soil, they foster and help sustain the growth of these helpful, necessary bacteria.

In addition to bacteria, the microecology of soil includes fungi, protozoa, and nematode worms. The protozoa and nema-todes feed on bacteria and, in the process, recycle nutrients and release nitrogen, which serves as a natural plant fertilizer. The fungi, which attach to plant roots, consume some of the plant's carbohydrates. But the relationship is symbiotic, and the fungi absorb hard-to-get soil nutrients and share them with the plants.[11]

In healthy agricultural soils and grasslands, the biomass of bacteria greatly exceeds that of fungi. However, high levels of agricultural production or overfarming stress the soil and increase the number of fungi. As fungi become the dominant soil microorganisms, crop productivity declines significantly, according to Elaine R. Ingham, M.S., associate professor of botany and plant pathology at Oregon State University, Corvallis.[12]

To preserve soil quality and this microenvironment, organic farmers rely on compost and manure as fertilizers and avoid synthetic pesticides. There is sound reason for this practice. According to Ingham, pesticides kill large numbers of bacteria, sometimes reducing their numbers to under a hundred thousand per gram of soil, or one-tenth that found in arid regions. As a consequence, crop yields drop and pesticide-sprayed soil can even show signs of nitrogen deficiency. The soil is, in effect, dead. Once this disruption in soil ecology occurs, the ecosystem becomes less capable of resisting disease and more dependent on conventional fertilizers and synthetic pesticides, which further stifle any opportunity for the soil to recover.[13,14] In a bizarre way, the soil becomes addicted to drugs.

Conventional farmers often contend that organic farming is labor intensive and unprofitable. Careful comparison, however, suggests the opposite. A four-year study in New Zealand looked at the differences between seven organic farms and nine conventional farms. The organic farms relied on compost and manure as fertilizers and on crop diversification to maintain healthy soils. Earthworms, essential to soil health, were eight times more common in the soil of organic farms compared with conventional farms. Topsoil also formed much faster and was thicker at the organic farms, a consequence of greater bacterial activity.

Economically, the organic farms fared as well as their soil. Their higher labor costs turned out to be less expensive than the pesticides, fertilizers, and herbicides used by conventional farms. Describing the study, environmentalist Edward Flattau wrote that "the New Zealand organic farms had less fluctuations in their profit margins than conventional operations did in bad weather years. . . . The explanation: Soil on organic farms is generally healthier and thus better able to withstand the often unwelcome vagaries of seasonal climate change."[15]

Organically grown crops better resist drought as well. At the Rodale Institute Experimental Farm in Kutztown, Pennsylvania, researchers have been growing the same species of corn organically and conventionally for years. During most years, crop yields have been virtually equal. During a 1988 drought, the organic corn yielded more grain. During another drought, in 1995, the organic corn grew normally, but the conventionally grown corn was stunted.[16]

And what of the inevitable insect pests? How can they be kept from destroying crops? Conventional farmers have become addicted to a broad range of pesticides to control insect pests during each stage of food production. This is in sharp contrast to organic farmers (and many home gardeners) who often use "good" insects to control the destructive ones. The simplest examples are using ladybugs to eat aphids and praying mantises to kill grasshoppers.

Grain farmers typically fumigate silos and storage sheds to eradicate insects in harvested grain. But researchers at the USDA's Agricultural Research Service in Manhattan, Kansas, have found that a type of wasp can efficiently seek out the larvae of the maize weevil beetle, which grow inside corn kernels. The wasp lays its eggs in the beetle larvae, and the hatching wasp larvae eat the beetle larvae. The wasps are washed away during grain processing, so they don't end up in cereals. The USDA also found that wasps control different beetle species that attack wheat. In one experiment, wheat bins treated with wasps had one-third the beetles of untreated bins. Because the reduction of beetles was so significant, the bins did not have to be fumigated.[17]

Other insect-control techniques work as well. An agricultural experiment in India found that planting more seeds, changing sowing times, and rotating crops also protected against insect damage without harming the soil or the environment.[18] But strange as it might sound, a little insect damage may actually be good for plants. Melvin I. Dyer, Ph.D., of the University of Georgia, Athens, recently identified six proteins in the mouths of grasshoppers that stimulate plant growth. In an experiment with sorghum plants, Dr. Dyer found that shoots exposed to the proteins grew faster than when they were exposed just to auxin, a plant growth hormone.[19] Although a grasshopper might take a bite, it leaves a chemical that promotes plant growth.

Plants grown in a nutrient-rich environment also seem to flourish and be more resistant to insects. Dale M. Norris, Ph.D., of the University of Wisconsin, Madison, discovered that plants contain stress-monitoring proteins that warn plants of environmental challenges, including drought and insects. In response, the plant releases a number of biochemical defenses, much the way your immune system responds to infection. If these proteins become damaged, however, the plants become defenseless.

As it turns out, free radicals can damage these stress-monitoring proteins. But Dr. Norris was able to protect the proteins by adding small amounts of vitamins C and E to the soil, much the way many people take these vitamins to protect their bodies against free radicals.[20] Of course, it makes sense to minimize the stresses before reaching for more vitamin supplements. One stress, apparently, is conventional nitrogen fertilizer, which USDA researchers found reduced the vitamin C content of some crops by as much as one-third. So one of the keys to low-stress, insect-resistant plants seems to be organic farming methods, which yield higher vitamin levels in crops.[21]

Organic Meats and Dairy Products

Like organically grown produce, meat from organically raised animals is often distinguished by what it does *not* contain. Conventionally raised farm animals—chickens, cattle, hogs, and sheep—are routinely fed low levels of antibiotics as growth stimulants. In addition, cattle receive injections of growth-promoting hormones, and their feed contains pesticides to discourage insects. Some meat products, such as sausages, are treated with nitrites and nitrates, which the heat of cooking turns into cancer-causing nitrosamines. It's enough to make a person a vegetarian, but devoted meat eaters do have alternatives to eating meat from conventionally raised farm animals.

One of the champions of organic ranching and meat production is Mel Coleman Sr., chairman of Coleman Natural Meats in Denver. Coleman's great-grandfather began ranching in southern Colorado in 1875, and the family's herds continue to graze on this land, which has never been treated with pesticides or herbicides. Like many other organically minded ranchers, Coleman steadfastly avoids giving growth hormones or growth-promoting antibiotics to the animals. "I think it's absolutely wrong to use medicine for the sake of production," Coleman explained in an interview. He prefers to raise animals of good genetic stock—such as Black Angus and Herefords—instead of using drugs to boost production of cattle from poor genetic stock. When an animal does become sick, Coleman separates it from the herd, treats it with antibiotics, and sells it to a conventional rancher.[22]

Ranchers who raise cattle organically may also have fewer problems with the virulent *E. coli* 0157:H7 strain. No actual studies have ever compared *E. coli* 0157:H7 in organically and conventionally raised cattle. But based on her experiences, Kay Weedon, who oversees quality control at Coleman Natural Meats, believes *E. coli* 0157:H7 is less of a problem in organically raised animals.[23] Coleman concurs and believes the lower levels of *E. coli* 0157:H7 are the result of slower and safer meat processing than in larger, high-production meat plants.[24] It's also possible that *E. coli* 0157:H7 gains a major foothold in the digestive tracts of cattle only when they have been fed antibiotics that destroy the resident beneficial bacteria.

Coleman, a member of the Nature Conservancy Board, shares the enthusiasm of organic farmers when it comes to sustainable agriculture. "Grass is my passion," he said, adding that healthy grasslands form the basis for sustainable ranching and a clean watershed. He says that moving herds of cattle through rangelands serves the same ecological role as buffaloes in the past, breaking up the ground and helping native grass seedlings germinate.

Alternatives to conventionally produced milk, which may contain traces of antibiotics and bovine growth hormone (rBGH), also exist. In fact, the largest single surge in organic food purchases occurred after the FDA's November 1993 approval of Monsanto's rBGH in dairy production. Many consumers switched to organic milk from dairies that guaranteed the absence of rBGH. Sales of organic dairy products jumped 125 percent from $11 million in 1993 to $24 million in 1994.[25]

Availability and Price of Organics

Only about 1 percent of the U.S. food supply is produced using organic methods, but the organic foods industry has grown steadily by 20 percent annually since 1989.[26] The expansion and profitability of natural food supermarket chains, such as Whole Foods and Fresh Fields, have made organics more accessible to the average consumer. Larger supermarket chains, including Kroger, Publix, and Fred Meyer, also sell pesticide-free or organic produce and are helping to make it a mainstream commodity. During the summer and early autumn, farmers markets typically include vendors selling organic produce.

According to Dennis Blank, editor of the trade newsletter *Organic Food Business News,* consumers may at times pay a 25 to 35 percent premium for organic produce and meat. But this may be a small price to pay given the health risks of eating conventionally produced fruit, vegetables, meat, and dairy products. But higher prices aren't always the case with organics. Mothers and Others for a Livable Planet, a consumer advocacy group in New York City, recently compared the prices of organic and conventional foods. Some organic products cost more and others less than conventional packaged foods, but a random selection of organic foods—including cereal, yogurt, and juice—

turned out to be slightly less expensive than comparable conventional foods. The same foods purchased at a food co-op were substantially cheaper than at either a supermarket or health food store.[27]

One other benefit of organic foods is that they often come with a legal pesticide-free guarantee. Many state agriculture departments have legal definitions of organic foods, and trade organizations, such as the Organic Trade Association, have helped organic farmers and processors police their own quality. The watchwords here are *certified* and *transitional*. Certified organic foods contain no detectable pesticides, and transitional foods denote those grown on land undergoing a three-year transition between conventional and organic farming methods.

Other "Natural" Improvements to the Food Supply

While the bulk of the food industry has not embraced organic farming or ranching, it *is* researching natural and sensible methods of controlling the supergerms in meat. Some of these efforts were accelerated after *E. coli* in fast-food hamburgers sickened 540 people in Washington state.

A number of studies have reported that veterinary vitamin and mineral supplements can help control disease-causing bacteria in farm animals and reduce the need for antibiotic treatment. In one experiment, researchers found that magnesium sulfate supplements significantly reduced the numbers of *E. coli* bacteria in the intestine and skin of broiler chickens.[28] Similarly, a combination of vitamin E and beta-carotene improved the ability of chickens to resist infections and normalized livers enlarged by *E. coli* infections.[29] In sheep, vitamin E alone has been found to stimulate white blood cells, and one researcher has reported that vitamin E supplements do more for the animals' immunity than do conventional vaccines.[30] In dairy cows, supplements of vitamin E and selenium activate white blood cells and protect against mastitis, an infection of the udders typically treated with antibiotics.[31]

In February 1995, the USDA proposed an overhaul of its antiquated eighty-eight-year-old system of visual meat inspection. A new meat-inspection program will ultimately rely on scientific analysis to assess—and, more importantly, to minimize—the risk of microbial contamination at various steps during meat processing. The USDA plans to establish specific standards for sanitation, refrigeration, and antimicrobial sprays (e.g., chlorine or hot water) to reduce the risk of *E. coli* 0157:H7 and *Salmonella* contamination at slaughterhouses.[32] Such changes are long overdue—the USDA estimates that 25 percent of meat is contaminated by disease-causing bacteria and hopes to reduce that number by half.

When meat processors try, they can accomplish a lot. Before the USDA proposed its new regulations, Pederson's Fryer Farms voluntarily adopted chlorine rinses and improved refrigeration at its Tacoma, Washington, slaughterhouse. Independent laboratory tests by Washington State University found that Pederson's brought broiler contamination down to only 5 percent.[33]

USDA researchers have also been exploring how to keep disease-causing bacteria out of farm animals before they become a problem during processing at slaughterhouses. One team of USDA researchers found that a mixture of twenty-nine species of beneficial intestinal bacteria effectively crowded out *Salmonella* from the digestive tracts of chicks. This bacterial cocktail, which is being patented, was sprayed on newborn chicks and added to their drinking water. Such a technique, if implemented widely, could reduce the need for prophylactic antibiotics on the farm, as well as reduce the level of *Salmonella* contamination in slaughterhouses.[34]

Still other researchers have found that stress and erratic eating habits, both associated with transport to the slaughterhouse, lead to an overgrowth of *E. coli* 0157:H7 and *Salmonella* bacteria in sheep and cattle. According to Mark A. Rasmussen, Ph.D., a researcher at the USDA's National Animal Disease Center in Ames, Iowa, well-fed and unstressed animals were much less likely to become hosts for E. coli 0157:H7.[35,36] He and other researchers have suggested that animals be consistently fed as long as possible—in a sense, that they not be treated like a bunch of animals.

Recommendations

Good nutrition and the avoidance of immune-depressing pesticides establish an excellent foundation for protection against supergerms. We recommend that you eat produce, legumes, and grains that have been grown organically whenever possible—hopefully, most of the time. Organic foods have other benefits as well. Because organics (canned and packaged, as well as fresh) tend to receive less processing, they are often higher in dietary fiber, which protects against cancer and heart disease. Packaged organic foods, such as vegetables or cereals, also tend to be lower in refined sugars, such as sucrose and high-fructose corn syrup, which interfere with the body's ability to fight bacteria.

If you eat meat, obtain it from organically raised farm animals. You may not entirely eliminate your risk of ingesting a food-borne pathogenic bacteria, but you will probably lower it substantially. (Careful handling of meats is paramount as well—which we discuss in Chapter 17.) By eating organic meats, you also eliminate a source of antibiotics, growth hormone, and pesticide residues. Under the circumstances, we also recommend pesticide-free organic baby foods for infants.

Where do you buy organics? While some of the large supermarket chains sell pesticide-free and organic foods, the most diverse source is probably a natural foods or health food store. Over the past few years, natural food supermarket chains have established strong footholds in Austin, Boston, Chicago, Dallas, Los Angeles, New York, Seattle, and other major cities. They sell organic produce, meats, dairy products, juices, cereals, and packaged foods similar to (but generally more nutritious than) what's found in conventional supermarkets.

At the very least, most cities have independent natural food stores and co-ops. All of these stores are supplied by a thriving, growing national network of organic farmers and food processors. Even health food stores in small towns can often order organic grains, breads, produce, and frozen organic meats from suppliers. Look under health food stores in the yellow pages. Another option is buying organic foods by mail. The Appendix of this book lists some sources for mail-order organic foods.

10

PROBIOTICS: GOOD BACTERIA THAT FIGHT THE BAD

⌘

Just as the evening news reports more bad than good news, people usually hear more about bad rather than good bacteria. As it turns out, only about a hundred species cause the majority of bacterial infections in people. Meanwhile, tens of thousands of bacterial species and strains exist in nature, and more than five hundred species inhabit the gastrointestinal tract,[1,2] skin, mouth, and genitals of people. Most of these bacteria do no harm, and some actively promote health. You can enhance your defense against supergerms by maintaining the health of your beneficial bacteria.

The number of individual bacteria in the body is simply astounding. A healthy adult carries around ten quadrillion (10,000,000,000,000,000) bacteria in the gastrointestinal tract alone. According to George Weber, Ph.D., an industrial microbiologist in Portland, Oregon, this number is at least ten times greater than the total number of cells in the human body. (Bacteria are much smaller than cells, which is why they don't weigh more than the body.) That fact gives credence to the idea that beneficial bacteria function as an actual organ of the body.[3] Indeed, intestinal bacteria collectively weigh two to four pounds—about the same weight as the brain, liver, or lungs.

These bacteria exist on two planes. First, they live, feed, compete, and reproduce within their own delicate but dynamic microecology—their own neighborhood, so to speak. This environment is dynamic because it changes in response to diet, stress, and antibiotic therapy. Second, the relationship between bacteria and their hosts—people like you—is often symbiotic. That means both the bacteria and the host derive benefit from the relationship. For example, bacteria in the mouth and intestine eat some of the carbohydrates we ingest. They also compete against disease-causing microorganisms and, in the process, protect us against many infections. In a sense, you and your bacteria are analogous to a good landlord-tenant relationship.

Natural Defenders Against Infection

Most people are colonized by beneficial bacteria at birth when they pass through the *Lactobacillus*-rich birth canal. Almost immediately, *Bifidobacteria* establish themselves and acidify the infant's intestine, which discourages the growth of most disease-causing bacteria. Within several days of birth, an infant's gastro-intestinal tract also cultivates large numbers of *Lactobacilli*, *Enterobacter*, *Streptococci*, *Staphylococci*, *Bacteroides*, and *Clostridia* bacteria.[4] Although some of these species, such as *Clostridia*, can be harmful, their presence is not usually a problem in a healthy intestine. For all practical purposes, the infant's colony of intestinal bacteria is a smaller but functional version of what exists in an adult.

Newborn babies acquire additional bacteria while cuddling with their mothers and by consuming breast milk. Not surprisingly, these bacteria take longer to establish themselves in infants delivered by cesarean section,[5] premature infants who spend time in an incubator, or infants treated with antibiotics.[6] It is likely that the routine hospital habit of whisking away newborns and bathing them with antibacterial soaps shortchanges babies by delaying the natural process of bacterial colonization. One study found that a month after delivery, *Lactobacillus* species were present in large amounts in the feces of full-term infants, reflecting the population of their intestines. Among preterm infants, however, *Lactobacillus* numbers were lower and *E. coli* numbers were comparatively high.[7]

BENEFICIAL BACTERIA ON THE SKIN AND IN THE MOUTH

An estimated one trillion (1,000,000,000,000) bacteria make their home on the surface of the skin, the outermost barrier to infectious microorganisms. Twenty years ago, Sydney Selwyn, M.D., of the Westminster Medical School, London, identified 139 strains of *Staphylococcus* and *Micrococcus* bacteria that inhibit the growth of disease-causing bacteria on the skin. Dr. Selwyn found large numbers of beneficial bacteria on the skin of approximately 20 percent of all people, but he also noticed that healthy skin provided only a so-so environment for beneficial bacteria.

During infections, however, bacterial populations change. Disease-causing germs may gain an initial foothold, but their grip is not guaranteed. In fact, the presence of disease-causing germs sometimes prompts the growth of large numbers of beneficial bacteria. Dr. Selwyn found that people with eczema, skin ulcerations, or surgical infections actually had twice the number of beneficial bacteria on their skin that healthy people did. These bacteria are a potent lot, producing their own types of antibiotics, so they can limit the damage caused by pathogens. Selwyn reported that hospitalized patients with large numbers of "antibiotic-producing" beneficial bacteria were far less likely than other patients to develop secondary infections around their surgical incisions.[8] It's very possible that the disease-causing bacteria on the skin excrete substances that attract the attention of beneficial bacteria.

Dr. Selwyn also noted that an extremely dangerous strain of *Staphylococcus aureus*, resistant to seven pharmaceutical antibiotics, *was* controlled by the natural antibiotics released by beneficial bacteria on the skin. In urging that doctors harness good bacteria to fight infections, Dr. Selwyn sadly observed, "In contrast to the modern enthusiasm for studying and administering antibiotic extracts, natural antibiosis in man has been almost completed ignored."[9]

Good and bad bacteria live and compete in the mouth as well. Some *Streptococcus* species attach to the teeth and produce acids that lead to dental cavities. Sticky, sugary foods give these bacteria a ready food supply—and prevent white blood cells from killing them. Similarly, *Actinobacillus* and *Porphyromonas* species cause periodontal diseases, which involve infection of the supporting structure of the teeth. Other types of bacteria compete against these species and protect against infections in the mouth.

BENEFICIAL INTESTINAL BACTERIA

The vast majority of the body's bacteria live in the intestine. In adults, *Bacteroides* tend to dominate, followed by *Eubacteria*, *Bifidobacteria*, *Peptococcacceae*, *Enterobacter* (which include *E. coli*), *Enterococci*, and *Lactobacilli*.[10] Most of the beneficial intestinal bacteria are referred to as "lactic acid" bacteria, not because they are found in milk but because they excrete lactic acid. Perhaps the best known of these bacteria is *Lactobacillus acidophilus*, one of the species used to culture yogurt.

In the 1980s, researchers at Tufts University discovered a particular strain of *Lactobacillus* called *L. casei* GG in the upper part of the small intestine. This type of *Lactobacillus* has received considerable attention in medical journals because it aggressively shoves many other species of bacteria out of the way and quickly colonizes the intestine.[11] (At the moment, *L. casei* GG is found in some European but not American-made dairy products.) Many *Lactobacillus* species also produce large quantities of the B vitamin folic acid, as well as modest amounts of vitamins B_1, B_2, B_6, and B_{12}. In yogurt, *Lactobacillus* predigests some of the protein, making it more absorbable than the protein in milk.[12]

Bifidobacteria, another group of well-known beneficial bacteria, perform many of the same roles as *Lactobacillus* species, but they do so in a different location. *Bifidobacteria* adhere to the walls of the lower portion of the small intestine and the large intestine, where they excrete lactic acid to discourage the attachment and growth of disease-causing bacteria. *Bifidobacteria* also produce respectable amounts of B vitamins and vitamin C.[13]

Various beneficial *Streptococcus* species live in the intestine as well, including *S. faecium* strain 68 (not to be confused with pathogenic strains of *S. faecium* and *S. faecalis*). *S. faecium* 68 grows rapidly in the upper part of the small intestine, suppressing disease-causing bacteria and aiding the growth of *Lactobacillus.* Unfortunately, many people have confused *S. faecium* 68 with dangerous species of *Streptococcus,* and some manufacturers are phasing out their use of this bacterium in probiotic dietary supplements to avoid what is essentially a public relations problem.

Lactobacillus, Bifidobacteria, and other species of lactic acid bacteria crowd out disease-causing bacteria in a number of ways. They excrete lactic or acetic acids, which reduces the pH of the intestine and creates an inhospitable environment for many other bacteria, such as *Staphylococcus.* (*E. coli,* however, can survive in acidic environments.) Bacteria also excrete antibiotic-like chemicals, called bacteriocins, which discourage the growth of other strains or species. Some bacteria produce microcins, chemicals that work against a broad range of microorganisms, including bacteria viruses, fungi, and protozoa.[14]

Generally stable and resilient, these remarkable defenses against infection are disrupted more significantly by antibiotics than by any other substance. Even the most specific antibiotic slaughters trillions of beneficial intestinal bacteria in its wake, and when these guardians of health are injured, opportunistic bacteria quickly fill the void. That's why people taking or completing a course of antibiotic therapy become highly susceptible to *Candida* infections and to secondary infections by antibiotic-resistant supergerms, such as *E. coli*.

Probiotics to Prevent Infection

The therapeutic use of *probiotics*—that is, beneficial bacteria—to combat infections dates to 1877, when Louis Pasteur and Jules François Joubert described how harmless soil bacteria suppressed anthrax (caused by *Bacillus anthracis*) in livestock. Later, the Ukrainian bacteriologist Elie Metchnikoff, who developed the theory of phagocytosis in 1884, pioneered research on probiotics while working at the Pasteur Institute in Paris. In 1906, Metchnikoff published *The Prolongation of Life* (G. P. Putnam and Sons, New York), in which he theorized that lactic acid bacteria could prevent putrefaction in the digestive tract and consequently extend the life span. Two years later, he was awarded the 1908 Nobel prize for physiology and medicine for his work related to phagocytosis. Metchnikoff's antiaging research remained controversial, and he died at age seventy-one.

For almost a century, research on probiotics either languished or was interrupted by catastrophic events, such as World Wars I and II. In 1921, Leo Frederick Rettger, professor of bacteriology at Yale, published the first of two major treatises on the therapeutic uses of lactic acid bacteria. And in 1938, A. D. Burke, head of the dairy department at the Alabama Polytechnic Institute, published a book on the commercial manufacture of fermented milk products, including yogurt and kefir. The increasing use of antibiotics in the 1940s and 1950s further sidetracked researchers from the antibacterial properties of probiotics. By the early 1960s, research on the anti-infective role of probiotics began to increase, and today the benefits of probiotics are well documented.

STIMULATION OF IMMUNE FUNCTION

The health benefits of eating yogurt and other fermented foods are generally attributed to their ability to reinforce the army of normal intestinal bacteria against species that cause disease. Some researchers have theorized that the presence of intestinal bacteria stimulates a low level of immune system activity— keeping the immune engine idling, so to speak. However, it now appears that some species of intestinal bacteria produce proteinlike substances that directly enhance the immunity of their hosts.[15,16] Destroying intestinal bacteria, such as with antibiotic therapy, stops production of these substances and reduces T-cell and white blood cell activity.[17,18] The consequence is greater susceptibility to infection.

Animal experiments have found that common strains of *Lactobacillus* and *Streptococcus thermophilis*, both found in yogurt, help white blood cells kill disease-causing bacteria[19,20] and increase T-cell activity.[21] In a controlled study on the effects of yogurt on people, Georges M. Halpern, M.D., of the University of California, Davis, asked sixty-eight healthy people to eat two cups daily of either "live-culture" *L. bulgaricus* and *S. thermophilus* yogurt or pasteurized yogurt for four months. (The heat of pasteurization kills both good and bad bacteria.) One-third of the group, eating no yogurt at all, served as a control group. Only the people eating the live-culture yogurt benefited from a significant boost in interferon, an antiviral substance produced by the immune system.[22,23]

TREATMENT OF DIARRHEA

Antibiotic therapy often causes diarrhea and gastrointestinal problems, such as flatulence and cramps. This diarrhea sometimes results from an overgrowth of the toxin-producing *Clostridium difficile*, not the antibiotic itself. Yogurt has long been used as a folk remedy for antibiotic-related diarrhea, but a study of sixteen healthy men found a big difference between live-culture and pasteurized yogurts.

Heikki Vapaatalo, M.D., of the University of Tampere, Finland, gave the men erythromycin, an antibiotic known to cause diarrhea, for one week. At the same time, half of the men ate two cups daily of live-culture L. casei GG yogurt, and the other half ate two cups of pasteurized yogurt. Stool samples indicated that the live L. casei GG yogurt rapidly colonized the intestines during antibiotic therapy, but no intestinal colonization occurred in people eating the pasteurized yogurt. Furthermore, the men eating the live-culture yogurt suffered diarrhea for an average of two days, compared with eight days in the other group. They also suffered less stomach pain and nausea than those eating the pasteurized yogurt.[24]

Similar antidiarrheal benefits were achieved in a study of seventy-one infants suffering from acute diarrhea. The infants received either L. casei GG in a fermented milk product, L. casei as a freeze-dried powder, or pasteurized yogurt, along with a normal diet. On average, diarrhea ceased about thirty-six hours after the first administration of L. casei GG, regardless of whether it was in fresh or freeze-dried form. Infants getting the pasteurized yogurt suffered diarrhea for a day longer—a serious issue considering the risk of dehydration and death.[25]

Doctors at Mount Washington Pediatric Hospital, Baltimore, recently reported that baby formula with B. bifidum and S. thermophilus dramatically reduced the incidence and spread of infant diarrhea caused by viral infections. Of twenty-nine hospitalized infants treated with the probiotic baby formula, only two (7 percent) suffered from diarrhea. In contrast, eight of twenty-six infants (31 percent) given regular formula developed diarrhea. José M. Saavedra, M.D., observed that the probiotic formula likely reduced the number of viruses shed in the feces, thereby lowering the risk of hospital-acquired infection for other infants in the nursery.[26]

Probiotics can sometimes prevent "Montezuma's revenge" and other types of travelers' diarrhea, though it makes far more sense simply to drink bottled water when traveling in developing nations. A study of several hundred people traveling from Finland to Turkey found that freeze-dried *L. casei* GG protected almost 40 percent of those taking the supplement from travelers' diarrhea.[27] As Marc Lappé, Ph.D., observed in *Germs That Won't Die*, "Even the worst cases of infections of the intestinal tract can be self-curing, self-limiting diseases—if you provide an environment that rapidly leads to the recolonization of your intestinal tract with natural flora."[28]

PREVENTING VAGINAL AND CANDIDA INFECTIONS

Lactobacillus species dominate in the normal vagina but are less likely to be present in vaginal infections caused by *Gardnerella vaginalis* and other pathogens. The first medical use of *L. acidophilus* in the treatment of vaginal infections dates to 1933, but only in the past few years have physicians conducted controlled studies. The results have been impressive.

Alexander Neri, M.D., of the obstetrics and gynecology department of Beilinson Medical Center, Israel, asked thirty-two women with bacterial vaginosis to apply yogurt intravaginally twice daily for a week, skip a week, then repeat the applications. Within two days, all of the women were free of symptoms, and after two months, twenty-eight of the women were still symptom free. About half of the women treated with acetic acid, a byproduct of *L. acidophilus*, improved. Without any treatment at all, only one of a group of twenty women was free of symptoms after two months.[29]

A similar experiment relied on vaginal suppositories containing a strain of *L. acidophilus*. Sixteen of twenty-eight women treated with the *L. acidophilus* suppository improved, whereas none of the twenty-nine women treated with a placebo got better.[30] Doctors also reported in *Lancet* the case of a thirty-three-year-old woman who had suffered from recurrent bladder and vaginal infections for four years. Tests found that *S. faecalis* was the predominant microorganism in the woman's vagina. The use of just one intravaginal suppository containing a strain of *L. casei* cured the woman of her bladder and vaginal infections.[31]

Eating yogurt with *L. acidophilus* is an effective treatment for vaginal *Candida* infections as well. Eileen Hilton, M.D., of the Long Island Medical Center, New Hyde Park, New York, asked twenty-one women with vaginal *Candida* yeast infections to eat eight ounces of yogurt daily for six months. They improved so dramatically that eight of the women refused to stop eating the yogurt for the second half of the experiment! According to Dr. Hilton, there was a clear relationship between the colonization of *L. acidophilus* in the rectums and in the vaginas of the women. How did the good bacteria help? Dr. Hilton theorized that the bacteria migrated from the rectum to the vagina.[32]

PREVENTING SALMONELLA INFECTIONS

In the 1970s, researchers demonstrated that "germ-free" laboratory animals were far more susceptible to infection than were animals with a normal complement of intestinal bacteria. One experiment showed that only ten *Salmonella* bacteria were needed to kill germ-free mice, whereas one million *Salmonella* bacteria were needed to kill mice with normal intestinal bacteria.[33]

A number of studies have demonstrated that *L. acidophilus* increases resistance to *Salmonella* infections. Anthony D. Hitchins, Ph.D., of the USDA's Agricultural Research Service, Beltsville, Maryland, found that laboratory rats fed freeze-dried yogurt were more likely to survive an infection with *Salmonella* than were rats given plain milk. The yogurt did not prevent salmonellosis, but it substantially reduced death and weight loss following infection.[34] Likewise, a German researcher has reported that drinking milk with *L. acidophilus* made asymptomatic *Salmonella* carriers less contagious.[35] The same researcher also found common yogurt to "very effectively" inhibit the growth of *Salmonella* and *Shigella* bacteria, even if the yogurt has been moderately heated.[36]

Recommendations

When you look at the scientific evidence, as we have, it's very clear that probiotics are essential for optimal immunity and protecting against dangerous germs. Enhancing your intestinal health, however, requires more than occasionally eating some yogurt. Large numbers of ingested bacteria perish in the stomach, a generally inhospitable environment for these microorganisms. Some, of course, do make it to the small or large intestine, where they can reproduce. Based on the evidence, the bacteria in live-culture dairy products, such as yogurt or kefir, colonize the digestive tract more effectively than do whatever might be left in pasteurized products. Be sure to look for "live culture" on the label.

Furthermore, blends of multiple bacterial species are better than products containing a single species. Complementary microorganisms create a stable, faster growing matrix of beneficial bacteria. For example, *L. bulgaricus* and *S. thermophilus* produce far more lactic acid together than they do individually, and mixed cultures are more resistant to contamination.[37]

Fermented foods have been used for thousands of years in Egypt, China, and Southeast Asia to reduce spoilage and risk of food poisoning, improve taste, and enable long-term storage, an important hedge against famines. It's also possible that probiotics in such foods stimulated the immune system at times when dietary deficiencies from famines would have impaired it.

Today, occasionally eating "ethnic" foods can help inoculate the digestive tract with a wide variety of beneficial, lactic acid–producing bacteria. While some of these foods are exotic, others are so common that we often don't think about them as fermented foods: cheeses, sourdough bread, sauerkraut, dill pickles, soy sauce, and wine.

Diced cabbage fermented first by *Leuconostoc mesenteroides* and then by *Lactobacillus plantarum* creates sauerkraut. Kimchi, the Korean equivalent to sauerkraut, is produced by the action of *Leuconostoc mesenteroides, S. faecilis, L. brevis, L. plantarum,* and *Pecicoccus cerevesiae* on Chinese cabbage and radishes. Likewise, the making of Japanese miso and soy sauce requires *Aspergillus oryzae* and *A. soyae,* and a variety of yeasts. Variations in essentially the same process yield sake, a rice wine. Tempeh, an Indonesian food, is produced by the fermentation of soybeans by various *Leuconostoc, Lactobacillus, Pediococcus,* and *Streptococcus* species. Nham, a Thai dish made from pork and rice, depends on *L. plantarum* and *P. cerevesia* as starter cultures. Researchers have documented that the number of pathogens, such as *Enterobacteria* and *Staphylococcus aureus,* often decrease during fermentation.[38]

Beneficial bacteria also discourage the growth of pathogenic bacteria, viruses, protozoa, and fungi in your gastrointestinal tract. Fermented dairy products with live bacteria or freeze-dried probiotic supplements (which include *Lactobacillus* and *Bifidobacteria* species) should be a regular part of the diet—even just a cup of yogurt or a glass of kefir daily. To consume a broad selection of beneficial bacteria, we recommend that you occasionally eat fermented foods from a variety of ethnic cuisines.

If you have recently taken antibiotics, or suffer from *Candida* yeast infections, you may have to take extra steps to restore a healthy intestinal environment. In this circumstance, consider adding freeze-dried probiotic supplements for a month. If you have ongoing problems, and the freeze-dried capsules seem to help, by all means take them for longer periods. We do have a warning, though. Having seen independent analyses of some probiotic supplements, we realize that some companies have had serious manufacturing and quality control problems. This observation has been confirmed by more methodical analyses of commercial probiotic products.[39] Quality can be erratic, but companies currently making and marketing probiotic supplements are working hard to improve their products.

So how should you select a probiotic supplement? Makers

of probiotic supplements typically date their products, and we urge you to buy only the freshest, highest potency products at your health or natural foods store. Bacteria die off, and most companies only guarantee the numbers of bacteria on the·day they are packaged—not for several months. The clerk at your local health or natural foods store can probably recommend the best brand based on feedback from other customers.

Recently, a number of companies have introduced "*pre*biotic" supplements containing sugars called fructo-oligosaccharides (FOS).[40,41] These are quite literally foods for bacteria because people cannot digest and absorb these prebiotics. Furthermore, these sugars are foods for only a few species of beneficial bacteria, and they do not aid disease-causing bacteria. Recent studies have confirmed that FOS supplements encourage the growth of *Bifidobacteria* in the intestine.[42]

Still, FOS is a pretty arcane supplement—it feeds only one species of your bacteria, not you. But FOS may be of benefit to some people with serious gastrointestinal problems. The richest food sources of FOS are garlic followed by onions, and in general, we prefer these food sources of FOS because they cost less, taste good, and provide other nutrients. We also recommend live-culture yogurts and other cultured dairy products sold in natural foods stores over the well-known supermarket brands of pasteurized yogurt. Many of the best live-culture yogurts are made by small, regional companies. Again, your local natural foods store can recommend specific brands.

11

GARLIC: A NATURAL ANTIBIOTIC

—————— ✥ ——————

Very few foods or herbs have acquired the medical lore of garlic. Even fewer have lived up to the superlatives attributed to them. Garlic has done both. Known scientifically as *Allium sativum*, garlic belongs to the lily *(Liliaceae)* family, along with onions, aloe, shallots, chives, and saffron. These plants share many chemical similarities, but garlic stands out as being particularly potent.

Garlic functions as a natural antibiotic that stimulates the immune system and increases the effectiveness of white blood cells and T cells. It also possesses broad-spectrum bacteriostatic and bacteriocidal properties, meaning that it either stops the growth of or kills bacteria. Remarkably, it exerts similar activity against viruses, fungi, and parasites. While garlic should never take the place of appropriately prescribed antibiotics, it is a key to achieving optimal immunity and protecting against infections. Tariq H. Abdullah, M.D., of Panama City, Florida, may have best described the value of garlic when he wrote, "Garlic is the best example of the philosophy that your medicine should be your food, and your food should be your medicine."[1]

Garlic Anecdotes and Active Ingredients

The Chinese have used medicinal teas from garlic or onions for more than four thousand years, and numerous references to the therapeutic uses of garlic and other *Allium* species appear in the Egyptian *Codex Ebers* papyrus, written around 1550 B.C. Hippocrates lauded garlic in 460 B.C., as did Aristotle in 384 B.C. In the first century A.D., the Greek physician Dioscorides recommended that Roman soldiers use garlic to treat intestinal and lung disorders. Pliny the Elder's *Natural History*, written about the same time, contained many references to the therapeutic uses of garlic.

According to one often-repeated story, four criminals were ordered to bury the dead during a plague in Marseilles in 1721. The gravediggers protected themselves by drinking garlic in vinegar—a still-popular concoction known as *vinaigre des quatre voleurs*, or Four Thieves. Whether or not the story has a factual basis, science began confirming the benefits of garlic in 1858, when none other than Louis Pasteur described its antibacterial properties.

During World War I, the French army used garlic to prevent wound infections, and later Albert Schweitzer, M.D., recommended garlic for the treatment of amoebic dysentery.[2,3] A landmark study published in 1944 documented the broad antibacterial properties of garlic,[4] and in 1952, one researcher contended that garlic was more effective than penicillin in the treatment of some throat infections.[5] Indeed, researchers used an antibiotic-like term—allicin—to describe the first antibacterial compound identified in garlic. Were it not for Fleming's accidental discovery of penicillin in 1928, it's conceivable that modern antibiotics might have been based on the chemistry of garlic instead of a mold.

Although conventional medicine does not officially embrace garlic as an antibiotic, the food clearly remains a medical curiosity. In a 1978 commentary on the historical significance of garlic, Winifred Spray, a British nurse, wrote in *Nursing Times*:

It is easy to accept these claims if ever you enter a building where large quantities of onions or garlic are stored. I recently returned from holiday to find my house smelling very strongly indeed of disinfectant. I was sure that a bottle of Jeyes fluid [a disinfectant] had been spilt during my absence. This was not so and the smell did not disappear until I had removed all the onions and garlic which had been harvested and left to dry indoors before my departure.[6]

Physicians, too, have long been intrigued by garlic, both professionally and personally. Gordon E. Rich, M.D., of Adelaide, Australia, related an incident in which family members developed ringworm (*Microsporum canis*) lesions from a stray cat. Dr. Rich treated his family with a pharmaceutical antifungal agent. But a teenage daughter, unimpressed with the drug, had heard from a friend that garlic worked better. Dr. Rich talked his daughter into volunteering for an informal experiment: one arm was treated with garlic, the other with the antifungal drug. The lesions on the garlic-treated arm healed in ten days; those on the arm treated with the antifungal drug took four weeks to heal.[7]

What makes such anecdotes more than a series of quaint tales are the 1,800 scientific studies detailing garlic's chemical complexity and multifaceted roles in preventing or treating disease.[8] At least two hundred compounds have been identified in garlic cloves,[9] including more than seventy sulfur compounds.[10] In addition, the cloves contain vitamins A, B_1, and C; the minerals calcium, copper, iron, magnesium, potassium, selenium, and zinc; vitamin-like flavonoids; and the eight essential amino acids and nine nonessential ones.[11,12] Many of these micronutrients contribute to immunity, although the amounts in a single garlic clove would be minute.

The health benefits of garlic derive principally from its sulfur-containing amino acids and non-amino acid sulfur compounds. Ironically, most of these compounds do not exist in raw garlic. They are formed when slicing, cooking, crushing, chewing, drying, aging, or "damaging" the garlic clove in other ways initiates a cascade of chemical reactions. The process begins when the interior of the clove is exposed to oxygen and begins oxidizing. This activates the enzyme alliinase, which converts alliin into allicin, the substance that gives garlic its pungent odor. Like a snowball increasing in size as it rolls downhill, allicin triggers the production of still more compounds, including S-allylcysteine, gamma-glutamyl-S-allyl cysteine, diallyl sulfide, diallyl trisulfide, allyl methyl trisulfide, ajoene, and dozens of other compounds.

Allicin was isolated in 1944 by Chester J. Cavallito and John H. Bailey of the Winthrop Chemical Company, Rensselaer, New York.[13,14] For many years, they and other researchers thought it was garlic's principal active ingredient. Since then, improved analytical techniques have shown that allicin is a short-lived compound. Still, it possesses powerful antibacterial activity. Allicin may also serve as some sort of indicator of a garlic supplement's overall potency, but research increasingly points to the greater value of other, longer-lived garlic compounds, including S-allylcysteine and ajoene. Ultimately, garlic's real value may be in its chemical diversity rather than in any single chemical constituent.

Garlic as an Immune System Stimulant

Garlic's constituents directly and indirectly stimulate several aspects of immunity. A particular protein, known simply as F-4, seems to stimulate immunity. F-4 was identified by researchers at the Wakunaga Pharmaceutical Company, Hiroshima, Japan, makers of Kyolic® aged garlic supplements.[15] Several years ago, Benjamin H. S. Lau, M.D., Ph.D., of Loma Linda University, California, documented that the protein boosted the ability of white blood cells to capture and kill harmful bacteria.[16] It's also mitogenic—that is, it enhances the ability of T cells to reproduce.[17]

In 1987, Dr. Abdullah and O. M. Kandil, Ph.D., reported that daily consumption of either raw garlic or Kyolic garlic capsules for three weeks increased the activity of natural-killer cells in healthy people.[18] The significance of this finding was borne out in a follow-up study of ten AIDS patients, who had low killer-cell activity and fewer T-cell abnormalities. The patients were given 5 grams daily of an aged garlic extract for six weeks and 10 grams daily for another six weeks. Three patients suffered gastrointestinal or neurological problems that prevented their continued participation, and they died before the end of the experiment. Of the remaining seven who took garlic supplements, all regained normal killer-cell activity and four had improved T-cell activity after twelve weeks.[19]

In addition, the AIDS patients had fewer outbreaks of diarrhea (caused by *Cryptosporidia*), genital herpes, and *Candida* while taking the garlic. One patient suffered from a sinus infection that failed to respond to antibiotics for over a year, but his condition improved with the garlic. Another patient suffered from depressed numbers of blood platelet cells, a condition difficult to treat in AIDS patients. After taking garlic for twelve weeks, his platelet cells almost tripled in number.[20] While such clinical improvements are by no means a cure for AIDS, they do improve the patient's well-being.

ANTIBACTERIAL AND ANTIVIRAL PROPERTIES

Garlic's antimicrobial properties were documented in 1941 with an analytical technique otherwise used to measure penicillin's potency. In analyzing allicin, Cavallito and Bailey found that the compounds had about 1 percent of penicillin's activity against *Staphylococcus aureus*. Not much perhaps—but allicin was active against some strains of bacteria unaffected by penicillin.[21] The researchers reported that very dilute allicin solutions (one part in 125,000) inhibited the growth of fourteen of fifteen species of bacteria, including strains of staph, strep, and *Shigella*, as well as *Vibrio cholerae*, which causes cholera. A slightly stronger allicin concentration was effective against all fifteen species.

With the passage of fifty years, Cavallito and Bailey's experiments could be retrospectively criticized for using antiquated analytical equipment and showing weaknesses in methodology. But other experiments have largely confirmed their findings and the important role garlic plays in defending against infection. Several years ago, researchers at the University of Dhaka, Bangladesh, related that garlic completely cured rabbits of *Shigella* infections (which cause severe diarrhea) in three days, compared with untreated rabbits that died in two days. In laboratory experiments, garlic also showed antibacterial activity against other *Shigella* species and against a toxin-producing strain of *E. coli.*[22]

Recently, Karen S. Farbman, M.D., and Elizabeth D. Barnett, M.D., of the Boston University School of Medicine, confirmed the broad antimicrobial properties of garlic, specifically allicin. They were motivated by the fact that "little regard" had been given to the antibacterial properties of garlic—at a time of rapidly increasing antibiotic resistance.[23]

Drs. Farbman and Barnett prepared liquid extracts of fresh garlic—what they referred to as garlic juice—and incubated it with fourteen strains of bacteria, including *E. coli, Haemophilus influenzae, Klebsiella pneumoniae, Pseudomonas aeruginosa, Staphylococcus aureus, Streptococcus* Group A, and *Streptococcus pneumoniae.* Although the garlic concentrations were weaker than those Cavallito and Bailey had used, they inhibited the growth of all fourteen strains. The garlic juice even worked against antibiotic-resistant *S. aureus,* currently the most dangerous antibiotic-resistant bacterium in hospitals.

Another early study on the antimicrobial properties of garlic was recently confirmed. In 1946, researchers at the Indian Institute of Science related in the journal *Nature* that a garlic extract prevented the growth of *Mycobacterium tuberculosis.*[24] In 1993, doctors at the Morehouse School of Medicine, Atlanta, described an experiment in which an extract of fresh garlic inhibited the growth of twenty strains of *Mycobacterium avium,* a closely related microorganism and a common cause of lung disease in AIDS patients.[25]

Unlike conventional antibiotics, garlic can kill some viruses. One team of researchers determined that the ajoene, allicin, allyl methyl thiosulfinate, and methyl allyl thiosulfinate components of garlic were capable of killing the herpes simplex, parainfluenza (which causes respiratory illness in children), and rhinovirus (which causes the common cold).[26]

PROTECTION AGAINST PARASITES

Each year, the *Entamoeba histolytica* amoeba infects an estimated four hundred million people worldwide, often causing diarrhea, nausea, and weakness. In a letter to the *Journal of Infectious Diseases*, a group of researchers from the Weitzmann Institute of Science, Israel, reported that allicin extracted from fresh garlic rapidly inhibited—and, at higher doses, killed—*E. histolytica* in just fifteen minutes.[27]

Hymenolepsis nana, a type of tapeworm, and *G. lamblia* are other nasty parasites. Egyptian researchers reported in 1991 that both "crude extracts" of garlic—essentially mashed-up garlic cloves—and commercial supplements quickly cured groups of children with *H. nana* or *G. lamblia* infections. They observed that "*A. sativum* [garlic] was found to be efficient, safe and shortens the duration of treatment."[28] Belgian researchers have also described allicin's ability to control *E. histolytica* and *G. lamblia*.[29]

One of the most remarkable studies on garlic demonstrated garlic's ability to control a type of malaria that infects rodents—with obvious implications for people. It's particularly noteworthy because garlic has long been used as a folk remedy to discourage mosquito bites, which is how *Plasmodium* parasites are transmitted. Hilda A. Perez. Ph.D., of the Instituto Venezsolano do Investigaciones Científicas, Caracas, Venezuela, found that a single injection of sulfur-containing ajoene suppressed the growth of *Plasmodium berghei* in mice. This would have been an exciting discovery in itself because many *Plasmodium* species are now resistant to the drug chloroquine. More remarkable, however, was Dr. Perez's discovery that ajoene makes *P. berghei* more susceptible to chloroquine, extending the usefulness of the antimalarial drug.[30]

CONTROL OF YEAST AND FUNGAL INFECTIONS

Garlic also acts as a broad-spectrum antifungal agent. In a very simple experiment, Dr. Lau added an extract of Schilling garlic powder—the type found in any grocery store—to a number of fungal cultures in test tubes. As the amount of garlic increased, fungal growth progressively decreased.[31]

In a more rigorous experiment, Dr. Lau infected two groups of mice with *Candida albicans.* He then treated them with injections of either a saline (salt) solution or garlic extract. After twenty-four hours, the saline-treated control mice had an average *Candida* colony count of 3,500 in the blood. Mice treated with garlic had an average colony count of only four hundred. After forty-eight hours, the *Candida* colony count in the saline-treated mice had dropped to 1,000, but by this time no *Candida* organisms could be detected in the blood of garlic-treated animals. The garlic rapidly and efficiently removed *Candida* from the blood, stemming what could have easily become a systemic fungal infection. Dr. Lau documented that the lower *Candida* numbers among garlic-treated mice were the result of more efficient destruction of the yeast by white blood cells.[32]

Another type of fungal infection, *Cryptococcus,* can involve the entire body or any single organ, and sometimes causes respiratory or kidney disease. It has a predilection for the brain, and this type of infection, called cryptococcal meningitis, is usually fatal. For some reason, *Cryptococcus* infections tend to infect men forty to sixty years old in the southeastern United States. People with AIDS and Hodgkin's disease are also susceptible, regardless of where they live, most likely because of their depressed immune systems.

In the 1950s, Chinese physicians treated cryptococcal meningitis and other fungal infections with a combination of garlic tea and pharmaceuticals, but for some reason the individual role of garlic was not pursued. Interest in garlic was renewed when physicians at the Hunan Medical College Hospital successfully treated a case of cryptococcal meningitis with garlic tea in 1972, and the following year, the hospital pharmacy began preparing garlic extracts for intravenous and oral use.[33] Over the next five years, physicians at the hospital treated a number of cases of cryptococcal meningitis with garlic or a combination of garlic and drugs. Of sixteen patients treated exclusively with garlic, eleven (two-thirds) improved. Six were completely cured—they had no remaining neurological symptoms— and five had greatly reduced symptoms. The Chinese doctors observed that garlic is "obviously cheap, plentiful and causes no major side effects."[34]

This research has also been brought up-to-date. In a recent collaborative study, Larry E. Davis, M.D., of the University of New Mexico School of Medicine, Albuquerque, and Yan Cai, M.D., of the Ren Ji Hospital, Shanghai, treated five meningitis patients with an intravenous garlic preparation. Two of the patients had been diagnosed with cryptococcal meningitis, two with viral meningitis, and one with chronic meningitis of an unknown cause. After the patients received garlic, antifungal immune factors in their blood and cerebrospinal fluid increased significantly. Antifungal factors in the blood of two healthy individuals also doubled after treatment with garlic, suggesting that garlic can enhance the immune system of people who are healthy.[35]

Although garlic exerts specific activity against many microorganisms, its real value is as a generic immune system stimulant, heightening the body's surveillance and response against a broad range of pathogens. Dr. Lau and Moses A. Adetumbi, M.D., once observed that "garlic extract has broad-spectrum antimicrobial activity against many genera of bacteria and fungi. . . . Because many of the microorganisms susceptible to garlic extract are medically significant, garlic holds a promising position as a broad-spectrum therapeutic agent."[36]

Garlic, Cancer, and Heart Disease

Garlic provides many other benefits to health, particularly in the prevention of cancer and heart disease. Indeed, frequent minor infections contribute to the risk of cancer and heart disease. Preventing infections and shoring up the body's response to them lower the risk of these devastating diseases.

One specific link between infections and cancer is found in free radicals, considered a principal cause of aging and many degenerative diseases. Free radicals oxidize cells (much the way oxygen rusts iron) and cause mutations in DNA. As more and more cells and DNA are damaged, aging accelerates and the risk of all diseases increases.[37] In a well-nourished person, many of these free radicals are mopped up by antioxidants, including superoxide dismutase, glutathione peroxidase, and vitamins C and E. But the body cannot quench all of these free radicals, and so their damage accumulates.[38] (We'll discuss the link between infection and heart disease in the next chapter.)

Recently, John A. Milner, Ph.D., of Pennsylvania State University, University Park, recently studied how aged garlic powder protected against cancer-causing nitrosamines, a class of chemicals formed when processed meats, such as bacon and bologna, are cooked and eaten. Dr. Milner found that garlic dramatically reduced the number of DNA adducts—that is, the chemical bonds that attach nitrosamines to DNA. Once tied to DNA, the adducts disrupt the genetic blueprint, causing mutations and precancerous changes.

Dr. Milner determined that laboratory animals that were fed large amounts of garlic had up to 80 percent fewer adducts than did animals not given garlic.[39] In experiments with another cancer-causing chemical, Dr. Milner found that a high-garlic diet slowed the development and reduced the numbers of breast cancers by 56 percent in animals, again compared with animals not fed garlic. Another benefit was that levels of glutathione-S-transferase, one of the antioxidant enzymes that helps the liver detoxify carcinogens and other dangerous chemicals, were 42 percent higher among animals eating garlic.[40]

Garlic also lowers blood levels of cholesterol,[41] possibly by inhibiting its production by the body.[42] Adesh K. Jain, M.D., of Tulane University School of Medicine, New Orleans, compared cholesterol levels among people receiving a garlic supplement (Kwai® brand) and those getting a placebo. After twelve weeks, total blood cholesterol levels dropped by an average of 6 percent among those taking the garlic tablets, but by only 1 percent among those taking the placebo. Those who took garlic tablets also benefited from an 11 percent decrease in the LDL form of cholesterol, whereas the placebo group had only a 3 percent reduction in LDL.[43]

Garlic also functions as an anticoagulant—a natural blood thinner.[44] H. Kiesewetter, M.D., of the University of Saarlandes, Hamburg, Germany, has described how garlic helps patients suffering from peripheral artery occlusive disease, characterized by blood clots in the legs. Dr. Kiesewetter was able to detect the benefits of garlic after patients took a *single* capsule.[45]

Recommendations

It's hard not to notice the heavily advertised garlic supplements sold in supermarkets, drugstores, and natural foods stores. A lot of people are simply confused about how to take garlic. According to Dr. John Milner, one of the top garlic researchers, just about any form of garlic provides *some* health benefits.[46] We wholeheartedly agree, but add that some forms will be more potent than others— fresh and supplements, for example, being better than garlic powder.

Our first choice is for the use of generous amounts of freshly prepared garlic as a food condiment because it's potent, tasty, and inexpensive. Some of the advertising, and at least one book on the benefits of garlic, warns people about the so-called dangers of eating raw garlic. Nothing could be further from the truth.

In our opinion, it is one thing to promote a garlic product—and quite another to scare people away from a reasonable food source. We don't know of anyone who swallows raw garlic cloves, and we don't recommend consuming garlic this way. Slicing, dicing, and cooking the clove are needed to create many of the beneficial compounds in garlic.

If you don't like the taste of garlic, or if you want a concentrated source to boost your immune system, then consider taking garlic supplements. The major brands are Kyolic, Garlicin®, Kwai, and Pure-Gar®, and each has its advocates and supportive studies. Wakunaga, the maker of Kyolic, seems to edge out the other companies in terms of scientific backing for its product.

Competition among these products makes it difficult to pick one over the other, and our impression is that the different manufacturing processes select for some of garlic's active ingredients over others. For example, Kyolic touts the product's S-allylcysteine content; Garlicin promotes allicin content; and Kwai promotes allicin "potential." It's a little like comparing apples and oranges, so exact comparisons are difficult. All of these products seem to be good, but they also have their drawbacks. For example, none cite their content of ajoene, one of the most powerful antibacterial components of garlic.

There's only one contraindication for garlic supplements. Garlic is an anticoagulant, and because of this, may reduce your need for blood thinners, such as aspirin or Coumadin®. If you have a tendency toward excessive bleeding, have heavy menstrual periods, or are a hemophiliac, it would be wise to first discuss the use of garlic supplements with your personal physician. In all other respects, garlic has passed the test of time—for at least four thousand years.

12

VITAMIN C: IMMUNE
BOOSTER SUPREME

———————— ✣ ————————

Vitamin C is a potent immune system stimulant, and medical studies describing its infection-fighting properties date back more than sixty years. But in 1970, when Nobel laureate Linus Pauling, Ph.D., publicly recommended vitamin C supplements to prevent and treat the common cold, he triggered a storm of protest from physicians and researchers.

Dr. Pauling, whose name quickly became synonymous with vitamin C, had by this time established himself as one of the most prominent and respected scientists of the twentieth century—and was eventually ranked second only to Albert Einstein. He had been awarded two Nobel prizes, one in chemistry for describing the nature of the chemical bond and one in peace for his efforts to control the spread of nuclear weapons. Dr. Pauling had laid the foundation of molecular medicine with his detailed explanation of sickle cell anemia and made countless contributions to chemistry, biochemistry, and medicine.

In light of his scientific stature, it was strange that controversy followed Dr. Pauling's advocacy of vitamin C. He was accused of being a gadfly, of possessing no proof that vitamin

C worked, and of having stepped outside his expertise in science and medicine. What Dr. Pauling had done to generate such criticism was simple: because of the importance of his message, he bypassed conservative scientific traditions and took his message about vitamin C directly to the public. He was, as he tended to be, ahead of his time.

A quarter of a century later, and despite overwhelming evidence confirming the value of vitamin C in treating colds and flus, medicine still remains largely apathetic toward the use of vitamin C. There are two reasons for this, aside from the general conservatism of the medical establishment. One is that physicians and dietitians wrongly perceive vitamin C as a micronutrient and have consequently undervalued the importance of vitamin C in health. The other reason is a frequently cited anti-vitamin C study—a study that has turned out to be fundamentally flawed.

We will describe the value of vitamin C step-by-step. The point to keep in mind is this: vitamin C *does* work against infectious diseases—and it works well. The precedent exists in studies in vitamin C and the common cold; the proof positive is in the treatment of much more significant infections, such as HIV infections and AIDS.

Why People Need Vitamin C

There is no controversy that vitamin C is an essential nutrient for people. The body needs it to produce bone, dentin in teeth, and collagen, a biological "cement" that holds tissues together. It is essential for the integrity of blood vessel walls, and mild deficiencies are marked by the skin bruising easily. Severe deficiencies of vitamin C, called scurvy, result in spontaneous ruptures of the skin and hemorrhaging: the body literally breaks apart at the seams. Until the eighteenth century, when Dr. James Lind discovered that citrus fruit (which is rich in vitamin C) prevented scurvy, more British sailors died from a lack of the vitamin than from battles at sea.

Vitamin C is found universally in plants, which produce it from dextrose (glucose), a simple sugar. Because dextrose ($C_6H_{12}O_6$) and vitamin C ($C_6H_8O_6$) are very similar chemically, the conversion is a relatively straightforward biochemical process that depends on the activity of several enzymes. Most mammals convert glucose, or blood sugar, to vitamin C in the liver or kidneys. For these animals, vitamin C is not an essential nutrient. Rather, it is an essential "metabolite" produced by the body. (Other metabolites include thyroid hormone, insulin, and adrenaline.) As a metabolite, vitamin C helps animals maintain homeostasis—biological equilibrium—in the face of stresses.

As it turns out, only a very small number of animals cannot manufacture their own vitamin C. These include the guinea pig, the fruit-eating bat of India, the red-vented bulbul songbird, and the Anthropoidea suborder of primates, which includes monkeys, chimpanzees, and gorillas. *Homo sapiens*—human beings—are also members of Anthropoidea and lack one enzyme, L-gulonolactone oxidase, needed to complete the conversion of glucose to vitamin C.

A GENETIC DEFECT AFFECTING VITAMIN C PRODUCTION

Of more than four thousand mammalian species, why do so few *not* produce their own vitamin C? In the mid-1960s, biochemist Irwin Stone, D.Sc., of San Jose, California, proposed an intriguing theory: because of a mutation an estimated twenty-five million years ago, a common evolutionary ancestor of Anthropoidea primates and *Homo sapiens* lost its ability to produce vitamin C. It is possible that the mutation arose in some sort of cataclysmic event, such as in the aftermath of an asteroid collision with Earth. Nonproducers of vitamin C had to obtain vitamin C from food. For them, this important metabolite became a dietary nutrient essential for survival.[1,2] Up to this point, Dr. Stone's theory was not controversial.

Dr. Stone then considered how much vitamin C people and other nonproducing animals need. He looked at how much some animals produced, how much veterinary scientists recommended for nonproducers, and how much was recommended for people. Throughout the animal kingdom, animals produce vitamin C at approximately the same rate, in the neighborhood of 86 milligrams per pound of body weight. As his principal benchmark, Stone used a 150-pound goat, which makes 13,000 milligrams (13 grams) of vitamin C daily—an amount 217 times higher than the human Recommended Dietary Allowance (RDA) of 60 milligrams. Under stressful conditions, such as when fighting an infection, the goat's production of vitamin C increases to even higher levels.

It can, of course, be argued that people are not goats and that people don't need massive amounts of vitamin C. So Dr. Stone considered the amount of vitamin C required by monkeys, a close relative of *Homo sapiens*. Laboratory guidelines for keeping monkeys healthy call for comparatively large amounts of vitamin C—up to several grams a day for a 150-pound animal. Dr. Stone concluded that people were not biological anomalies, as far as vitamin C requirements were concerned, and needed as much vitamin C as did other mammals. In fact, if we could produce vitamin C, we certainly would. That was aptly demonstrated in a proof-of-principle experiment in which L-gulonolactone oxidase from a chicken was inserted into a guinea pig. The guinea pig began producing prodigious quantities of vitamin C until the enzyme was exhausted.[3]

In his book *The Healing Factor: Vitamin C Against Disease*,[4] Dr. Stone elegantly described his theory and repositioned the role of vitamin C in health. People could not produce vitamin C, but they still required large amounts of it for health. By subsisting on meager dietary sources of vitamin C, people literally hobbled from one generation to the next suffering from an unrecognized genetic defect. The consequence was greater susceptibility to infectious and degenerative diseases, which people simply assumed were a natural part of life. But what would happen if people corrected this genetic defect by taking large doses of supplemental vitamin C? In citing hundreds of medical studies, Dr. Stone documented that vitamin C supplements enhanced resistance to and hastened recovery from infectious and degenerative diseases.[5] In other words, supplemental vitamin C could restore homeostasis.

In fact, Dr. Stone was instrumental in arousing Dr. Pauling's interest in vitamin C. During the speech in 1965, on the eve of his official retirement, Dr. Pauling offhandedly remarked that he wouldn't mind living another twenty-five years. Dr. Stone happened to be in the audience, and in a follow-up letter he described his evolutionary theory of vitamin C and suggested that Dr. Pauling could live longer if he took vitamin C. Dr. Pauling and his wife increased their intake of vitamin C and noticed an immediate improvement in their health. Those experiences helped shape Pauling's 1968 concept of orthomolecular medicine, which in part recommended the use of vitamins to achieve *optimal* health. The remarkable disease-fighting benefits of vitamin C make perfect sense if supplementation is seen as a way to correct a universal human genetic defect.

VITAMIN C AND THE COMMON COLD

If your vitamin C requirements are actually comparable to those of other animals, and if you obtained only a fraction of what you should, the health consequences would be profound. Among other things, inadequate vitamin C would leave you especially vulnerable to infections in general and, specifically, to supergerms. Conversely, supplementing with high doses of vitamin C would compensate for this genetic defect and protect against infection.

In his 1970 book, *Vitamin C and the Common Cold,*[6] Dr. Pauling recommended that people take 1,000 to 2,000 milligrams of vitamin C daily for general well-being. To fight a cold, he suggested that people increase that amount to 4,000 to 10,000 milligrams daily. The following year, in an article in the *Proceedings of the National Academy of Sciences of the USA,* Dr. Pauling analyzed several scientific studies of vitamin C used to prevent colds. He related evidence that 100 to 200 milligrams of vitamin C daily had little effect on colds, but that 1,000 milligrams daily reduced the incidence of colds by 45 percent and cold symptoms by 63 percent.[7]

Supplemental vitamin C remained controversial, however, and in 1975 Thomas C. Chalmers, M.D., of New York's Mount Sinai Medical Center, published a damning assessment of vitamin C. Dr. Chalmers argued that vitamin C had few if any benefits. He was sarcastic and mean-spirited in his criticism of vitamin C and Dr. Pauling, ending his analysis by writing, "The best way to conclude this review of the evidence for and against the efficacy of ascorbic acid [vitamin C] in preventing the common cold and amelioration of its symptoms is to state that I, who have colds as often and as severe as those of any man, do not consider the very minor potential benefit that might result from taking ascorbic acid three times a day for life worth either the effort or the risk, no matter how slight the latter might be."[8]

Over the next twenty years, Dr. Chalmers's analysis was cited in medical journals twice as often as Pauling's 1971 paper.[9] Physicians routinely accepted Chalmers's conclusions without reading or analyzing his paper and assumed his was the final word on the subject. Since the early 1970s, however, researchers have conducted more than a hundred studies on vitamin C and the common cold, and in 1992 Harri Hemilä, Ph.D., of the University of Helsinki, Finland, analyzed thirty-two studies involving people taking at least 1,000 milligrams of vitamin C daily. Thirty-one of these studies supported the use of vitamin C in treating colds; one showed vitamin C and a placebo to be equal.

Dr. Hemilä's meta-analysis (collective analysis) was a partial, though powerful, vindication of Dr. Pauling. He found that high doses of vitamin C consistently reduced the length and severity of colds, but not their incidence. The greatest reduction in cold duration and symptoms occurred when people took 4,000 to 8,000 milligrams of vitamin C daily. At times, the findings were dramatic. In one attempted double-blind study, patients were given 6,000 milligrams of vitamin C daily at the beginning of a cold, "The benefits," wrote Dr. Hemilä, "were so obvious that the physician could recognize the subjects receiving the vitamin by their clinical progress. Therefore the double-blind study was terminated, and a less-well-controlled study was performed."[10]

Two years later, Dr. Hemilä conducted another meta-analysis, this time narrowing his focus to twenty-one very well controlled studies. He found that people taking 1,000 milligrams of vitamin C daily had a 19 percent decrease in cold symptoms, and those taking 2,000 to 6,000 milligrams daily had an impressive 29 percent (almost one-third) decrease in symptoms. While the vitamin C did not completely relieve symptoms, the effect was anything but negligible.[11]

By any standard in medicine, twenty-one double-blind studies should have constituted a convincng body of evidence. So why, asked Dr. Hemilä the following year, did the medical community still reject the use of vitamin C? One reason was Dr. Chalmers's 1975 analysis.

Curious, Dr. Hemilä and Zelek S. Herman, Ph.D., took a close look at Dr. Chalmers's original data and discovered that his analysis was fraught with errors and omissions of data. Furthermore, Dr. Chalmers failed to account for a crucial variable: the amount of vitamin C given to subjects—that is, the difference between an effective and ineffective dose. For his recommendations, Dr. Pauling had relied on studies in which people were given at least 1 gram (1,000 milligrams) of vitamin C daily. Meanwhile, Dr. Chalmers's analysis had included studies in which people were given as little as 250 milligrams.[12]

Then, reanalyzing *all* of Dr. Chalmers's original data, Drs. Hemilä and Herman found that higher doses of vitamin C did consistently reduce the severity of symptoms and the length of common cold infections, whereas lower doses did not—confirming Pauling's argument in favor of vitamin C. The best results, based on Dr. Chalmers's original data, occurred when people took 2 to 6 grams of vitamin C daily.[13]

Vitamin C and Other Infections

Dr. Pauling's research on vitamin C did not occur in a vacuum. It was part of a scientific continuum that began in the 1930s, when vitamin C was discovered and researchers first described its role in controlling bacterial and viral infections[14]—and one that has continued with other researchers and clinicians.

In the 1940s, Frederick R. Klenner, M.D., of Reidsville, North Carolina, became the first physician to consistently use large doses of vitamin C to treat infectious and degenerative diseases. He often administered the vitamin intravenously or intramuscularly, rather than orally, and his average therapeutic dose was a little over four grams daily. For severe illnesses, he would administer twenty-five or more grams daily.[15]

Dr. Klenner had great success with vitamin C in reducing the symptoms and duration of encephalitis, viral pneumonia, and mononucleosis among his patients. But his most remarkable work may have been in the successful treatment of polio, for which he combined very large doses of vitamin C—often 25 to 30 grams daily—with vitamin B_1 and gentle leg massage.[16] Vitamin C was unfairly discredited in the treatment of polio by none other than Albert B. Sabin, M.D., developer of the oral live-polio vaccine. Dr. Sabin treated polio-infected monkeys with a meager 100 milligrams daily—less than 1/250th of Dr. Klenner's dose.[17]

DR. CATHCART'S TREATMENT OF INFECTIONS

Since the late 1960s, Robert F. Cathcart III, M.D., currently of Los Altos, California, has treated more than twenty thousand patients with vitamin C. Dr. Cathcart was a conservative orthopedist who had established a name for himself as the developer of an innovative hip prosthesis. He was skeptical about vitamin therapy, but he had also been plagued for years by regular colds and allergies to pollens and cats. When he heard about "megadoses" of vitamin C in 1969, he decided to experiment on himself. Supplements of the vitamin immediately diminished his allergy symptoms and increased his resistance to colds. The effect was so dramatic that he decided to give vitamin C to a few patients, and their responses were equally impressive.[18] Buoyed by these successes, Dr. Cathcart refined his vitamin C protocol over the next ten years.

One criticism of megadoses of vitamin C is that they often cause diarrhea. But Dr. Cathcart discovered that a person's tolerance of vitamin C generally increases relative to the seriousness of his infection. This was an original observation and one that lent credence to vitamin C's role in maintaining homeostasis—the greater the stress, the higher the vitamin C requirements.

According to Dr. Cathcart, a person who ordinarily developed diarrhea taking more than 1 gram of vitamin C might be able to consume 10 or more grams during a cold without getting diarrhea. Dr. Cathcart also determined that the therapeutic dose of vitamin C was typically just under the amount causing diarrhea. So he began coaching sick patients on how to titrate, or adjust, the dose of vitamin C every two hours to "bowel tolerance." The idea was to increase vitamin C levels until the onset of diarrhea, then to lower the dose slightly. As the patient recovered from the infection, bowel tolerance would decrease, and the vitamin C dose would have to be adjusted downward.

In a magazine interview, he explained:

> I discovered that about 80 percent of people can take between 10 to 15 grams of vitamin C as fine granules dissolved in water, divided up four to six times a day, before developing diarrhea. The astonishing thing was that the same person could take 50 grams if they had a mild cold, 100 grams if they had a more serious cold, 150 grams with the flu, or in excess of 200 grams with mononucleosis or viral pneumonia—without diarrhea. This illustrated the bowel tolerance concept. The sicker a person is, the more he can take.[19]

While the vitamin C might not "cure" the infection, it could often suppress up to 80 to 90 percent of the symptoms.[20] Dr.

❦

USUAL BOWEL TOLERANCE DOSES OF VITAMIN C[21]

CONDITION	GRAMS PER 24 HOURS	DOSES PER 24 HOURS
Normal	4–15	4
Mild common cold	30–60	6–10
Severe common cold	60–100	8–15
Influenza (flu)	100–150	8–20
Mononucleosis	150–200+	12–25
Viral pneumonia	100–200+	12–25
Bacterial infections	30–200+	10–25
Infectious hepatitis	30–100	6–15
Candida albicans	15–200+	6–25

Adapted from Cathcart, R. F, "Vitamin C, Titrating to Bowel Tolerance, Anascorbemia, and Acute Induced Scurvy," *Medical Hypotheses*, 1981;7:1359–1376. Reprinted with permission.

❦

Cathcart stressed that it was of paramount importance to quickly reach bowel-tolerance doses of vitamin C, because treating a 25-gram cold with only 5 grams of vitamin C daily would be ineffective and discouraging. Furthermore, inadequate amounts of vitamin C—either taking too little or not taking any at all—would wipe out the body's stores of vitamin C, leading to a scurvylike vitamin C deficiency. And that severe deprivation of vitamin C would increase the body's vulnerability to a secondary infection.

Dr. Cathcart has successfully treated many different types of bacterial and viral infections with high doses of vitamin C, including mononucleosis and viral pneumonia, for which recovery can be excruciatingly slow. Other than flatulence and diarrhea from exceeding bowel tolerance doses, Dr. Cathcart has found vitamin C to be remarkably safe.

To illustrate the vitamin's safety, he has related the story of a twenty-three-year-old, ninety-eight-pound librarian with mononucleosis who took two heaping tablespoons of vitamin C every two hours—almost a full pound in two days—without producing diarrhea. She felt reasonably well after several days, but had to take 20 to 30 grams daily for two months.[22] Sometimes Dr. Cathcart uses intravenous vitamin C to attain extremely high doses, which completely avoids bowel disturbances. Following Dr. Cathcart's approach ourselves, it's abundantly clear that such high doses of vitamin C promote rapid recovery and contribute to a sense of well-being among patients with infections.

VITAMIN C, AIDS, AND EBOLA

Vitamin C has also proved of value in the treatment of HIV infections and full-blown AIDS. In 1983, when physicians were just starting to appreciate the seriousness of HIV, Dr. Cathcart began using his vitamin C protocol on AIDS patients who had few if any medical options. He was able to dramatically extend the length and improve the quality of their lives.[23,24,25]

HIV, which is transmitted through the exchange of body fluids (e.g., semen and blood), infects and kills T4 "helper" cells, which are considered the brains of the immune system. In a healthy person, the blood contains 400 to 1,200 T4 cells in each cubic millimeter of blood. As the number of T4 cells decreases, the relative number of T8 "suppressor" cells increases. In healthy individuals, the T8 cells help prevent T4 cells from overreacting to an infection, but in AIDS too many T8 cells further stymie an effective immunological response to infection. AIDS is diagnosed when an HIV infection causes the T4 cell count to drop to 200 or less. At that point, immunity has virtually disappeared, leaving the AIDS patient vulnerable to any number of deadly infections, including pneumocystis pneumonia and Kaposi's sarcoma (an infectious cancer).

In treating these patients, Dr. Cathcart has focused on slowing the progression from HIV to AIDS and, when necessary, on reducing the signs and symptoms of AIDS. He generally recommends 60 grams of intravenous vitamin C three times weekly, along with 40 to 80 grams daily by mouth. Dr. Cathcart observes that patients often exhibit a renewed feeling of well-being within a few weeks. In addition, Kaposi's sarcoma lesions would often decrease in number and flatten, and enlarged lymph nodes would decrease in size and firmness during vitamin C supplementation.

Finally, while it is entirely speculative, vitamin C supplements might reduce the severity and increase survival among people suffering from hemorrhagic infections, such as Ebola and dengue fever. These viral epidemics have tended to occur in impoverished areas where malnutrition is common. The symptoms of these infections resemble the rapid onset of scurvy, in which collagen disintegrates and blood leaks through the body. Could it be that vitamin C deficiency increases the severity of the infection? Or that the inherent ferocity of these viruses depletes a person's vitamin C stores faster than any other virus? Unfortunately, no one has studied why 20 percent of Ebola victims survive. It's conceivable they are protected by sufficient dietary intake of vitamin C, and the similarity between some Ebola symptoms and scurvy deserves serious investigation.

How Vitamin C Works

How does vitamin C help protect against such a broad array of infectious diseases? Rather than working against specific germs, the vitamin enhances the body's physical and immune defenses against infection in general.

First, vitamin C is required by the body to synthesize collagen, which strengthens the integrity of tissues the way metal rebar reinforces some walls. Strong collagen strengthens the physical barriers against disease-causing germs. When collagen is inadequate, tissues become more permeable and allow bacteria and bacterial toxins to infiltrate and spread.[26]

Second, white blood cells require enormous amounts of vitamin C to efficiently attack and digest bacteria.[27] This role was
illustrated by a patient suffering from recurrent boils. His white
blood cells failed to attack and digest bacteria, but when he was
given 500 milligrams of vitamin C daily for a month, his white
blood cells behaved normally and he stopped developing boils.[28]
In a study of healthy people, researchers found that 2,000 to
3,000 milligrams of vitamin C daily stimulated white blood cells'
attacks on bacteria, but lower doses of the vitamin had no notice-
able effect.[29]

Third, vitamin C also increases the body's production of
glutathione, an antioxidant that further stimulates the immune
system and detoxifies bacterial waste products. Carol S. Johnston, Ph.D., of Arizona State University, Tempe, has reported
that 500 milligrams of vitamin C daily increases blood levels of
glutathione in people by 50 percent.[30]

Not surprisingly, inadequate vitamin C impairs the body's
defenses against disease-causing microorganisms. The numbers
of white blood cells and T cells do not always decrease with
vitamin C deficiency, but their responses to infection are seriously impaired.[31] For example, white blood cells in vitamin
C–deficient animals kill only 12 percent of *Actinomyces*, a species
of bacteria that causes periodontal disease, but vitamin C supplements decreased the numbers of bacteria, presumably by restoring normal white blood cell function.[32]

In addition, glucose interferes with vitamin C uptake by
white blood cells, most likely because the two chemicals are
similar. This may very well explain why many dietary sugars
reduce the ability of white blood cells to capture bacteria. To
some extent, vitamin C supplements can reverse this effect of
sugars.[33]

Immunity also decreases with age, as do blood and tissue
levels of most vitamins, either because of inadequate diet or
poor absorption. Blood levels of vitamin C are routinely below
normal in the elderly, impairing T cells. In a study of twenty

men and women age seventy and older, Belgian investigators found that regular injections of vitamin C substantially increased T-cell activity.[34]

Infections also rapidly deplete vitamin C levels. The normal level of vitamin C in white blood cells is approximately 20 micrograms (mcg) per 100 million cells. Within twenty-four hours of the start of a cold, vitamin C levels drop by half, indicative of a vitamin C deficiency. (It is only reasonable to assume that more severe infections deplete vitamin C levels faster and more profoundly.) Vitamin C levels increase gradually and return to normal by the end of the infection, suggesting that the most deleterious effect on the vitamin's levels occurs at the start of the infection.[35,36]

A Scottish study found that regular supplementation of 1 gram of vitamin C daily boosted vitamin C levels to a higher average of 30 micrograms per 100 million cells. When those who were given this supplement contracted colds and their vitamin C intake was immediately increased to 6 grams daily, their leukocytes did not suffer a significant drop in vitamin levels. On the "worst" day of the infection, vitamin C levels dropped to only 23 micrograms per 100 million cells—still above average.[37,38]

Vitamin C also increases the size of the "free radical burst," which white blood cells use to kill bacteria. Excessive radicals, however, can be toxic to white blood cells, T cells, and antibody-producing B cells. During an infection, free radicals are likely produced faster than ordinary numbers of antioxidants can quench them. Vitamin C, in addition to increasing the free radical burst, later mops up many of the leftover free radicals.[39,40,41]

In the case of HIV, vitamin C rolls out one more defense. Steve Harakeh, Ph.D., and Raxit J. Jariwalla, Ph.D., of the Linus Pauling Institute of Science and Medicine, Palo Alto, California, discovered that large, consistent doses of vitamin C suppressed reverse transcriptase—that is, the method HIV uses to replicate itself—by a remarkable 94 percent.[42] It may not be a coincidence that the two mammalian reservoirs of the AIDS virus are humans and higher primates, neither of which produces the vitamin that would stop its growth.

VITAMIN C REDUCES ANTIBIOTIC RESISTANCE

A number of studies have also shown that vitamin C supplements decrease antibiotic resistance and broaden the activity of "old" antibiotics, to which bacteria are commonly resistant. This role of vitamin C is important because antibiotics may be needed in severe bacterial infections, and vitamin C is an easy way to increase their potency. One Japanese researcher has reported that persistent antibiotic-resistant *Pseudomonas aeruginosa*, *Staphylococcus aureus*, and *Enterococcus faecalis* infections were eradicated only after vitamin C was added to the treatment program.[43]

These benefits have also been observed by Dr. Cathcart, who has found that large doses of vitamin C enhance the activity of penicillins against many bacteria that would otherwise be antibiotic resistant,[44] as well as reduce allergic reactions to antibiotics.[45] In addition to enhancing the body's response to infections, vitamin C appears actually to remove the antibiotic-resistant plasmids from some strains of *S. aureus*, and it may do the same in other species. Vitamin C also decreases the amount of antibiotics needed to kill bacteria.[46]

Vitamin C, Cardiovascular Disease, and Cancer

Over the past few years, researchers have established a clear link between the body's response to infections and the risk of cardiovascular diseases. As strange as it might sound, elevated numbers of white blood cells, specifically neutrophils, constitute a major risk factor for cardiovascular disease.[47] Vitamin C reduces this risk.

White blood cells contribute to cardiovascular disease in a number of ways. Being larger and stiffer than red blood cells, they easily become stuck in capillaries and cause blockages,

---

❦

**A POSSIBLE LINK BETWEEN LOW VITAMIN C,
INFECTIONS, AND CARDIOVASCULAR DISEASE**

Lower Seasonal Intake of Vitamin C
↓
25 to 30 Percent Higher Seasonal Risk of Infection
↓
Large Numbers of Activated White Blood Cells
↓
White Blood Cells Produce Large Numbers of Free Radicals
↓
(Insufficient Vitamin C for Quenching Free Radicals)
↓
Free Radicals Activate Blood-Clotting Factors
↓
Higher Seasonal Risk of Cardiovascular Diseases and Deaths

Based on Khaw, K.T. and Woodhouse, P., *British Medical Journal*, June 17, 1995;310:1559–1563.

❦

---

which grow in size. When activated by the immune system, white blood cells can also adhere to the endothelium, a layer of cells lining the heart and blood vessels, causing still more capillary blockages.

In addition, white blood cells release a number of chemicals, including free radicals and bacteria-attacking enzymes, that can damage red blood cells and trigger the leakage of blood-clotting chemicals. Antioxidants quench many of these free radicals, limiting the damage. However, patients suffering from cardiovascular diseases tend to have low dietary, blood, and tissue levels of protective antioxidant nutrients.[48]

In 1994, a team of British physicians led by Kay-Tee Khaw and Peter Woodhouse, both fellows of the Royal College of Physicians and professors at Cambridge University, reported that an annual

25 percent jump in cardiovascular deaths during winter months was strongly associated with a seasonal elevation in blood levels of fibrinogen, one of the compounds that causes blood clots. That increase in fibrinogen levels was, in turn, related to the wintertime increase in serious infections and white blood cell activity.[49]

Drs. Khaw and Woodhouse subsequently tightened the link between respiratory infections and cardiovascular disease. They contended that the entire process begins with a modest seasonal decline in the consumption of vitamin C–rich foods. They showed that people who ate less fruit during winter months had lower blood levels of vitamin C and a higher incidence of infections. These infections increased the number of white blood cells, which lead to higher blood levels of fibrinogen and a greater likelihood of blood clots.

In contrast, subjects who happened to take supplemental vitamin C had higher blood levels of the vitamin and much lower levels of fibrinogen and other blood-clotting substances. How does vitamin C help? Drs. Khaw and Woodhouse felt that vitamin C improves the body's response to infection.[50] We believe that a higher intake of vitamin C would substantially reduce the risk of infection and cardiovascular disease.

VITAMIN C AND CANCER

Just as chronic inflammation and infection are associated with cardiovascular diseases, they are also linked to cancer risk. Although the details are not yet well understood, vitamin C supplements do improve the well-being and life expectancy of cancer patients.

In the 1970s, Dr. Linus Pauling and a Scottish physician, Ewan Cameron, M.B., F.R.C.S., began exchanging ideas on how the body might fight cancer. They thought that vitamin C would provide a number of benefits, such as promoting collagen production to encapsulate the tumor and stimulating neutrophils and macrophages to seek out and destroy cancer cells. When

Dr. Cameron inquired about specific dosages, Dr. Pauling recommended 10 grams of vitamin C daily.

In 1972, Dr. Cameron began treating terminal cancer patients with large intravenous doses of vitamin C. Most of the patients lived two months, but those receiving large amounts of vitamin C lived fourteen months, seven times longer! A couple of the patients were actually "cured" of their cancers.[51,52]

Abram Hoffer, M.D., Ph.D., a psychiatrist in Victoria, Canada, took Dr. Pauling's vitamin C regimen for cancer patients a step further. He began treating cancer patients for anxiety and depression subsequent to their diagnosis. Because he had successfully used large doses of vitamins to treat schizophrenic patients, he adapted the regimen to cancer patients. The program, which includes large amounts of vitamin C, the B-complex vitamins, and vitamin E, improved survival of cancer patients even more. When Dr. Pauling analyzed the data about Dr. Hoffer's patients, he determined that this broader nutritional program increased life expectancy by twelve to twenty times.[53,54]

With such findings, it should come as no surprise that high vitamin C consumption is associated with longevity. James E. Enstrom, Ph.D., of the University of California, Los Angeles, analyzed the dietary habits of eleven thousand people recorded over a ten-year period. Dr. Enstrom found that men who consumed at least 300 milligrams of vitamin C daily from food or supplements suffered 41 percent fewer deaths compared with men who consumed only 50 milligrams of the vitamin. In fact, the men consuming 300 milligrams or more of vitamin C lived approximately six years longer than those eating very little vitamin C. Women consuming large amounts of vitamin C also lived longer than those who consumed less, although the difference was not as dramatic.[55]

Recommendations

Based on the theoretical, clinical, and experimental evidence, we wholeheartedly agree with Dr. Stone's view that vitamin C is an essential metabolite. Though humans cannot produce vitamin C in their bodies, they clearly need and benefit from large amounts of it. This has been demonstrated time and again when people take vitamin C supplements to prevent or treat disease.

We consider vitamin C to be the single most important supplemental nutrient for maintaining a strong, efficient immune system and recovering from infections. If you don't like taking supplements, or if money is tight, vitamin C is the one you *should* take.

As a preventive dose for adults, we recommend daily consumption between 1,000 to 10,000 milligrams daily, depending on your individual bowel tolerance and how much money you're inclined to spend on supplements. This is a very broad range, and you'll have to determine what works best for you. When you experience the first symptoms of an infection, increase your intake of vitamin C using Dr. Cathcart's bowel tolerance concept as a guide. Having mildly loose stools for a few days is preferable to suffering from an infection.

In general, we recommend that you divide your vitamin C so you take it at least twice daily, and four times daily would be even better. Doing so increases vitamin C's absorption, reduces its excretion, and maintains relatively steady blood levels of the vitamin. Time-release tablets are another option, but they're about twice the price of plain vitamin C. If you go the time-release route, read the label to ensure that the time-release method is based on a "wax matrix." Other types of time-release products tend to dissolve faster—that is, more like regular tablets.

Dr. Pauling used to take vitamin C by simply dissolving crystals in a glass of water. Some people have argued that the acidity of vitamin C could damage tooth enamel, but Dr. Pauling had his natural teeth until the day he died at ninety-three. If you tend to have weak enamel, you might do better with tablets or capsules. Buffered, nonacidic vitamin C is another option.

Should you buy natural or synthetic vitamin C? All of the vitamin C on the market is ascorbic acid, and most of it is synthesized from corn sugar. A few products contain ascorbic acid from sago palm or beets. So-called rose hips (the meat of rose fruit) products actually contain ascorbic acid with a small amount of added rose hips. A tablet containing 100 milligrams vitamin C exclusively from rose hips would be too large to swallow. There may be some nutritional value to the rose hips, but tablets just don't supply much of them, and so rose hips is more window dressing than anything else. On the other hand, vitamin C tablets with added flavonoids (sometimes called bio-flavonoids) are quite worthwhile. Flavonoids will be discussed in Chapter 16.

Several year ago, a company introduced an "esterified" vita-min C supplement. Often referred to generally as "ester C," this type of vitamin C is supposed to be able to be absorbed very well. Is it? Some respected researchers and physicians argue that it is, but the real question is whether the difference between Ester C® and plain old vitamin C is worth a price that is 25 to 50 percent higher.[56] In addition, Dr. Pauling, without question the most brilliant chemist of the century, pointed out that there is no such thing as a vitamin C ester (a chemical resulting from the reaction of an acid and an alcohol). Plain old vitamin C is an inexpensive and effective step toward achieving optimal immunity. We recommend that you stick with it.

13

VITAMIN A AND THE CAROTENES: THE "2-CENT SOLUTION"

———————— ✤ ————————

Discovered in 1913, vitamin A is well known for its essential roles in promoting healthy vision and skin. It also ensures proper cell differentiation—something that goes awry in cancer—and is one of the most powerful, fastest-acting immune stimulants. Yet newspaper and magazine articles that laud vitamin supplements routinely warn readers about the dangers of vitamin A overdose.

The body, with impressive efficiency, stores unused vitamin A in the liver. However, the risk of vitamin A toxicity is more theoretical than real. Vitamin A overdose *can* occur, and occasionally *does*. But vitamin A overdoses are actually quite rare, whereas inadequate consumption of vitamin A is common.

The medical emphasis on risks, instead of benefits, has been clearly misplaced, and if a vitamin has ever needed public relations, this is the one. Misconceptions about vitamin A abound even among people who work in the field of nutrition. Consider, for example, that the latest edition of the *Recommended Dietary*

Allowances, published by the federal government, describes vitamin A deficiency as "rare" in the United States.[1]

Despite the authority of this official pronouncement, dietary surveys suggest the very opposite. Half of Americans consume 19 percent *or less* of the RDA for vitamin A, and one-fourth of the population consumes no more than 11 percent of the RDA.[2] Under these circumstances, the majority of people are really walking wounded, immunologically speaking. Alarmist warnings about the dangers of vitamin A only serve to deprive large numbers of people of a profoundly important nutrient.[3]

The most dramatic recent research on vitamin A shows that one or two high-potency capsules can reduce the severity of infections, often preventing death, without even the most remote risk of toxicity. Vitamin A's value is especially well documented in the treatment of measles, but it also benefits children with chicken pox, respiratory infections, and AIDS. Clearly, it is an essential nutrient for optimal immunity.

The "Anti-Infective" Vitamin

As a group, vitamin A compounds are known to chemists as retinoids, and the form of vitamin A in the bloodstream is retinol. Mild dietary deficiencies of the vitamin result in night blindness, which prevents the eyes from adjusting rapidly to bright headlights or to the dark interior of a movie theater. The condition is easily treated with vitamin A supplements. More severe deficiencies cause xerophthalmia, an inflammation and drying of the eye that, if untreated, causes permanent blindness. In addition, dermatologists use a synthetic form of the vitamin to treat acne, psoriasis, age spots, and fine wrinkles.

The role of vitamin A in immunity has, over the years, taken a backseat to its application in visual and skin disorders. But the use of vitamin A in the treatment of infection dates back to at least the seventeenth century, when cod liver oil (which contains vitamins A and D) was used to treat tuberculosis.[4] In 1922, shortly after the vitamin was isolated, researchers discovered that it was essential for the normal development of epithelial cells, which form a protective barrier around many organs. This role, it turns out, is not the only way vitamin A helps immunity. The vitamin also stimulates the production of antibodies, and it primes powerful T cells into action against bacteria and viruses.[5]

In the 1920s, during the heady early days of vitamin discoveries, researchers followed the fashion of defining vitamins by what they cured. Thus, they described vitamin C as the antiscorbutic vitamin because it cured scurvy, and vitamin D as the antirickets factor because it prevented rickets. At that time, in the *British Medical Journal*, two researchers at the University of Sheffield, England, called vitamin A the "anti-infective" vitamin. They reviewed the human and animal research linking vitamin A deficiency to abnormal epithelial cells and to lowered resistance against infections. In experiments, the researchers found that laboratory animals lived for months in "fair health" despite eating a diet deficient in vitamin A. Then, their health took a sudden downturn and the animals died. Detailed postmortems found extensive infections of the internal organs.[6]

For reasons not entirely clear, infections prompt the rapid excretion of vitamin A, sometimes inducing deficiency states where none previously existed. In a study of twenty-nine men suffering from either pneumonia or sepsis (a blood infection), doctors noted that one-third of the men excreted 50 percent of the RDA and one-fourth excreted 100 percent of the RDA for vitamin A. Men receiving aminoglycosides (a class of antibiotics that includes streptomycin and gentamicin) also had high rates of vitamin A loss.[7] In contrast, healthy men excreted almost no vitamin A. Such extensive losses of vitamin A further compromise immunity and increase the risk of secondary infection and slow recovery. Of course, the situation would be even worse for people who had only marginal vitamin A intake before an infection.

VITAMIN A AND MEASLES

Interest in vitamin A as an anti-infective vitamin has been renewed, thanks largely to the research and eloquent arguments of Alfred Sommer, M.D., professor and dean at the school of hygiene and public health, Johns Hopkins University. About fifteen years ago, Dr. Sommer and his colleagues discovered that *occasional* vitamin A supplements could dramatically reduce the death rate of malnourished children, particularly those infected with measles.

A simple vitamin treatment for measles may not seem, at first, terribly significant in the United States, where immunizations have almost completely eradicated the disease. But it is important for several reasons. First, an immunization might improve resistance to measles, but it cannot correct an underlying vitamin A deficiency, which increases susceptibility to other infectious diseases. In fact, overreliance on immunization might instill a dangerous sense of complacency. Second, in developing nations, measles is far more than a nuisance childhood infection. It is a plague that kills millions of malnourished children each year—far more than does the occasional Ebola outbreak. Third, the successful treatment of measles provides further proof that the vitamin does offer a bulwark against infection. It is also, as Dr. Sommer has observed, a simple two-cent solution for protecting these children.[8] And fourth, the evidence suggests that the value of vitamin A probably applies to other infections as well.

In 1976, with Indonesian researchers, Dr. Sommer launched a study on the relationship between xerophthalmia and vitamin A deficiency in malnourished children. They collected the data in three years, and by 1981, most of it had been published.[9] But a much more dramatic finding lay buried in their statistics.

In December 1982, Dr. Sommer and his colleagues realized that large numbers of children with xerophthalmia, caused by a severe deficiency of vitamin A, were "dropping out" of the study. Puzzled, they ran their computer analysis in reverse. The children with xerophthalmia hadn't just dropped out. They had died at a rate much faster than those without the eye disease. Further analysis revealed that the most significant consequence of vitamin A deficiency was death from infection, not blindness.

The sequence of events was this: vitamin A deficiency led to the hardening of the epithelial lining of the respiratory and gastrointestinal tracts, weakening a key barrier to infection. Contracting an infection further depleted vitamin A levels and caused diarrhea. The diarrhea interfered with the absorption of fat-bound nutrients, including vitamin A. Poor nutrient absorption exacerbated the situation, resulting in further malnutrition, blindness, and death.

Based on the data, Dr. Sommer estimated that vitamin A supplements might reduce the death rate in children ages one through six by about 20 percent.[10,11] So with the approval of the Indonesian government, the researchers immediately began a follow-up study involving more than twenty thousand preschool children in 450 Indonesian villages. Half of the children received 200,000 IU of vitamin A once every six months. These children had a death rate one-third that of children not receiving the vitamin.[12]

Dr. Sommer and his colleagues knew that the measles virus attacked the body's protective epithelial cells and that a measles infection rapidly depleted the body's vitamin A stores. So in another study, he and his colleagues gave 200,000 IU of vitamin A on two successive days to Tanzanian children hospitalized with measles. The death rate of these children dropped by half.[13]

The medical response, wrote Dr. Sommer, was "the long silence of disbelief." He understood why. "With its vision fixed on the high-tech and high-cost frontiers of modern medical care," he explained, "the medical and research establishment found it difficult to accept that something as simple and cheap as a 2-cent capsule of vitamin A could represent such a breakthrough for human life and health."[14]

Reducing the death rate of children by one-third to one-half, however, was sufficient justification for the World Health Organization and UNICEF to incorporate vitamin A as part of its treatment for measles. By 1992, several other studies in Ghana, India, Indonesia, and Nepal supported the original observation that vitamin A supplements reduced death from measles by about one-third. Since then, a large number of African, Asian, and Latin American nations have adopted large-scale programs to supplement children with vitamin A.[15]

The benefits of vitamin A, however, extend beyond measles infections and to the life expectancy of children in general. Wafaie W. Fawzi, M.D., of the Harvard University School of Public Health recently reported that vitamin A supplements (200,000 IU), given once every six months, substantially decreased the risk of death from all causes among twenty-eight thousand Sudanese children. The vitamin had the most dramatic effect on children who were wasted, stunted, or with diarrhea or cough.[16]

Domestically, the American Academy of Pediatrics' infectious disease committee has recommended that U.S. physicians also consider vitamin A administration for the treatment of measles when signs of vitamin A deficiency are evident. In its guidelines, the academy suggested one dose of 200,000 IU of vitamin A for children over twelve months of age, followed by additional doses the next day and four weeks later. For infants ages six to twelve months, the academy recommended half the dose on the same schedule.[17]

VITAMIN A AND OTHER INFECTIONS

Because measles is partly a respiratory infection, physicians have begun investigating the protective role of vitamin A in other infections, particularly those of the lungs. Vitamin A–dependent epithelial tissues line the bronchial tubes and lungs, and the vitamin appears essential to many aspects of normal lung development and function.[18] Because infection interferes with vitamin A, the body will need, at least for a while, above average amounts of the vitamin to heal injured tissues.[19]

Barney S. Graham, M.D., Ph.D. of the Vanderbilt University School of Medicine, Nashville, measured the severity of respiratory syncytial virus (RSV) infections in twenty-three children by how much "mechanical" assistance they needed to breathe. RSV is a very serious infection affecting several hundred thousand children and hospitalizing some 4,500 annually in the United States. Dr. Graham found that children with lower vitamin A levels had greater difficulty breathing and needed more medical intervention. The likely benefits of vitamin A supplementation, Dr. Graham and his colleagues noted, were faster healing of epithelial tissues, less risk of secondary infections, and a stronger immune response to the infection.[20]

Another team of physicians has described how one single dose of vitamin A (200,000 IU) sped the recovery of forty-seven children infected with chicken pox. Unlike the children in many other studies, all of these apparently had adequate vitamin A intake. The doctors reported that crusting of the lesions, indicative of recovery, occurred sooner among the children given the vitamin A, compared with a group that did not receive the vitamin. The lesson, again, is that adequate or normal levels of vitamin A may not always be optimal levels.

When vitamin A supplements are given earlier—preventively—the results are even better. The doctors also gave vitamin A supplements to eight siblings of infected children during the incubation period for chicken pox. These children recovered faster than their siblings. None of the children receiving vitamin A suffered secondary complications, but five children in a control group had complications, including viral pneumonia, conjunctivitis, and gastroenteritis.[21]

Even children with AIDS seem to benefit from vitamin A supplements. Both measles and AIDS trigger a rapid decline in the number of T cells (although the effect in measles is usually temporary), and vitamin A supplements increase T cell counts and antibody responses.[22]

Anna Coutsoudis, Ph.D., of the University of Natal, South

Africa, gave vitamin A supplements to 118 infants of HIV-infected women. Both mothers and infants (at age one month) had normal vitamin A levels. Half of the infants received vitamin A supplements every three months until they reached fifteen months of age. (We do *not* recommend giving vitamin A to infants without guidance from a physician.) Eighty-five of the infants were later diagnosed with HIV infections. Infants receiving vitamin A supplements suffered fewer illnesses, ranging from simple rashes to respiratory infections, *regardless* of whether they were infected with HIV. The children with HIV suffered less diarrhea, helping them avoid a deadly cycle of infection, malabsorption, and malnutrition.[23]

The Carotenoids and Immunity

More than six hundred carotenoids occur in plants, and about forty are found in vegetables and fruits in the average American diet. They are associated with vitamin A because the body converts some beta-carotene and other carotenoids to vitamin A.

In plants, carotenoids function as pigments, adding color, and as antioxidants, quenching damaging free radicals generated during photosynthesis. Beta-carotene is a common plant carotenoid and, as an example, accounts for about two-thirds of the carotenoids found in carrots. When people eat these carotenoids, they also derive benefits from the carotenoids' antioxidant qualities. In fact, the carotenoids are very powerful antioxidants, whereas vitamin A is only a mild antioxidant.

Researchers reported back in the 1930s that dietary carotenoids protected against ear, bladder, and other types of bacterial infections. But until 1958, the medical community assumed the health benefits of beta-carotene were related strictly to its role as a vitamin A precursor.[24] Even after the relationship between beta-carotene and immunity was identified, the nutrient remained in the shadow of vitamin A. That changed in 1982, when the U.S. National Academy of Science's *Diet, Nutrition and*

Cancer report recommended diets high in beta-carotene and low in fat to reduce the risk of cancer.[25]

Practically overnight, beta-carotene was recognized as a nutrient in its own right. Around two hundred studies have reported that diets high in vegetables and fruit (and thus high in beta-carotene) lower the risk of cancer and heart disease.[26] Many of these studies have also shown a specific relationship between low dietary beta-carotene and the increased risk of heart disease[27,28] and cancer.[29,30] Finally, diets high in beta-carotene appear to be more protective against heart disease and cancer than do diets high in vitamin A.[31]

BETA-CAROTENE AND IMMUNITY

Like vitamin A, beta-carotene stimulates many aspects of immunity. While it does not always have the dramatic therapeutic benefits of vitamin A in treating infections, it does seem to be more protective on a long-term basis against cancer. Beta-carotene enhances the activity of T cells and antibody-producing B cells, and boosts the tumor-destroying ability of macrophages, natural-killer cells, and cytotoxic T cells.[32]

Beta-carotene's antioxidant properties make it an ideal complement to vitamin A. As you recall, white blood cells use large numbers of free radicals to kill bacteria. After an infection, many of these free radicals can damage healthy cells and DNA, contributing to cardiovascular disease and cancer.

Like vitamin C, beta-carotene plays a dual role in immunity. First, it helps white blood cells produce more free radicals to kill bacteria. Second, it helps clean up many of the excess free radicals during and after an infection, thereby reducing free radical damage to DNA.[33] This protective role was well illustrated in a study that found beta-carotene to protect against radiation-induced free radical damage to chromosomes.[34]

Unchecked, free radicals can also suppress immunity[35] and damage white blood cells.[36] Again, beta-carotene comes to the rescue by protecting neutrophils against free radical damage.[37]

Supplements of this nutrient also prevent immune depression triggered by excessive exposure to sunlight.[38]

Conversely, low intake of beta-carotene may predispose people to immune depression, particularly if their health has already been compromised by infection or other stresses. Magdy S. Mikhail, M.D., a gynecologist at the Albert Einstein College of Medicine, New York, has suggested that low beta-carotene in vaginal tissues might leave women susceptible to *Candida albicans* infections. Whether decreased levels of beta-carotene or the *Candida albicans* infection (which can depress immunity by itself) comes first is not entirely clear. But certainly, Dr. Mikhail has observed, low levels of beta-carotene in vaginal tissues impair the local immune response to *Candida albicans*. Even semen, which is immunosuppressive, can alter the local immune response, and beta-carotene may very well shore up a person's defenses.[39]

Beta-carotene supplements also increase the ratio between T4 and T8 cells.[40] This is especially important to people infected with HIV, because they have relatively few T4 cells. Given the relationship between beta-carotene and immunity, a number of researchers have investigated whether this nutrient might be of value in the treatment of HIV infections or AIDS. People with HIV are frequently deficient in, or have abnormal metabolism of, many nutrients essential for immunity, including vitamin A, vitamin C, vitamin E, vitamins of the B complex, selenium, and zinc.[41,42] AIDS patients also suffer from fat malabsorption and diarrhea, which further reduce beta-carotene levels in the body.[43]

As with measles, a vicious cycle of malabsorption and malnutrition develops in AIDS, and correcting it can be difficult but not necessarily impossible. Large doses of beta-carotene ensure that at least some of the nutrient is actually absorbed, helping the body restore some immune functions. Harinder S. Garewal, M.D., of the University of Arizona Cancer Center found that supplements of 60 milligrams (100,000 IU) of beta-carotene daily increase the number of natural-killer cells, which help defend the body.[44] Similarly, Gregg O. Coodley, M.D., of the Oregon

Health Sciences University, has reported that large supplemental doses of beta-carotene—180 milligrams, equivalent to 300,000 IU—boost T4 cells by an average of 13 percent.[45,46]

When it comes to HIV, though, beta-carotene is only the tip of the proverbial iceberg. Giving RDA levels of nutrients to people infected with HIV cannot compensate for the biochemical havoc created by the disease. Much higher doses are required. Marianna Baum, Ph.D., R.D., of the University of Miami School of Medicine, recently showed that people infected with HIV need five times the RDA for vitamin E; ten times the RDA for vitamin A, vitamin B_6, and zinc; and twenty-five times the RDA for vitamin B_{12} to achieve *normal* blood levels of these nutrients.[47]

Furthermore, carotenoids other than beta-carotene function as antioxidants and build resistance to disease. These other carotenoids include alpha-carotene, lycopene, lutein, zeaxanthin, cryptoxanthin, and gamma-carotene. The *diversity* of these antioxidants in the diet may be every bit as important as their amounts.[48] While some supplements contain large amounts of specific carotenoids, a diet with a diverse selection of vegetables and fruit provides many others.

Recommendations

Because vitamin A, beta-carotene, and other carotenoids have independent roles in immunity and other aspects of health, it only makes sense to consume *all* of them as part of a program to achieve optimal immunity. As a baseline, we recommend that you eat organically produced foods rich in these nutrients.

Liver, eggs, fish, and fortified whole-milk products are excellent sources of vitamin A. Vegetables and fruit contain the carotenoids, but ratios of individual carotenoids vary from food to food. For example, carrots contain a 2:1 ratio of beta-carotene to alpha-carotene. Pumpkins have more alpha- than beta-carotene but, ounce for ounce, fewer carotenoids than carrots. Cooking breaks down the cell walls of vegetables and provides 30 percent more carotenoids than raw carrots. All things considered, vegetable soup is one of the best sources of mixed carotenoids.

VITAMIN A SUPPLEMENT RECOMMENDATIONS

If you want to add supplements, how much vitamin A should you take? If you are prone to infections, we recommend 10,000 IU of vitamin A daily as a safe range for most adults. During an infection, *brief* high doses of vitamin A—50,000 to 100,000 IU *for a couple of days*—can strengthen epithelial cells and resistance in both adults and children.

In general, scare tactics about the dangers of vitamin A are an overreaction to a potential risk and discourage people from taking a supplement that has a profound, beneficial effect on immunity. Vitamin A toxicity generally doesn't occur unless someone consumes and stores more than 1,000,000 IU in a two- to three-week period.[49] Sometimes, overdoses can occur when people take 50,000 to 100,000 IU daily for several months. Symptoms include headache, vomiting, loss of hair, dryness of the skin and mucous membranes, bone pain, and liver damage. If you're taking vitamin A supplements and have any of these symptoms, stop until you and your physician determine whether they are related to the vitamin.

There's one other important caution with respect to vitamin A. In 1995, a researcher at the Boston University School of Medicine reported that vitamin A intake above 10,000 IU daily around the time of conception or during the first trimester of pregnancy increased the risk of delivering a baby with birth defects.[50] Vitamin A deficiency can also cause birth defects.[51] Our advice: if you're planning to have a baby or are pregnant, don't take supplements with more than 5,000 IU of vitamin A.

CAROTENE SUPPLEMENT RECOMMENDATIONS

In contrast to vitamin A, natural carotenoids are generally non-toxic, and the only effect of an overdose is a yellowing of the skin. If the yellowish tone isn't appealing to you, simply stop taking carotenoid supplements until the color goes away. The body safely stores carotenoids and converts them to vitamin A only as needed. The only exception appears to be heavy smokers who have smoked for years. Two studies have shown that high levels of *synthetic* beta-carotene supplements slightly increased the risk of developing lung cancer, although people in the same studies eating diets rich in beta-carotene had a low incidence of cancer.

Questions have also been raised regarding how much beta-carotene (and presumably other carotenes) from food is actually absorbed and converted to vitamin A. Saskia de Pee, M.Sc., of the Wageninen Agricultural University, Netherlands, found that an extra serving of dark green vegetables did not increase blood levels of vitamin A. In contrast, beta-carotene supplements *were* converted to vitamin A. Dr. de Pee suspected that the carotenoids in the vegetables were bound in a tight nutritional matrix, whereas beta-carotene supplements were far more easily absorbed.[52]

We recommend two natural carotenoid products. The most common one (Betatene®) contains beta-carotene from *Dunaliella salina* algae, grown in Australia. This product is available from a large number of vitamin companies, including Carlson, Solgar, and Twin, which sell through health and natural food stores. This beta-carotene product is also a mixed-carotenoid supplement because it contains 5 percent of numerous other important carotenoids, including alpha-carotene, lutein, zeaxanthin, cryptoxanthin and, in some formulations, lycopene. The other natural product (Caroplex®) contains about two-thirds beta-carotene and one-third alpha-carotene, plus small amounts of lycopene and gamma-carotene. It, too, is sold under a variety of brand names. We do *not* recommend supplements containing synthetic beta-carotene. Look for the word *natural* on the label.

For long-term prevention of disease and optimal immunity, we recommend 15 to 30 milligrams of natural beta-carotene or mixed-carotene supplements daily. Current smokers should not take any more than the modest doses of beta-carotene found in multivitamin supplements.

Sometimes, however, label doses of carotenoids can be confusing. In their research, scientists count carotenoids in milligrams, but most brands of beta-carotene describe their product in international units (IU). In many respects, identifying beta-carotene doses in IU is an anachronism, dating to when carotenoids were perceived as only vitamin A precursors. One milligram of beta-carotene is equivalent to 1,666 IU. To convert IU to milligrams, multiply the number of IU by 0.0006. For example, 25,000 IU equals 15 milligrams of beta-carotene.

In sum, for long-term prevention, eat a diet rich in fruits and vegetables and supplement it with mixed natural carotenoids. When fighting an infection, however, increase your vitamin A for a short period of time.

14

SELENIUM: PROTECTION AGAINST VIRAL MUTATIONS

———————— ✣ ————————

Of all the nutrients essential to immunity, none has suffered the peculiar and unfortunate history of selenium. For years, this mineral was considered nothing less than toxic, an opinion based on old studies passed through scientific generations like folklore. The belief in selenium's toxicity did have a foundation: cows, grazing on plants in the high-selenium soil of South Dakota, have been known to drop over from paralysis.

In 1980, selenium was officially judged as *essential* for the health of people,[1] and in recent years research on the health benefits of the mineral has been conducted at a rapid pace. Experts now acknowledge that the dangers of excessive selenium were greatly overstated.[2]

Most researchers have focused on the role of selenium as an essential component of a powerful antioxidant manufactured by the body. This antioxidant, called glutathione peroxidase, defends specifically against peroxides, a type of free radical that attacks fats. Like other antioxidants, glutathione peroxidase also reduces the risk of developing cancer and heart diseases and stimulates the immune system's response to infections.

In just the past couple of years, researchers have begun realizing that selenium's health benefits go beyond being part of glutathione peroxidase. It prevents the dangerous mutation of one type of common virus—and likely others—meaning that it can prevent the creation of some supergerms. Selenium also seems to slow the progression from HIV to full-blown AIDS. All in all, supplemental doses of selenium rank with vitamins C and A as a powerful promoter of immunity.

Selenium Deficiency and Virus Mutations

Historically, when immunologists and infectious-disease specialists addressed nutritional deficiencies, they thought only about how a grossly inadequate diet might impair a person's immune system. In the 1980s, Chinese researchers noticed a link between a number of viral diseases—including the Coxsackie virus and hepatitis B—and more subtle dietary deficiencies. Building on the Chinese research, a team of American scientists in 1995 reported one of the most remarkable and revolutionary discoveries in modern medicine: a common, relatively benign virus mutates into a deadly supergerm when it happens to infect a nutritionally deficient person or animal.[3]

Although the research focused on only one germ—the Coxsackie virus—the implications are profound and likely relevant to other viruses. Deficiencies of selenium might explain the frequent mutations that occur in the influenza and AIDS viruses, and researchers have begun investigating this possibility. Furthermore, if deficiencies of other nutrients also create supergerms (as well as weaken immunity), many outbreaks and epidemics might be prevented simply by ensuring that people eat adequate diets and take nutritional supplements.

The key researchers in this story, Melinda Beck, Ph.D., a virologist at the University of North Carolina at Chapel Hill, and Orville Levander, Ph.D., a nutritional chemist with USDA's Agricultural Research Service, Beltsville, Maryland, carefully documented how deficiencies of either selenium or vitamin E in animals lead to permanent genetic changes in the Coxsackie virus. Although you may never have heard of the Coxsackie virus, it is far from being an obscure germ. Coxsackie viruses annually infect some twenty million children and adults in the United States, causing sore throats, diarrhea, and a form of the common cold. It is part of the family of viruses that causes polio in people and foot-and-mouth disease in livestock.

Drs. Beck and Levander's research grew out of a medical detective story in China. In many regions of that country, large numbers of peasants have developed Keshan disease, characterized by an enlarged heart and heart failure. By the mid-1980s, Chinese researchers had traced Keshan to a dietary deficiency of selenium, a consequence of eating food grown in selenium-deficient soils. In fact, the Chinese research is what led to selenium being deemed essential to human health.

But while Keshan disease was clearly linked to selenium deficiency, the incidence of the disease was worse in some seasons than in others, so Chinese and American researchers suspected an associated microorganism. They discovered that the Coxsackie virus was involved, but they did not initially understand how or why it became virulent—that is, more dangerous.

In their initial experiments on mice, conducted in the early 1990s, Drs. Beck and Levander determined that animals deficient in either selenium[4,5] or vitamin E[6] transformed the Coxsackie virus from a relatively innocuous germ into one that attacked the heart. Their observation paralleled what researchers saw in Chinese peasants. They also discovered that the virulent form of the Coxsackie virus could subsequently attack heart tissue in healthy animals that were consuming adequate amounts of selenium and vitamin E.

In one of their most significant experiments to date, Drs. Beck and Levander fed mice diets either with or without selenium. After several weeks, they infected all of the mice with the run-of-the-mill Coxsackie virus and, a week later, began comparing hearts from both groups of mice. The Coxsackie virus in animals eating a selenium-rich diet did not mutate. Only those mice eating selenium-deficient diets displayed signs of heart disease. Furthermore, the selenium-deficient mice contained larger numbers of the Coxsackie virus, indicating that it had become more virulent. The mutated virus could also infect healthy mice eating diets with adequate amounts of selenium.

What distinguished this study in the eyes of their fellow scientists was Drs. Beck and Levander's description of the genetic details. By comparing the genes of the benign "parent" Coxsackie virus with that of its virulent descendants, they pinpointed six specific changes. Although it's not yet clear whether one or all of these genetic changes led to a more aggressive virus, the genetic evidence unquestionably demonstrated a clear link between nutritional deficiency and viral mutation.[7]

Both selenium (as part of glutathione peroxidase) and vitamin E function as powerful antioxidants, and this fact did not escape Beck and Levander's attention. These nutrients protect cells and genetic material (DNA and RNA) against damage from free radicals. A deficiency of either nutrient would leave genes, including the genes of the Coxsackie virus, more vulnerable to mutations caused by free radicals.

Selenium and vitamin E also stimulate the immune system, and the Coxsackie virus infection becomes more dangerous when the immune system is incapable of fighting it. This means the virus goes unchecked and can reproduce faster. Furthermore, the Coxsackie virus is an RNA type of virus, meaning that it lacks the ability (found in DNA) to proofread and correct genetic errors. So in the end, the viruses mutate faster and faster and with more and more mutations.

It sounds like science fiction, but it's not. And the health implications are not limited to nutritionally deprived populations, such as the Chinese peasants. "In theory," Drs. Beck and

Levander explained, "it would take only one selenium-deficient person or animal to produce a new family of virus mutants." These mutant viruses could then jump from one species to another and spread throughout the world.[8] Selenium deficiency may very well explain the yearly emergence from China of new influenza strains that originate in ducks, jump to pigs, and then spread to people around the world. In some years, influenza is virulent and deadly enough to be considered a supergerm.

It's also likely that even minor deficiencies of other nutrients contribute to mutations in both viruses and bacteria. But until recently, scientists had not even considered this possibility. "Perhaps virus evolution does depend on what we eat or what we *do not* eat," observed Charles Gauntt, Ph.D., of the University of Texas Health Sciences Center, Austin, and Steven Tracy, Ph.D., in the journal *Nature Medicine*.[9]

Selenium Deficiency and AIDS

Some people live with an HIV infection for a decade before the virus completely destroys the immune system. Others die within a couple of years. Strong theoretical evidence suggests that selenium deficiency triggers, in a variety of ways, the progression of HIV infections into full-blown AIDS. HIV of course, stands for the *h*uman *i*mmunodeficiency *v*irus, which causes AIDS, or the *a*cquired *i*mmuno*d*eficiency *s*yndrome.

In an extraordinarily detailed paper on the genetics of HIV, Ethan Will Taylor, Ph.D., of the College of Pharmacy at University of Georgia, Athens, theorized how this deadly virus might rob the body of selenium and weaken immunity.[10] Dr. Taylor believes that several previously unnoticed genes in HIV create proteins that require selenium. If true, HIV would stress the body's store of selenium—which is typically only about 10 milligrams.

According to Dr. Taylor's theory, when the virus uses all of the selenium in an HIV-infected T cell, it reproduces faster and starts attacking other T cells in search of more selenium. More viruses would further increase the demand for selenium. In addition, HIV and the Coxsackie virus share some genetic similarities, and selenium deficiency might also account for the rapid mutation of HIV. (This rapid mutation rate is one reason why an HIV vaccine has been elusive.) The infection spirals out of control, destroying immunity and leaving a body vulnerable to other infections and cancers, which actually kill AIDS patients.

One would think, though, that a nutritional deficiency would inhibit rather than prompt the replication of HIV. That doesn't seem to be the case here. Indeed, a similar paradox exists with another nutrient, arginine, a deficiency of which stimulates viral replication. Like a hungry lion, HIV doesn't seem to sit around— it aggressively attacks in search of more food.

Ultimately, the entire body's stores of selenium are wiped out by the spreading and selenium-hungry virus. As one consequence, the body cannot produce sufficient quantities of glutathione peroxidase. So as the immune system vainly tries to combat HIV, its vestiges (mostly white blood cells) produce large amounts of free radicals in a last-ditch effort to kill the virus and associated bacterial infections. Without glutathione peroxidase and other protective antioxidants, these free radicals become toxic to the immune system, and the body becomes less able to defend itself.

It would seem to be a no-win situation for the person with AIDS, and nearly every time it is just that. But in theory, supplemental selenium would do two things to limit the damage caused by an HIV infection. First, supplemental selenium would provide what the HIV virus needs, so the virus would stay put and not attack other cells. This is a little like throwing a steak to a hungry animal so it doesn't eat your leg. Second, selenium would keep the person's overall immune system functioning at a reasonable level. That would be analogous to giving you the strength to run away from the animal.

HOW SELENIUM FIGHTS INFECTIONS

Deficiencies of selenium and other nutrients are common among patients with HIV infections or AIDS. Until recently, most researchers assumed that these deficiencies occurred because associated diarrhea prevented normal nutrient absorption. That's not the case, though. Brad Dworkin, Ph.D., of the New York Medical College, has pointed out that the decline in selenium levels parallels the decline in T cells—and the progression from HIV to AIDS—regardless of whether patients suffer diarrhea or malabsorption.[11] The mineral is used up or excreted extremely fast.

Selenium seems to stem supergerm infections in a number of ways apart from its apparent roles in placating hungry viruses. For example, supplements of the mineral directly boost immunity, even in healthy individuals. In an experiment with college students, researchers found that selenium supplements significantly enhance the body's production of white blood cells and specialized infection- and cancer-fighting T cells.[12,13] Conversely, selenium deficiency diminishes the activity of white blood cells and decreases T-cell numbers.[14]

Selenium deficiencies are exacerbated because HIV infection and AIDS create exceptional demands for the mineral. AIDS patients have a very high turnover of T4 cells, with billions of new cells destroyed and replaced daily.[15] These T cells contain selenium, and their loss further depletes selenium levels. Each T4 cell is a potential incubator for HIV—and a potential source of selenium to be raided. All these demands on selenium could divert enough selenium to interfere with the body's production of glutathione peroxidase,[16] which would explain why HIV-infected people are routinely deficient in this powerful antioxidant.[17,18]

Such a profound depletion of glutathione peroxidase would greatly weaken the body's defenses against free radicals, and this is exactly what happens. People infected with HIV are "oxidatively stressed"—that is, their bodies are literally overrun by dangerous free radicals.[19] Incredibly, these free radicals fan the virus like a flame, promoting the activation and reproduction of more HIV.[20] A number of free radicals seem to be involved,[21] but the chief culprit seems to be the peroxide type of free radical that glutathione peroxidase (containing selenium) specifically protects against. Indeed, laboratory experiments have shown that glutathione peroxidase inhibits the replication of HIV.[22,23] In a nutshell, free radicals excite the virus, whereas antioxidant nutrients calm it.

While neither selenium nor any other antioxidant supplement can actually cure an HIV infection, laboratory experiments and clinical studies show that selenium supplements do slow the virus and improve the well-being of infected patients.[24] One of the best studies was conducted by Juliane Sacher, M.D., of Frankfurt, Germany. Dr. Sacher gave fifteen HIV-infected men 200 micrograms of selenium daily for a year. During this time, the patients gained weight and skin conditions related to the infection improved. Some of the men even benefited from an increase in protective T4 cells.[25]

Not surprisingly, supplements of other antioxidant nutrients help control the free radicals that arouse HIV. In a study of 281 HIV-positive men, Alice M. Tang, Ph.D., of Johns Hopkins University, found that a high intake of vitamins A, C, B_1, and B_3 over seven years dramatically slowed the progression of HIV to AIDS. The men consuming larger amounts of these nutrients were 40 to 48 percent less likely to develop full-blown AIDS.[26,27] Vitamins C and A are antioxidants, and B_1 and B_3 help the body produce antioxidants. In addition, the body uses B_3 to repair damaged DNA—something that might be helpful considering that HIV burrows into the DNA of T cells.

Has Selenium Deficiency Fueled the Ebola Virus?

During the spring 1995 outbreak of Ebola hemorrhagic fever in the African nation of Zaire, Dr. Taylor began studying the genetic structure of this virus. He found that, like HIV, Ebola has the potential to create several proteins requiring selenium. In the case of Ebola, though, the selenium content appears much higher than in HIV—perhaps as much as ten times higher.[28] If these selenium-demanding proteins really do exist in Ebola, they may partly account for the speed with which the virus kills, presumably as it ravages the body in search of the mineral. But as savage as the Ebola infection is, 20 percent of the disease's victims do survive. Could the reason be that they have more selenium in their diets?

According to Dr. Taylor's theory, the Ebola virus behaves very much like HIV. When selenium levels in infected cells drop, or are low to begin with, Ebola reproduces and aggressively searches for cells with more selenium, spreading the infection throughout the body. Adding to the gravity of the situation, much of the population of Zaire may be immune compromised and highly vulnerable to infection. Zaire is where both the Ebola and HIV-1 viruses first appeared.[29] In addition, Kaposi's sarcoma, which commonly afflicts AIDS patients, also affects large numbers of central and western African farmers without AIDS.[30]

Why has Zaire become such a viral hot zone for HIV and Ebola, two of the most deadly supergerms? The soils in this part of Africa are deficient in selenium,[31,32] and people are commonly deficient in this mineral.[33] "This raises the possibility that selenium deficiency in host populations may actually foster viral replication," observed Dr. Taylor, "possibly triggering outbreaks and perhaps even facilitating the emergence of more virulent viral strains."[34] And once again, normal immune defenses against the virus would be handicapped by selenium deficiency.

Although the role of selenium deficiency in mutating and fueling Ebola is theoretical, the situation does parallel that of China, where selenium deficiency and the Coxsackie virus together cause Keshan disease. It's also supported by another intriguing piece of evidence. Selenium deficiency has been linked to hemorrhaging—pathological bleeding—in livestock and in people. A number of agricultural and veterinary reports have specifically noted gastrointestinal hemorrhaging, the site of massive bleeding in typical Ebola cases, according to Dr. Taylor.[35]

While there are many types of hemorrhagic fever besides Ebola (e.g., dengue hemorrhagic fever), the underlying mechanism may be the same. In 1993, Chinese doctors described how they used 2 milligrams of selenium daily (no drugs) to treat an outbreak of hemorrhagic fever affecting more than eighty people. The death rate dropped from 22 percent to zero in most infected people and from 100 percent to 36 percent in the most serious infections.[36] The hemorrhagic fever wasn't Ebola—but the parallels and benefits of selenium are too strong to ignore.

There's still one more factor influencing the nutritional availability of selenium—air pollution. "Because sulfur dioxide [a pollutant] reacts with selenium compounds in soil, making it more difficult for plants to absorb, it has long been suspected that fossil-fuel burning and acid rain may be contributing to a gradual decrease of selenium in the food chain," observed Dr. Taylor. "Thus, like deforestation in jungles and rain forests, the resulting alterations in global selenium cycling and distribution may be yet another example of how human activity possibly contributes to the emergence of new viral diseases."[37]

Dr. Taylor has always stressed the theoretical nature of his work. But there is laboratory evidence to support him. Just recently, Bernard Moss, Ph.D., a researcher at the National Institutes of Health, reported that the molluscum contagiosum virus (MCV), a member of the vaccina group of viruses, contains a gene that actually does create selenium-hungry proteins. Taylor suspects the MCV virus acquired this gene from the cell of a mammal, something large viruses commonly do.[38] If viruses can do that, then just about anything is possible.

Recommendations

As an essential component of glutathione peroxidase, selenium provides benefits similar to many other antioxidants—namely, it reduces the risk of cancer and heart disease. Although the area around Rapid City, South Dakota, has often been noted for its high soil and water levels of selenium, as well as the mineral's toxic effect on livestock, the city has the lowest incidence of cancer in the United States. In contrast, Ohio has low selenium levels and an incidence of cancer twice that of South Dakota.[39,40]

The RDA for selenium is 70 micrograms for adult men and 55 micrograms for adult women. Good dietary sources of the mineral include broccoli, fish and shellfish, and grains. Of course, mineral levels in foods reflect mineral levels in the soil and water, and organically grown produce and grain contain higher amounts of selenium than do conventionally grown foods. (See Chapter 9.)

For those people who don't live in South Dakota, selenium supplementation might be a good idea. To maintain optimal immune function, we recommend taking a 200 microgram capsule or tablet of selenium every other day. This is a safe amount.

If you seem to catch every infection that goes by, try increasing your selenium intake to 400 micrograms daily, then reduce the dose to 200 micrograms after a few months. If you are infected with HIV, start with 800 micrograms of selenium daily for a month, then reduce the dosage to 400 micrograms daily. If you travel through Africa or Asia, where outbreaks of various hemorrhagic fevers occur with regularity, selenium supplementation should be de rigueur.

People can consume up to 750 to 850 micrograms of selenium daily without side effects.[41] The symptoms of selenium overdose include the smell of garlic on the breath (when you haven't eaten garlic), loss of hair, and thick but brittle fingernails.

15

COENZYME Q$_{10}$: ONE MORE KEY TO OPTIMAL IMMUNITY

❧

Despite the unusual name, coenzyme Q$_{10}$ (or simply CoQ$_{10}$) is a vitamin-like nutrient that plays one of the most fundamental roles in immunity and overall health. Discovered in 1957, relatively late as vitamins go, CoQ$_{10}$ was for years considered unremarkable. The drug giant Merck, Inc., the first to synthesize CoQ$_{10}$, sold off the process for making it to the Japanese. Then researchers—in Japan, not surprisingly—discovered that CoQ$_{10}$ was essential for heart function.

Today, hundreds of medical journal articles document the benefits of CoQ$_{10}$. It is one of the top five heart medications prescribed in Japan and widely used in Europe as well. But in the United States, CoQ$_{10}$ has been a sad victim of scientific apathy, medical politics, and economic competition. Most American physicians don't have the foggiest notion of what it is, what it does, or how it should be used. Those who have heard of it are skeptical of its use in treating heart failure, cancer, muscular dystrophy, blood infections, and AIDS. Similarly, the Food and Drug Administration has dismissed CoQ$_{10}$ as being worthless—even while the agency ponders approval of a CoQ$_{10}$ "drug" for the treatment of AIDS.

Our description of CoQ$_{10}$ research begins with a necessary but brief discussion of what might strike you at first as being nothing more than arcane science. Bear with us. The significance of CoQ$_{10}$ grows with accumulating and fascinating research on its role in treating heart disease, cancer, and, of course, supergerm infections.

CoQ$_{10}$, CELLULAR ENERGY, AND HEALTH

Shortly after its discovery, CoQ$_{10}$ was saddled with a name that meant little, if anything, to the average person or physician. In retrospect, this unfathomable name—coenzyme Q$_{10}$—has hindered its recognition. The term vitamin is better understood, and the scientists who gave CoQ$_{10}$ its name now regret not simply calling it a vitamin.[1] The substance's chemical name, ubiquinone, is equally esoteric to most people, but more familiar to biochemists. Ubiquinone belongs to a class of common chemicals called quinones that are ubiquitous in plants and animals. Vitamin K, which helps your blood clot after a cut, is a quinone derivative. (And at this point, you probably know more about quinones than your doctor does!)

CoQ$_{10}$ is made in your body when ubiquinone's vitamin, mineral, and amino acid building blocks are present. It's also produced by all other animals and plants, including the broccoli and carrot sticks you snack on, which makes it a nutrient. CoQ$_{10}$'s scientific stature increased measurably when researchers discovered that it is essential for "bioenergetics," that is, energy production in plants and animals.

The generation of energy—to keep your heart beating, wake up in the morning, go to work, and even turn this page—occurs in biological furnaces called mitochondria. These mitochondria, which even contain their own DNA, are highly specialized components of cells. In very simple terms, here's what happens: glucose (blood sugar) is burned in the mitochondria much the way gasoline is burned in a car to release energy, though much more gently. The burning of glucose requires two molecules of a chemical called adenosine triphosphate (ATP). ATP functions like a "portable battery" in that it moves around in the mitochondria and provides an initial jolt of energy wherever needed. ATP cannot provide that burst of energy unless CoQ_{10} is present.

In 1975, Peter Mitchell, Ph.D., theorized that CoQ_{10} works by moving around in a circle picking up and depositing electrons involved in energy production.[2,3] Dr. Mitchell called the process the "Q cycle," and he was awarded the 1978 Nobel prize in chemistry for describing this and other aspects of cellular energy production.

The implications of this seemingly arcane bit of biochemistry are quite significant. You are composed of billions of cells, and your energy as a human being depends on the collective energy output of all of your individual cells. Just as a car engine starts to ping and misfire when it has energy (fuel) problems, a body also starts to ping and misfire when it also has energy problems. And just as inadequate fuel or a weak battery impair the function of an engine, similar problems in people's cells can hurt the entire body. We call the symptoms diseases, and both cars and people have been known to expire under such circumstances.

But CoQ_{10} has an important additional role in the body. It functions as a powerful antioxidant, much like other antioxidant nutrients, such as vitamins C and E. The difference is *where* it works—specifically in the mitochondria. This is significant because over the past several years, researchers have focused on the mitochondria as the place where aging and disease actually originate.

Doctors who study the aging process increasingly believe that aging and age-related diseases are ultimately related to two factors. The first is inadequate bioenergetics in the mitochondria, resulting in large part from a CoQ_{10} deficiency. The second is free-radical damage to mitochondrial DNA, resulting from inadequate levels of CoQ$_{10}$ and other antioxidants.[4,5] Until very recently, researchers assumed that CoQ$_{10}$ levels decreased as a result of aging and disease. But now, some scientists are thinking that aging may occur because of inadequate dietary intake and cellular production of CoQ$_{10}$.

So one of the paradoxes is that CoQ$_{10}$ has not been widely known, and it has been disparaged by the FDA, but its fundamental role in energy production was one of the major discoveries of the twentieth century. This is only one of many CoQ$_{10}$ paradoxes as confounding as its name.

CoQ$_{10}$ and Heart Failure

How is bioenergetics related to fighting infections and supergerms? One of the leading CoQ$_{10}$ researchers, Emile Bliznakov, M.D., has observed that the process of fighting an infection requires a tremendous amount of cellular energy[6]—and consequently, large amounts of ATP and CoQ$_{10}$. In a sense, serious infections drain energy from all of the body's cells.

The basis for this idea comes from studies of CoQ$_{10}$ and cardiomyopathy, a severe weakness of the heart muscle that leads to heart failure. Of all the body's organs, the heart seems most dependent on CoQ$_{10}$. Japanese researchers were the first to notice this relationship in the mid-1960s, and in 1972 a team of American and Italian researchers documented that people with heart disease routinely suffered from low CoQ$_{10}$ levels.

Since then, it has become clear that CoQ$_{10}$ concentrates in the myocardium, or heart muscle. (Heart, an organ meat that few people eat anymore, is by far the richest dietary source of CoQ$_{10}$.) Given CoQ$_{10}$'s role in bioenergetics, the nutrient's role in the heart makes perfect sense. The heart easily qualifies as the body's most energetic organ, beating approximately a hundred thousand times a day and thirty-six million times a year. Without sufficient bioenergetics in the cells of the heart, the organ stops beating.

In the early 1980s, Karl Folkers, Ph.D., then director of the

Institute for Biochemical Research at the University of Texas, and the late Per H. Langsjoen, M.D., conducted the first well-controlled medical study of CoQ_{10} in the treatment of cardiomyopathy. To compensate for the heart's difficulty in pumping blood, the organ enlarges in size, as if bigger were better. The effect of CoQ_{10} supplementation on nineteen patients was simply astounding. All were expected to die from heart failure, but they rebounded with an "extraordinary clinical improvement." The size of their hearts decreased and their pumping ability increased.[7]

Betty Dwyer of Dallas, Texas, was one of the patients in this early study. She was diagnosed at age fifty with cardiomyopathy; her heart was enlarged and weak, pumping only a fraction of the blood her body needed. As a consequence, she was practically an invalid and could barely walk from her bedroom to the bathroom. After two years of conventional treatment, Dr. Langsjoen, Betty's cardiologist, asked her to participate in a research study on CoQ_{10}. Within a few months of taking CoQ_{10} supplements, she noticed a definite improvement. Her heart had become smaller, stronger, and more efficient.[8] Sixteen years later—an astounding length of survival—Betty technically still has cardiomyopathy, but she hardly notices it as long as she takes CoQ_{10}. She now takes 240 milligrams of CoQ_{10} daily, a little more if she's stressed.

The truly curative role of CoQ_{10} in cardiomyopathy was not a minor discovery. But it has gone virtually unnoticed in the United States. Why? Medicine is wedded to high-priced surgery, technology, and drugs. A heart transplant, costing more than $150,000, is considered the ideal surgical treatment for advanced cardiomyopathy and heart failure, and it must be followed with lifelong drug treatment to prevent organ rejection (which sharply increases the risk of infection and other diseases). Furthermore, the two thousand hearts that become available for transplant each year are only a fraction of those needed to help patients with cardiomyopathy or heart failure, which is why people hear so many calls to become organ donors.

CoQ$_{10}$, however, could eliminate the need for many, perhaps even most, heart transplants. It's a natural substance and relatively inexpensive—perhaps $10 a month for a preventive dose and $100 a month for a therapeutic dose. Even a lifetime supply would cost considerably less than a transplant. Used widely, CoQ$_{10}$ could help reduce health care costs.

Hundreds of published medical journal articles, dozens of well-controlled clinical trials (involving thousands of patients), and eight international symposia have demonstrated the value and safety of CoQ$_{10}$. The studies have been published in such mainstream journals as the *American Journal of Cardiology, Clinical Investigator, Biochemical and Biophysical Research Communications,* and the *Japanese Heart Journal.*[9,10]

Today, Peter Langsjoen, M.D., (son of Per) is probably the most seasoned American cardiologist using CoQ$_{10}$ in the treatment of cardiomyopathy and other diseases of the heart muscle. Langsjoen, who practices in Tyler, Texas, used to practice conventional cardiology using such quasi-surgical procedures as balloon angioplasty. He acknowledges that many people do need and benefit from such high-tech procedures, but he prefers CoQ$_{10}$ in his own clinic. "CoQ$_{10}$ is the backbone of my practice—it makes such a dramatic improvement," he said. "It's unthinkable for me to practice medicine without it."[11]

What has kept CoQ$_{10}$ out of the medical mainstream? Langsjoen contends that pharmaceutical companies provide a major share of physicians' post-medical school education, and they are unlikely to promote CoQ$_{10}$ when it can be purchased inexpensively over the counter.[12]

CoQ$_{10}$, Immunity, and Cancer

Research on CoQ$_{10}$ in immunity has followed two general themes: the treatments of cancer and infection. Although there are differences in how the body responds to these two diseases, there is also a common denominator: many components of the immune system scavenge for both cancer cells and germs. For example, CoQ_{10} boosts the activity of various immune system cells that seek out and destroy both cancer cells and bacteria. Sometimes, the line between fighting cancer and infection gets very fuzzy: for example, CoQ_{10} protects against a type of leukemia caused by a virus.[13]

Studies have shown that cancer patients tend to have abnormally low blood levels of CoQ_{10}. The use of CoQ_{10} as an adjuvant cancer treatment began with animal studies and quietly percolated up to include a small number of human patients. Dr. Folkers, one of the pioneers in CoQ_{10} research, began treating a small number of cancer patients in the late 1970s.

At first, the justification was the treatment of heart failure, not cancer. Some of the patients suffered from heart failure as a side effect of chemotherapeutic drugs. In 1993, Dr. Folkers broke his public silence on the matter and described ten cancer patients treated with CoQ_{10}. The one who lived the longest was a forty-eight-year-old man who had been diagnosed with inoperable lung cancer in 1977. He began taking CoQ_{10} the following year, and had a complete remission. When Dr. Folkers wrote his medical paper in 1993, he noted the patient's "exceptional survival for 15 years." In the same paper, Dr. Folkers described nine other cancer patients successfully treated with CoQ_{10}.[14]

Several months later, at the Eighth International Symposium on Biomedical and Clinical Aspects of Coenzyme Q_{10} in Stockholm, Knud Lockwood, M.D., described how CoQ_{10} helped a number of his breast cancer patients.[15] Lockwood, a cancer specialist in Copenhagen treated thirty-two breast cancer patients with daily supplements of antioxidants, essential fatty acids, and 90 milligrams of CoQ_{10}. After two years of treatment, none of the patients had died and all expressed a feeling of well-being, according to an article by Drs. Lockwood and Folkers in *Biochemical and Biophysical Research Communications*. Ordinarily, the researchers wrote, they would have expected to see six deaths.

Six of the thirty-two breast cancer patients had partial tumor remissions, and two had total remissions. In one case, the tumor stabilized at about one-half inch in diameter. When Lockwood boosted the woman's CoQ$_{10}$ intake to 390 milligrams daily, the tumor completely disappeared, and its absence was confirmed by mammography. The other woman had a complete remission of her cancer after taking 300 milligrams of CoQ$_{10}$ daily. Lockwood, who has treated an estimated seven thousand cases of breast cancer over thirty-five years, wrote that until using CoQ$_{10}$, he had never seen a spontaneous or drug-induced remission of breast cancer tumors of one-half to three-quarters of an inch in size.

In a subsequent medical journal article, Drs. Lockwood and Folkers stated that 90 milligrams of CoQ$_{10}$ was probably too low of a dose for most cancer patients. They described three more breast cancer patients who had complete remissions after taking 390 milligrams of CoQ$_{10}$ daily. The response of one forty-four-year-old woman was particularly noteworthy. Her cancer had metastasized to the liver, which is generally a sign of imminent death. She was given CoQ$_{10}$ plus the drug tamoxifen and had a complete remission of her breast and liver cancers.[16]

CoQ$_{10}$ and Infections

Much of the early research on CoQ$_{10}$ and immunity was conducted by Dr. Bliznakov, then president of the New England Institute and, later, head of the Lupus Research Institute. He reported that CoQ$_{10}$ marshaled the body's immune system against infectious organisms—just like it did in the treatment of cancer.

In one experiment, three groups of mice were infected with the parasite that causes malaria. All of the untreated mice died within three weeks. During the same time, even 80 percent of the mice treated with antimalarial drugs died. But when CoQ$_{10}$ was combined with the antimalarial drug, only 42 percent of the mice died. Dr. Bliznakov reported similar benefits in laboratory animals infected with *E. coli, Pseudomonas,* and *Klebsiella* (one type of pneumonia) infections. He emphasized that CoQ_{10} did not act directly against the germs and that it did not produce more immune cells. Rather, CoQ_{10} supercharged immune cells, making them more efficient germ killers.[17,18]

CoQ_{10} can also be of value in the treatment of sepsis, the bacterial infection and poisoning of the blood. This is one of the deadliest supergerm infections, striking 500,000 and killing 175,000 people each year in the United States.[19] The most common causes are two bacteria, *E. coli* and *Staphylococcus aureus.* Even with the use of powerful antibiotics, 35 percent of patients with sepsis die. When the condition degenerates into septic shock, which includes the rapid onset of heart failure, up to 80 percent die.

In a recent experiment, Arnold G. Coran, M.D., and his colleagues at the University of Michigan, Ann Arbor, infected three groups of dogs with lethal doses of live *E. coli* bacteria. One group of dogs was not treated, and two groups received CoQ_{10} (20 milligrams per kilogram of body weight) ten minutes before being infected. All of the untreated dogs died. Although the dogs given CoQ_{10} became extremely ill from the infection, and their heart function was compromised, they survived.[20]

Severe infections stress the immune system, and extreme fatigue (and chronic fatigue syndrome) sometimes follows infections of influenza, Epstein-Barr, and other viruses.[21] The association may be more than coincidence. It's very possible that fighting the infection wipes out the body's store of CoQ_{10} and other nutrients involved in mitochondrial energy production. If this is the case, the road back to health can be very long without heroic efforts to replenish these nutrients. The precedent for treating such fatigue with CoQ_{10} certainly exists with the treatment of hereditary exercise intolerance and fatigue.[22,23]

CoQ$_{10}$ and AIDS

In the mid-1980s, a University of Texas team led by Dr. Folkers and the Langsjoens treated seven HIV patients with CoQ$_{10}$. Four of the patients had full-blown AIDS. The rationale was that AIDS patients often have heart problems, low levels of CoQ$_{10}$, and, obviously, depressed immunity.

All of the HIV patients felt better soon after starting CoQ$_{10}$ supplements, according to a report in *Biochemical and Biophysical Research Communications*. One case history illustrates the value of CoQ$_{10}$. A twenty-two-year-old man with AIDS had suffered from various symptoms including fever, weight loss, and *Candida* yeast. After regularly taking CoQ$_{10}$ supplements, his appetite improved, he suffered less fatigue, and he felt good enough to return to work.[24] Four of the original patients eventually died, and the researchers lost track of two others. The seventh, the one who cooperated the fullest with the treatment program, was still alive and in reasonably good health in 1996.

Before the publication of that medical paper in 1988, the University of Texas, which sponsored the study, applied for a use patent covering the use of CoQ$_{10}$ in the treatment of patients with AIDS and related viruses. Use patents are a type of patent in which people or organizations can obtain rights to the use of a common, natural substance, if they demonstrate that the *use* is original. The use patent, which was granted in 1991,[25] gave the university exclusive rights to sell CoQ$_{10}$ for the treatment of AIDS, assuming the FDA also approved the use of CoQ$_{10}$ for this purpose.

In 1994, the university sold the use patent to Ryan Pharmaceuticals for approximately $200,000. Ryan Pharmaceuticals was soon acquired by Receptagen, a U.S./Canadian biotechnology firm. Receptagen is currently developing *prescription* versions of CoQ$_{10}$ for the treatment of AIDS. Depending on the ultimate value of Receptagen stock, Ryan will make an estimated $2 million from the deal.[26]

Ordinarily, this type of pharmaceutical wheeling and dealing would not be an issue, and to be fair, there are two ways of looking at the issue. On the one hand, CoQ_{10} is a nutrient and a substance produced by every living animal—even lowly protozoa. It is currently sold as a dietary supplement, without a prescription, in health food and natural foods stores. Everyone has access to it and should continue to. Classifying a nutrient or a natural substance like CoQ_{10} as a drug would be tantamount to putting vitamin C, broccoli, or hamburgers on prescription. Its cost would inevitably be higher than without a prescription, and people would not be able to purchase it freely.

On the other hand, Charles Morgan, Ph.D., president of Receptagen, has stated that the company is working on more absorbable forms of CoQ_{10}, which are better suited to medical treatment. He has also indicated that he has no problem competing against over-the-counter CoQ_{10}. A higher grade of prescription CoQ_{10}, he said, would be more acceptable to physicians than a supplement bought at health food stores.[27] He contended, and he may be right, that the stewardship of a pharmaceutical company might bring the benefits of CoQ_{10} to larger numbers of people.

There aren't any easy answers here. And it might not even be an issue were the FDA not so hostile toward CoQ_{10} supplements. Several years ago, in testimony before Congress, FDA commissioner David Kessler, M.D., singled out CoQ_{10} as an unsubstantiated dietary supplement. And encouraged by the FDA, the Texas state department of health briefly banned CoQ_{10} sales. Considering the role of CoQ_{10} in biochemistry, health, and the 1978 Nobel prize in chemistry, these acts were as absurd as trying to ban drinking water. After a few weeks, the state agency backed down in a storm of protest from consumers.

We see a definite need for more powerful CoQ_{10} products where heroic treatments are really required, such as in AIDS. But we believe there is a need to curb excessive profiteering from a common nutrient—and to keep CoQ_{10} on the market as a nonprescription dietary supplement (even if some forms are eventually treated as prescription drugs). Because CoQ$_{10}$ levels in the body decrease with age, it may be worthwhile to take it preventively, the way people take vitamins, instead of waiting until the onset of serious disease.

Recommendations

So, is CoQ$_{10}$ really a vitamin? And how much of it should you take?

Vitamins have traditionally been defined as essential substances that must come from the diet. Because the body can make its own CoQ$_{10}$, it is officially considered nonessential and not a vitamin. But nonessential does not mean unnecessary, and it's reasonable to assume that some people do not produce it as efficiently as others do. It's often simpler to view vitamins and vitamin-like substances as biochemicals, not nutrients.

And so, like other vitamins and biochemicals, CoQ$_{10}$ is essential for life. It also functions at a fundamental level in the body, which accounts for why it has such profound and diverse benefits. People suffering from serious diseases, such as cancer and heart disease, routinely have below normal levels of CoQ$_{10}$. Do they produce less CoQ$_{10}$ because they are sick? Or do they become sick because they produce less CoQ$_{10}$?

The answer, which has relevance to all people, can be found in studies of "mitochondrial" diseases. These conditions include hereditary forms of exercise intolerance and cardiomyopathy, in which the mitochondria fail to produce adequate amounts of energy. Researchers have traced the causes of mitochondrial diseases in part to defects in CoQ$_{10}$ metabolism. Not surprisingly, CoQ$_{10}$ supplements usually help these patients.[28] Researchers have even suggested that aging itself is a mitochondrial disease,[29,30] and CoQ$_{10}$ levels in the body do decrease with age.

Virtually every unprocessed food contains CoQ$_{10}$ or closely related molecules, but the amounts vary greatly. The richest dietary sources of CoQ_{10} are organ meats, particularly heart but also liver and kidneys. Abram Hoffer, M.D., Ph.D., of Victoria, Canada, recently related the case of a patient who obtained a therapeutic intake of CoQ_{10} by eating a diet rich in organ meats.[31] Unfortunately, organ meats are not appetizing to most Americans, who miss out on this source of CoQ_{10}. By comparison, vegetables and fruits contain CoQ_{10}, but in very small amounts.

Can the body make enough to compensate for inadequate dietary levels of CoQ_{10}? Dr. Folkers has expressed doubts. The body's production of CoQ_{10} depends on numerous vitamins and minerals being in the right place at the right time, metabolically speaking. Dr. Folkers recently observed that "many Americans do not have adequate levels of all the vitamins, coenzymes and trace elements for the multistep biosynthesis of CoQ_{10} even for limited health and survival apart from optimum health and survival."[32]

To maintain general health and to reduce your risk of disease, we suggest 10 to 30 milligrams of CoQ_{10} daily. Don't be surprised by CoQ_{10}'s bright orange color—it's the natural color of the molecule. To enhance its absorption, take it with a small amount of oily or fatty food—oil and vinegar dressing on a salad, a piece of bread with butter, some peanut butter, or a regular meal.

The therapeutic dose for the treatment of cardiomyopathy, heart failure, and cancer ranges from 200 to 400 milligrams daily (in divided doses), ideally under the supervision of the physician already treating you for one of these serious diseases. CoQ_{10} will reduce the cardiotoxicity of some of the chemotherapeutic drugs used in cancer treatment.

CoQ_{10} is exceptionally safe, but there are some situations you should be aware of. If you are taking ACE inhibitors, beta-blockers, or digitalis to treat a heart condition, you may be able to reduce your dose of these drugs after starting CoQ_{10}. With a serious condition, don't experiment with yourself—*insist* that your doctor work with you. Some cholesterol-lowering drugs, such as lovastatin, inhibit the body's production of CoQ_{10}, so they might actually set the stage for heart failure and increase the need for supplementation.[33]

In the treatment of HIV and full-blown AIDS infections, we recommend 200 to 400 milligrams daily. The lower range should be sufficient for people with asymptomatic HIV infections. The higher range might benefit people with AIDS, especially if they also suffer cardiovascular complications.

In his experiment on dogs with a life-threatening *E. coli* infection, Dr. Coran administered 20 milligrams of CoQ$_{10}$ per kilogram of body weight.[34] If we had a serious food-borne infection, such as *E. coli*, we would certainly take large amounts of CoQ$_{10}$ as part of a broader treatment regimen. CoQ$_{10}$ happens to be one of the safest nutrients ever discovered.[35]

16

MORE NUTRIENTS THAT BOOST IMMUNITY

By now, you should appreciate the value of organic foods, probiotics, and garlic in laying the foundation of a healthy immune system. Likewise, you should have gained considerable respect for the roles of vitamins C and A, selenium, and CoQ_{10} in jump-starting the immune system and maintaining a high level of readiness to ward off bacteria and viruses. However, many people struggle day in and day out to feel better but succumb frequently to common colds and flus—and fear the consequences of a supergerm encounter.

If you're one of these "fragile" people who just can't seem to get the upper hand against infections, you may have to do a little more to identify the right combination of nutrients to optimize your immunity. A great many nutrients are involved in the immune system, and a number of scientists have found that something as simple as a multivitamin or multimineral supplement can do wonders for people, such as the elderly, who routinely have weak immune systems. Often, the key is not the amount of a nutrient so much as the *diversity* of immune-stimulating nutrients.

But let's assume you've followed all or most of our advice and you want to do more. This chapter describes a large number of nutrients, some easily available in foods as well as supplements, which we also consider important for optimal immunity. From a biological standpoint, some of these nutrients, such as the B vitamins, are of fundamental importance to immunity. Others, such as bee propolis, contain various building blocks for the immune system. We provide some guidelines for taking these nutrients and fine-tuning your immunity.

Amino Acids and Peptides

Amino acids are the building blocks of protein. Twenty are required in human health, and eight of these are considered essential nutrients because the body cannot make them. All of the other twelve amino acids are considered *non*essential because the body can ordinarily make them from the essential ones. Not all people make the nonessential amino acids efficiently, and the often dramatic benefits of single amino acid supplements suggests that amino acid problems may be common.

One amino acid, lysine, improves the body's ability to fight infections. Carnitine, a nutrient composed of two amino acids (lysine and methionine) also helps, and a related substance, glutathione, is an especially powerful immune stimulant. Glutathione is considered a tripeptide because it consists of three amino acids. Peptides are more complex in structure than amino acids, but they are not quite proteins.

LYSINE

Lysine has become a modern-day folk remedy for herpes simplex infections, and there is sound evidence to support its anti-infective role. A study of forty-three patients in the 1970s found that lysine supplements (300 to 1,200 milligrams per day) accelerated recovery from herpes infections and reduced their recurrence.[1]

In a follow-up study, more than 1,500 people were queried after taking about 1 gram of supplemental lysine daily for six months. These people suffered from cold sores, canker sores, and genital herpes. Eight-four percent said that supplemental lysine reduced the frequency of their herpes outbreaks. The herpes lesions of those who took lysine generally healed in less than five days, compared with six to fifteen days among those not taking the amino acid.[2]

In contrast, the amino acid arginine seems to promote replication of the herpes virus. Lysine might work in part by suppressing arginine activity. In addition to taking lysine supplements, consider increasing foods high in lysine (such as potatoes and pork) and decreasing foods high in arginine (such as nuts and chocolate). There's no hard evidence showing that lysine is of benefit in other infections, but we think it might be.

CARNITINE

Carnitine, composed of two amino acids (lysine and methionine), works closely with CoQ_{10} and transports fats into the mitochondria where they are burned as fuel. Infections appear to deplete carnitine levels, whereas supplements seem to restore the immune response. In one study, doctors gave 2 grams of acetyl-L-carnitine (a more biologically active form of the amino acid) daily to ten patients with full-blown tuberculosis. After thirty days, their T cells showed more antibacterial activity.[3]

The most dramatic recent findings relate to the use of carnitine in the treatment of AIDS. Several years ago, a team of Italian researchers suspected that AIDS patients were deficient in carnitine because of muscle weakness and cardiac symptoms. Nearly three-fourths of the patients tested had carnitine levels substantially below normal. The researchers found that 6 grams of carnitine daily for two weeks significantly increased the activity of AIDS patients' white blood cells and other measures of immunity.[4,5]

GLUTATHIONE

Several glutathione-containing compounds are involved in immunity, detoxification of hazardous compounds (such as alcohol, cigarette smoke, and pollutants), and quenching free radicals. One of the more important compounds, glutathione peroxidase, requires selenium to function as an antioxidant. (See Chapter 14.) Another related compound, glutathione-S-transferase, helps the body break down toxic substances.

Although the body produces glutathione, it may not make enough, particularly when fighting infections. One of the building blocks of glutathione is cysteine, an amino acid. Both glutathione and cysteine contain sulfur molecules, which are essential for immunity, and the remarkable immune-stimulating properties of garlic may be partly due to all the sulfur it contains.

A number of medical journal articles have reported that glutathione or glutathione-S-transferase can protect against infections. Animal studies have reported that glutathione can help defend against the malaria parasite and worms that infect the livers of sheep. At least one drug company is investigating glutathione "mimics"—chemicals that function similarly.

Recent studies have demonstrated that glutathione supplements have impressive effects on immunity in very young and elderly people, both of whom commonly have weak immune systems.[6] Considerable attention has focused on the role of glutathione in slowing the progression of HIV infections and AIDS. Free radicals stimulate HIV replication, whereas increases in glutathione peroxidase slow the virus.[7] Indeed, one experiment found that reverse transcriptase activity—the method HIV uses to reproduce—decreased by 80 to 90 percent after treatment with various forms of glutathione or cysteine.[8] Another recent study suggests that glutathione or N-acetylcysteine, a form of cysteine, might prevent T cells from being destroyed by free radicals, particularly in AIDS.[9]

RECOMMENDATIONS

Individual amino acid supplements are sold through health food stores, though some of them are expensive. Still, if they lead to a significant improvement in your health, they may be worth the price. There are also indirect and less expensive ways to increase amino acid levels. Lysine, which is comparatively cheap, is one of the building blocks of carnitine. Taking it can help your body produce more carnitine on its own. Similarly, modest amounts (500 milligrams per day) of supplemental vitamin C increase blood levels of glutathione by 50 percent.[10] Likewise, N-acetylcysteine supplements boost the body's glutathione levels.

These individual amino acid supplements are often referred to as "free" amino acids because they are not bound to others in a protein matrix. If they are consumed with protein, the amino acids end up competing with each other, and their effectiveness will diminish. Because of this, individual amino acids are best taken twenty to thirty minutes before you eat or drink anything in the morning.

B-Complex Vitamins

The B-complex vitamins are necessary for some of the most fundamental aspects of life and, therefore, for immunity and overall health. For example, DNA (the complex molecule that forms our genetic blueprint) is made from different arrangements of four compounds called bases, adenine, guanine, cytosine, and thymine. The body must have various B vitamins to make and repair these bases. For example, thymine depends on vitamins B_3 and B_6, guanine and adenine need folic acid, and cytosine must have B_3. Impair the body's production of any of these bases and everything falls like a house of cards. For example, a deficiency of folic acid leads to DNA damage and potentially cancer.

B vitamins promote the normal activity of various parts

of the immune system, such as white blood cells, T cells, and antibodies. Some, such as folic acid, do double duty in that they are required for more than one aspect of immunity. In this respect, vitamin B_6 (also known as pyridoxine or pyridoxal 5' phosphate) may be the master B vitamin. Deficiencies hurt the immune system, such as by reducing the numbers of white blood cells and T cells and antibody production. Its deficiency can be induced with isoniazid, one of the antibiotics used to treat tuberculosis.[11]

In a study of eight healthy adults, Simin N. Meydani, D.V.M., Ph.D., of Tufts University found that a B_6-depleted diet significantly reduced the numbers and activity of T cells within three weeks. Short-term supplementation restored much of the immune function, but not entirely, and Dr. Meydani suggested that the elderly in particular might benefit from higher intake of B_6.[12] HIV patients tend also to suffer low B_6 levels.[13] In addition, a recent animal experiment found that excessive exposure to sunlight suppressed immunity, but that vitamin B_6 reversed the effect.[14]

RECOMMENDATIONS

Although vitamin B_6 appears to be the most significant of the B vitamins in terms of immunity, we do not recommend taking this vitamin by itself. We may be overly cautious, but there have been some medical reports suggesting that very high doses of B_6 taken for years can cause nerve damage.

Furthermore, the B-complex vitamins really do work best as a team. They are found in most protein foods, such as meat and fish, as well as grains. If you would like to take the B-complex, we generally recommend "Super B" formulas containing ten milligrams to twenty-five milligrams of the major B vitamins, which include B_1, B_2, B_3, and B_6.

Stress burns up the B vitamins, and if you face a lot of stress at home or work, you might even consider a "super B50" supplement, which contains 50 milligrams of the major B vitamins. If you're already taking a more general multivitamin supplement with B vitamins in these potencies, there is no need to add more. But we also have a caution. In our opinion, many of these B-complex supplements do not contain the proper ratios of B vitamins. For our idea of a balanced formula, refer to the Appendix near the end of this book.

Vitamin E

Vitamin E is probably better known for its role in preventing coronary heart disease than for stimulating immunity. But after conducting an animal experiment in the 1980s, Adrianne Bendich, Ph.D., perceptively observed that the first signs of vitamin E show up as immune problems.[15]

The reason is that white blood cells and T cells are highly susceptible to damage from free radicals, and as a potent antioxidant vitamin E quenches the radicals. As if to guard against this damage, immune cells contain higher levels of vitamin E than do other types of cells. According to Moshen Meydani, Ph.D., of Tufts University, vitamin E "is one of the few nutrients for which higher than recommended amounts have been shown to enhance the immune response and might be needed to maintain the optimum immune response."[16]

To evaluate immune responsiveness, doctors sometimes use what's called a "delayed-type skin hypersensitivity" test. This test involves injecting a small amount of common allergens under the skin to trigger an immune response. Swelling at the injection site indicates a good immune response, whereas a lack of swelling or a slow response is indicative of a weak immune response.

Sluggish immune responses are common among the elderly, but vitamin E supplements can improve immune function in as little as a month. In one experiment, Simin N. Meydani, D.V.M., Ph.D., of Tufts University gave vitamin E to a group of elderly men and women. Numerous aspects of immunity improved, including increased T-cell activity. At the same time, free-radical damage decreased.[17] In a separate and preliminary study, Dr. Meydani found that vitamin E supplements also improved immune function in otherwise healthy young adults.[18]

One of the major litmus tests for supplements, however, is how they modify activity of HIV. In studies, vitamin E has been shown to indirectly inhibit HIV replication by quenching free radicals (which promote HIV replication) and by stimulating various aspects of the immune system.[19] One type of vitamin E, d-alpha tocopheryl succinate, can also stop the growth of cancers, including those caused by retroviruses similar to HIV.[20]

RECOMMENDATIONS

Vitamin E is found in whole wheat grains and bread, wheat germ oil, nuts, sunflower seeds, and minimally processed vegetable oils (such as Hain and other brands sold in natural foods stores). But the dramatic benefits of vitamin E cannot be obtained solely through foods. Supplements are necessary, partly to compensate for high-fat diets. For example, people who eat large amounts of fat have higher requirements for vitamin E to prevent free radical damage to those fats. And people with elevated cholesterol levels seem to benefit the most from vitamin E supplements.

Shopping for vitamin E can be more confusing than for other vitamins. One reason is that the natural sources of this vitamin yield a nutrient more potent than its synthetic form. Thus, we believe you should always purchase the natural form of the vitamin. You can tell the difference by looking closely at the chemical name, tocopherol, on the label. Natural-source vitamin E is referred to as d-alpha tocopherol, d-alpha tocopheryl acetate, or d-alpha tocopheryl succinate. The key here is the "d-alpha," which indicates the molecular rotation of the molecule. The synthetic vitamin E is labeled as "dl-alpha."

There are many different brands of natural vitamin E sold in natural foods stores, but we recommend those marketed by Carlson Laboratories (see the Appendix), which has built a thirty-year reputation on its high-quality vitamin E. The company offers a broad line of natural vitamin E products, including capsules, tablets, ointments, suppositories, and sprays. As for specific supplements, we recommend d-alpha tocopheryl acetate, d-alpha tocopheryl succinate, or a natural blend that contains the d-alpha, beta, delta, and gamma forms of natural vitamin E.

Alpha-Lipoic Acid

Scientists have known for years that alpha-lipoic acid assists in the production of energy, along with CoQ_{10} and carnitine. In only the past few years, however, has its value as a powerful antioxidant been recognized. Alpha-lipoic acid also plays a role in stimulating immunity and inhibiting replication of HIV.

According to Lester Packer, Ph.D., a leading expert in free radicals and antioxidants and professor of biochemistry at the University of California, Berkeley, the body synthesizes its own alpha-lipoic acid for use in energy production. However, the body is "very stingy" in that it makes only trace amounts of alpha-lipoic acid with none to spare.[21]

As an antioxidant, alpha-lipoic acid normally helps the body recycle other antioxidants, including vitamin E, CoQ_{10}, and glutathione. But Dr. Packer believes that alpha-lipoic acid serves as a super-antioxidant only when there is an abundance of this substance, which can only happen with supplementation. Studies have demonstrated that alpha-lipoic acid prevents free-radical damage in diabetic nerve damage, cataracts, and the brain, where free radicals contribute to Alzheimer's and Parkinson's diseases. One study even found that alpha-lipoic acid improves thinking ability of mice and, presumably, people.[22]

Alpha-lipoic acid helps defend against infections in a number of ways. As an antioxidant, it helps the body clean up the excess free radicals produced to kill bacteria. It also boosts glutathione levels in T cells, which also helps the body fight infections. For example, glutathione slows HIV replication. Perhaps most interesting is that alpha-lipoic acid prevents a specific protein in DNA, NF-kappa B, from activating HIV.[23]

RECOMMENDATIONS

As a dietary supplement, alpha-lipoic acid is relatively new to the marketplace. Most supplements contain 50 milligrams, and this appears to be a reasonable and safe daily dose.

Zinc and Copper

In the late 1970s, a girl with leukemia, also suffering from recurrent colds and sore throats, was asked to suck on zinc tablets as if they were lozenges. Although zinc has long been known to be essential for immune function, no one could have anticipated her astounding response: she became symptom free in a matter of hours. Intrigued researchers followed up by investigating the health benefits of zinc lozenges.

Their findings turned out to be mixed. Some studies confirmed the benefits of zinc lozenges and others didn't. Then, in 1992, John C. Godfrey, Ph.D., figured out the reason. Saliva was probably reacting with some of the zinc compounds and rendering them unabsorbable. Dr. Godfrey developed his own zinc formulation and, in a study at the Dartmouth College Health Service, confirmed that it worked.

Dr. Godfrey and his colleagues used zinc lozenges that looked and tasted like a hard candy. It contained about 23 milligrams of zinc gluconate-glycine in a base that included astringent tannins. (Tannins also contain a number of beneficial flavonoids—see the following section in this chapter.) In a well-controlled study, Dr. Godfrey and his colleagues encouraged students to begin taking the zinc lozenges at the first appearance of cold symptoms. Those who took zinc lozenges right away had colds for an average of four days. Those who took lozenges identical except for the zinc had colds lasting an average of nine days.[24] Once the infection had passed, the students stopped taking the lozenges—until the next cold.

It makes sense not to overdo the zinc. Important as it is, too much zinc can suppress the body's copper levels. This is not desirable because copper also helps the body fight infections. In a recent study, researchers at the USDA's Western Human Nutrition Research Center in San Francisco placed eleven men on a copper-deficient diet for three months. The copper deficiency altered their immune function in a number of negative ways— T cells decreased and antibody-producing B cells increased in number.[25]

RECOMMENDATIONS

After news about the benefits of zinc lozenges began to spread, companies marketed numerous products. Unfortunately, we've found through personal experience that most of these zinc lozenges don't work very well. Some quickly break apart in the mouth, so their ingredients don't saturate mouth and throat tissues the way a lozenge should. Others simply taste awful.

There are, however, two zinc lozenges we wholeheartedly recommend. Formulated by Dr. Godfrey—a man who obviously knows something about these things—Cold-Eeze™ is a tasty, effective lozenge that tastes like a hard candy. It's available from the Quigley Corporation in Doylestown, Pennsylvania. The other product is Fast Dry™, marketed by George Eby, father of the girl with leukemia (who, by the way, recovered). (Their addresses and phone numbers are in the Appendix.)

If you're already taking a multimineral supplement, you're probably already getting adequate zinc and copper. The zinc lozenges are meant to be taken only during a cold. Taking them for long periods of time could upset copper levels, and taking too much zinc at one time could also cause nausea. There's one other concern with steady long-term intake of zinc: recent studies have found that zinc, of value in mental function, might harm people with AIDS or Alzheimer's disease (or people at risk for developing it).

Flavonoids

The flavonoids, sometimes referred to as bioflavonoids, have long been associated with vitamin C, although they are unrelated chemically. Both are common in fruits and vegetables—for example, vitamin C predominates in the edible fruit of citrus whereas the flavonoids are richer in the rind. Both nutrients were discovered in the 1930s by Nobel laureate Albert Szent-Györgyi. The flavonoids were initially termed vitamin P because they reduced the *p*ermeability (or leakage) of blood vessel walls in ways that vitamin C did not.

The flavonoids are no longer officially referred to as vitamin P. One reason is that they are not considered essential nutrients. Another reason is that more than four thousand flavonoids have been identified in plants, an extraordinary chemical diversity that precludes their classification as a single vitamin. Although the flavonoids are not considered essential nutrients, they are clearly beneficial nutrients and should be part of any well-rounded diet—especially a diet for optimal immunity.

Numerous studies have shown that people eating high-flavonoid diets have a lower-than-average risk of developing heart disease and cancer. These nutrients also enhance the activity of white blood cells and boost the body's defenses against a broad range of bacterial and viral infections, from urinary tract infections to HIV.

CRANBERRIES

Cranberry juice, bright red and acerbic, has long been a folk remedy for treating urinary tract infections, which are typically caused by a strain of *E. coli*. People have generally believed that cranberry juice works because it acidifies the urine, creating an unpleasant environment for many bacteria, or because of its vitamin C content. Cranberry juice does work but not for these reasons. The principal antibacterial flavonoid in cranberries (and blueberries), methyl alpha-D-mannopyranoside, works by making the urinary tract slippery for bacteria, which prevents them from adhering and establishing an infection.[26]

A few years ago, Jerry Avorn, M.D., of the Harvard Medical School, asked 153 elderly women to drink a large glass of cranberry juice or a look-alike noncranberry drink with vitamin C every day for six months. After only two months, the women drinking cranberry juice had half the incidence of urinary tract infections.[27] In a review of the research on cranberry juice, James C. Fleet, Ph.D., of Tufts University, observed that "out-of-hand dismissals of folk remedies are common in the cynical research communities. . . . This study provides a good example of how the research and medical communities should address the validity of folk remedies in the future."[28]

GREEN TEA

Green tea, a common beverage served with Japanese meals, contains a group of diverse flavonoids, including tannins, gallic acid esters, and catechins. Many of these compounds fight infections by acting directly against bacteria and by stimulating the immune system. For example, some of the flavonoids promote the body's production and activity of white blood cells, T cells, and antibodies.[29]

Green tea and many of its individual flavonoids inhibit the activity of *Streptococcus mutans*, the bacterium that causes dental cavities. While *S. mutans* does not pose a life-threatening infection, it is at the very least a nuisance. In one experiment, a group of Japanese researchers found that simple green tea reduced the number of cavities in laboratory rats, even when they ate a high-sugar diet.[30]

Green tea prevents cavities in a couple of ways. It inhibits *S. mutans*'s production of glycans, a sticky material that helps the bacteria attach to teeth. In a recent experiment, Isao Kubo, Ph.D., of the University of California, Berkeley, determined that hexanes, a chemical component of many flavonoids, are also quite capable of killing *S. mutans*. Dr. Kubo believes that green-tea toothpastes and mouthwashes may be a way to bring the benefits to those who do not drink tea. But similar hexanes occur in coriander, sage, and thyme.[31]

It's not surprising that the Japanese, who drink large quantities of green tea, are most interested in its health benefits. Various researchers have reported that the tea's flavonoids inhibit the influenza virus,[32] diarrhea-causing rotaviruses and enteroviruses,[33] *Bordetella pertussis* (whooping cough),[34] and *Mycoplasma pneumoniae* ("walking pneumonia").[35] The gallic acid flavonoids, in concentrations comparable to those found in green tea, also stop the reproduction of antibiotic-resistant *Staphylococcus aureus*, the most dangerous bacterium found in hospitals today.[36,37]

Numerous other flavonoids also possess antibacterial and, especially, antiviral properties. For example, grape seed extract, a popular type of flavonoid supplement, contains a number of proanthocyanidins, which have anti-herpes virus properties. (More than 250 proanthocyanidins have been identified in plants.) Grape seed extracts also contain gallic acid esters similar to those found in green tea.

Quercetin, one of the most powerful flavonoids, is well documented for its anticancer and antiallergy properties. It also stops reverse transcriptase, the method by which HIV and some other viruses reproduce.[38] Quercetin also acts against the herpes simplex I, polio, and influenza viruses. Other common flavonoids, such as naringin, hesperetin, and catechin also possess antiviral properties.[39]

RECOMMENDATIONS

The most *diverse* source of flavonoids is a diet containing many different kinds of fruits and vegetables. Health food stores sell a variety of flavonoid supplements, including rutin, hesperidin (closely related compounds have different spellings), green tea, and grape seed extract. As a general rule, select flavonoid-containing foods (fruits and vegetables) to build immunity and prevent disease, and consider flavonoid supplements when actually fighting an infection.

Bee Propolis and Honey

Bee products such as propolis have tended to attract a quirky and eccentric following. That's unfortunate because the antimicrobial properties of honey and propolis are reasonably well documented in medical journals. In fact, using honey as a medicine dates back to ancient Egypt, Rome, Greece, and China. All of these bee products contain antimicrobial substances, some apparently obtained from the flowers bees visit.

Renewed medical interest has resulted in a number of surprising and positive studies. Two British researchers recently observed in the *Journal of the Royal Society of Medicine*, "The therapeutic potential of uncontaminated, pure honey is grossly underutilized. It is widely available in most communities and although the mechanism of action of several of its properties remains obscure and needs further investigation, the time has now come for conventional medicine to lift the blinds off this 'traditional' remedy and give it its due recognition."[40]

HONEY

A number of recent studies have shown that externally applied honey can prevent a broad range of bacterial infections and promote healing in surgical and burn patients (who are at high risk of infection). Most but not all of these studies have been conducted in developing nations. While it might be easy for Westerners to dismiss the benefits, it's clear that honey often works—sometimes better than antibiotics.

In one instance, a physician at the medical college in Maharashtra, India, used honey-soaked gauze to treat forty burn patients. These patients healed in about half the time and with half the scar tissue of twenty-four patients treated conventionally.[41] In Nigeria, doctors at the University Teaching Hospital reported that unprocessed honey "inhibited most of the fungi and bacteria" causing surgical and wound infections. The researchers concluded, "Honey is thus an ideal topical wound dressing agent in surgical infections, burns and wound infections."[42]

Just as remarkable was the use of honey in the treatment of gastric ulcers, now known to be caused by the *Helicobacter pylori* bacterium. Because honey has been a folk remedy for dyspepsia (stomach upset), a team of researchers from the University of Waikato, New Zealand, conducted a controlled experiment. Honey stopped the growth of *H. pylori* colonies in only three days.[43] Various other studies have reported that honey also inhibits the growth of much more dangerous bacteria, including *E. coli, Staphylococcus aureus, Salmonella, Shigella,* and *Vibrio cholera.*[44]

PROPOLIS

Propolis is essentially weather stripping for beehives. Bees create it by collecting a resinous sap from trees, then mixing it with wax. Chemically, propolis is exceedingly complex and contains a rich variety of potent polyphenols and flavonoids, including terpenes and benzoic, caffeic, and cinnamic acids. The flavonoids alone may account for many of the benefits attributed to propolis, and some researchers have even referred to propolis as a type of flavonoid.

Research suggests that propolis is a powerful natural antibiotic. Chinese researchers reported that propolis extracts stopped the growth of *S. aureus.*[45] European scientists have found that propolis enhanced the antistaph activity of some pharmaceutical antibiotics, including streptomycin.[46] Like green tea, propolis inhibits the activity of several streptococci species involved in dental caries.[47] It probably works by preventing bacterial cell division and by breaking down bacterial walls, which is exactly how some antibiotics work.[48]

In independent assays, Southern Testing & Research Laboratories, Inc., of Wilson, North Carolina, evaluated the antibiotic properties of propolis. The lab analyzed propolis from the C C

Pollen Company of Phoenix, Arizona, and found it to be either equal to or slightly more effective than two common antibiotics, erythromycin and amoxicillin, in killing *Staphylococcus aureus* and *Streptococcus faecalis* bacteria.[49] Although the tests involved cell cultures, not living animals, they did demonstrate the antibiotic potential of propolis.

Unlike antibiotics, though, propolis also acts against viruses. Numerous medical journal reports have discussed the role of propolis in fighting upper respiratory infections, such as those caused by the common cold and influenza viruses.[50] Some of the flavonoids in propolis might also play a role in preventing colon cancer, which kills sixty thousand Americans each year. Researchers at the American Health Foundation, Valhalla, New York, reported in *Cancer Research*, one of the top cancer journals, that propolis extracts prevented the formation of precancerous tissues in rats after exposure to cancer-causing chemicals.[51]

Why would bees need to surround themselves with antimicrobial substances with broad antibacterial and antiviral properties? Any beekeeper will tell you the answer. As social insects, bees are very susceptible to bacterial and viral infections, which can destroy hives the way the bubonic plague ravaged Europe in the seventeenth century.

RECOMMENDATIONS

We can learn a lot from bees that eat honey and seal their hives with propolis. By eating these bee products, we can preventively help protect ourselves from many bacterial and viral infections and perhaps reduce our risk of developing cancer.

Perhaps it's the way we grew up or how we learned about medicine, but we'd be reluctant to treat serious (i.e., life-threatening) burns and injuries with honey-soaked gauze. We do think, however, that raw honey dressings are appropriate for minor burns. In addition, we're convinced that you can derive the antimicrobial benefits of honey by using it as a sweetener. Too much sugar, of course, interferes with the body's defense against infection, but a little honey goes a long way and it's difficult to consume large quantities of this sweetener.

As with the flavonoids, try to use bee products as close to their food form as possible. A number of companies market tasty spreads and sweeteners containing honey, propolis, and royal jelly. (You can find such products at health food stores.) If you feel as though your immunity isn't what it should be after following our advice in Chapters 9 through 15, consider taking propolis capsules as a concentrated natural antibiotic.

We have one warning, though. Do not, under any circumstances, give honey or any other bee food to an infant under one year of age. Honey contains dangerous spores that an infant's immature immune system cannot fight. These spores are not a problem for the immune systems of older, healthy children and adults.

Melatonin

Over the past year or so, several books and countless magazine articles have touted melatonin as a "miracle" antiaging drug. Before this surge of interest, melatonin was recognized as the hormone that induced restful sleep, helped insomniacs, and fixed jet lag. Made in the pineal gland, melatonin is the hormone that controls your biological clock.

Despite what has often seemed like hype, there's a lot to be said in favor of melatonin. According to Russel J. Reiter, Ph.D., and Jo Robinson, authors of *Melatonin: Your Body's Natural Wonder Drug* (Bantam, 1995),[52] melatonin's hormonal properties may be actually secondary to its role as a powerful antioxidant. A substance that works as both an antioxidant and a hormone would have nothing less than a profound impact on the body.

Like many other key biochemicals in the body, melatonin levels decrease with age, and this decline seems to accelerate the aging process. It becomes a vicious cycle, ending in disease or premature death. But melatonin supplements, like essential nutrients, seem to slow aging and the development of age-related diseases.

The immune system, of course, deteriorates with age, which is why the average elderly person is more vulnerable to infection and cancer. On the basis of research by Dr. Reiter and others, melatonin supplements can boost immune function in the young, middle-aged, and elderly. Why would melatonin do all this? Melatonin levels normally increase in the evening, signaling the body to rest and renew itself against the day's stresses. But melatonin levels also increase during the autumn and winter. The reason, some researchers suspect, is to compensate for the stresses historically associated with winter—cold and less food—which would impair immunity.[53,54]

Melatonin dramatically improves the immune response to both cancers and infections. In a study of cancer patients, supplemental melatonin substantially increased the number of T cells, natural-killer cells, and other types of white blood cells.[55] Researchers have also reported that melatonin enhances antibody production.[56] Georges J. Maestroni, Ph.D., who directs the Center for Experimental Pathology in Locarno, Switzerland, observed that "melatonin seems to have an immunoenhancing effect that is particularly apparent in immunosuppressive states." Indeed, melatonin specifically counters the immune suppression associated with cortisone-type drugs.[57]

In an animal experiment, researchers discovered that melatonin supplements reduced the severity of viral infections of the brain and increased the survival rate by almost 50 percent.[58] Under the circumstances, it's not surprising that melatonin can slow the replication of HIV and improve immune function in patients with AIDS.[59]

RECOMMENDATIONS

By most measures, melatonin is extraordinarily safe. If you take too much melatonin, or take it at the wrong time of day, you may feel groggy the next day. If you're contemplating taking melatonin, it's important to read up on it. One doctor, in New York City, has found that melatonin exacerbates depression.

The beneficial amount varies from person to person, so you'll have to experiment a little. Some people feel well taking only 0.5 milligram whereas others do better taking several milligrams daily. As with anything else, if you feel worse rather than better, stop taking it.

Herbs

Although the effects of herbs can be pharmacologic rather than nutritional, we want to include them because they have a respectable history—and sometimes impressive scientific documentation—for boosting immunity and fighting infections. Many conventional physicians dismiss herbal therapy, but 38 percent of all commercial drugs are based on plant medicines. For example, quinine originally came from the bark of a tree, and digitalis is still made from the crushed leaves of the foxglove plant.

Some herbs work because they provide important nutrients, such as the flavonoids. For example, a recent study found that anacardic acid, which is found in cashews, apples, and nuts, destroys antibiotic-resistant *Staphylococcus aureus*.[60] You'd have to eat a lot of cashews to get a clear antibacterial effect, but in moderate amounts such foods contribute to a good, immune-enhancing diet.

Most herbs, however, seem to function as natural drugs—foxglove is clearly not nutritional and can be highly toxic. Each year, dozens of studies describe the antibacterial or antiviral properties of dozens of plant species from around the world. In fact, there is actually far too much information on plant chemistry and immunity for us to comprehensively cover it here. So with an eye to practicality, we'll focus on a few of the better documented immune-stimulating herbs that you can purchase at natural foods stores. For detailed and referenced studies on plant medicines, we recommend *Botanical Influences on Illness,* by Melvyn R. Werbach, M.D., and Michael T. Murray, N.D. (Third Line Press, 1994—see the Appendix.)

ECHINACEA

Perhaps the best-known and best-documented immune-enhancing herb is echinacea. A member of the sunflower family, echinacea was once the medicinal herb used most commonly by Native Americans. Physicians started using echinacea in the 1880s, but it faded into oblivion by the early part of the twentieth century. In the 1930s, German doctors rediscovered the herb, and since then it has remained popular overseas.

More than 350 scientific studies have described the chemistry or benefits of echinacea. The most commonly sold species are *Echinacea angustifolia, E. purpurea,* and *E. pallida,* and the principal active ingredient in them appears to be a very complex sugar molecule called a polysaccharide. Echinacea extracts boost the immune system's response to colds, flus, and many other types of infections. A German study, published in 1992, reported that 900 milligrams of echinacea significantly reduced flu symptoms. Lower doses, however, were no better than dummy pills.[61]

Scientists have reported that echinacea stimulates the activity of white blood cells, making them more potent killers of bacteria and other microorganisms. A number of studies have found that echinacea boosts the body's ability to fight *Listeria,* a bacterium that causes a deadly form of food poisoning, and *Candida* yeast.

OTHER HERBS

A number of other herbs have either a respectable scientific or folk medicine track record in enhancing immunity and fighting infections. Goldenseal *(Hydrasis canadensis),* barberry root bark *(Berberis vulgaris),* and Oregon grape root *(Berberis aquifolium)* contain berberine, a bitter compound with antibacterial, antiprotozoal, and antifungal properties. Astragalus *(Astragalus membranaceus)* is a Chinese herb historically used to treat viral infections, and elderberry *(Sambucus nigra)* has been shown to have similar benefits. The roots of osha *(Ligusticum porteri)*, a member of the parsley family, have long been used by Hispanics in the southwestern United States as a remedy for infections.

RECOMMENDATIONS

Many herbs are now available in capsule form, and while more expensive than the raw herbs, they sidestep the common problem of bitter or unpleasant taste. If you opt for capsules, such as echinacea, it's probably best to follow label directions. Also, with echinacea in particular, its immune benefits are strongest when it is used no more than a couple of weeks at a time. For most other plant medicines, seek out the advice of an expert herbalist (check your phone book or get a referral from your health food store), who can provide you with guidance and the appropriate part of the plant.

Through the past nine chapters, you have learned about some relatively simple dietary changes and easy-to-take supplements that can dramatically improve your body's defenses against infections. There is still a little more you need to know, and a few additional steps you can take to defend yourself against supergerms and many other infections. In the final chapter, we explore the value and limitations of immunizations, when and how antibiotics can be optimally used, as well as some guidelines for avoiding (rather than preparing to defend yourself against) supergerms and other infections. We also describe several generic vitamin regimens.

17

A Rational Approach to Optimal Immunity

———— ✤ ————

In this final chapter, we address in a little more detail several issues related to immunity. Among them are the benefits and limitations of immunizations and the prudent use of antibiotics. We also make recommendations regarding hygiene, sanitation, and traveling—in other words, how to avoid flirting with danger. We also provide some general recommendations for immune-enhancing vitamin/mineral regimens.

What Immunizations Can and Cannot Do

Controversies about abortion, gay rights, and guns have split political parties and commanded countless headlines. They are among the hottest political issues today. But another highly volatile issue is emerging in medicine and politics, and it's one that might surprise you—immunizations.

Many people take immunizations for granted, and for them it's not controversial at all. After all, immunizations have been credited with stopping or curbing the spread of many dangerous diseases, including diphtheria, influenza, measles, pertussis, and smallpox. But there is a growing number of people, often parents of young children, who are simply uncomfortable with or firmly opposed to government-mandated immunizations.

There's a lot to be said in favor of immunizations, and a few things to be said against them. But first, let's begin with some basics. The material used in immunizations generally consists of either dead or attenuated (weakened) microorganisms or molecular fragments from the germs. The idea of using trace amounts of germs originated in nineteenth-century homeopathic medicine, in which physicians prescribed extremely minute, almost undetectable amounts of drugs. Theoretically, these dilute substances trigger the immune system's reaction, but not an overreaction. The concept made sense to Louis Pasteur, the great French bacteriologist, and to many other nineteenth-century scientists who promoted the concept of immunization.

How immunizations work is very complicated, and in many respects still not completely understood. Essentially, a vaccination tricks the body into believing it is being attacked by an actual disease-causing microorganism. The immune system mounts a response, including antibodies tailored specifically to counter the germ. Because the immune system remembers many types of germs, people often gain lifelong immunity after a single exposure, either during an infection or an immunization. This does not mean you'll never get infected by the germ again. Rather, you won't notice subsequent infections because the immune system quietly and efficiently mops up the germs before they cause symptoms.

For all their benefits, the value of immunizations has also been overstated. A number of physicians have pointed out that the incidence of many infectious diseases began to decline just before the widespread use of immunizations. Improved sanitation and personal hygiene also probably helped stem infectious diseases.[1] As a defense against supergerms and other types of infections, immunizations have a more mundane limitation: they are simply outnumbered by the opposition. Only about two dozen vaccines are commonly in use, but there are several hundred types of bacteria, viruses, and parasites that can cause serious infections.

Why aren't there immunizations for more types of infections? In the case of HIV, the virus mutates so rapidly that it has stayed a step ahead of the most promising approaches to immunizations. In general, though, the manufacture of vaccines and other drugs is driven by profit, not public welfare. That's why a vaccine that protects against Ebola will probably not be pursued unless the virus kills considerably more than three hundred people every twenty years. In an era of federal budget cutbacks, the government is funding less, not more, immunization research.

Aside from money, there are also a number of practical issues limiting the development of immunizations. Is science, for example, even capable of catching up to and controlling germs—particularly when one or more new supergerms is now discovered each year? Even given the money and the manpower, it's doubtful. In addition, would extensive immunizations be in the best interest of a person's health? We are not sure that getting dozens of immunizations would be. It may be best to reserve immunizations for preventing the deadliest diseases, instead of squandering this resource on relatively innocuous and nuisance diseases, such as chicken pox.

What really gets some people stirred up—and has led to organized opposition to immunizations—is seeing or hearing about two-month-old infants who become sick or permanently disabled after receiving immunizations. There is a basis for these concerns. By conservative estimates, the oral polio vaccines cause five to ten cases of paralysis a year, and the pertussis vaccine causes brain damage in one out of every three hundred thousand children in the United States. The numbers may be higher, and interestingly enough, one study found that physicians were more worried than parents about children becoming "pincushions from immunizations."[2]

⌘

INFECTIONS FOR WHICH IMMUNIZATIONS ARE COMMONLY AVAILABLE

BACTERIAL

Cholera
Haemophilus meningitis
Meningococcal meningitis
Pertussis (whooping cough)
Plague

Pneumonia *(S. pneumoniae)*
Rocky Mountain spotted fever
Tuberculosis
Typhoid fever

VACCINATIONS AGAINST VIRUSES

Chicken pox
Hepatitis B
Influenza
Measles
Mumps

Polio
Rabies
Rubella
Smallpox
Yellow fever

VACCINATIONS AGAINST BACTERIAL TOXINS*

Tetanus
Diphtheria

---

*The vaccination protects against toxins produced by the bacteria, not the bacteria themselves.

⌘

There is evidence that the stress of immunizations may affect the breathing of some infants, and the incidence of sudden infant death syndrome (SIDS) in Japan decreased dramatically after physicians stopped giving infants DTP (diphtheria, tetanus, pertussis) shots.[3] In addition, the number of pertussis cases often increases after mass DTP shots.[4] There is also a strong association between measles vaccination and inflammatory bowel diseases.

It's not fair to dismiss such findings out of hand, so what's the problem? Harris Coulter, Ph.D., a medical historian in Washington, D.C., has pointed out that while medicine adopted the homeopathic concept of using minute amounts of germs in im-

munizations, it neglected the homeopathic principle of individualizing treatment. The reason, believes Coulter, is that
individualizing treatment simply takes too much time and
work.[5] But there's a practical problem. It's one thing to individualize homeopathic remedies for allergies and other mild conditions, and quite another to individualize immunizations. And,
of course, this line of discussion assumes you accept homeopathy
as a legitimate approach to medicine when, rightly or wrongly,
most medical doctors do not.

Many of the controversies surrounding immunizations re-
surfaced in 1995 with the approval of a new vaccine for chicken
pox, a viral infection related to herpes. The vaccine was expensive and many people wondered whether it was really necessary
for the treatment of a common infection that's generally no more
than a nuisance. Some people suggested, probably correctly, that
the vaccine would be worthwhile to parents who did not want
to be inconvenienced by their children's illnesses.

One of the deans of American pediatric medicine, Lendon
H. Smith, M.D., of Portland, Oregon, used to routinely give his
patients every recommended immunization. In retrospect, he
thinks that was a mistake. Dr. Smith believes that most infections
can be easily treated, and he now favors giving immunizations
only to prevent tetanus, caused by a germ found in soil. What
made him change his mind? Two events, he says. One was seeing
some of his patients become very sick from the immunizations.
The other was reading *Every Second Child*,[6] by Archie Kalokerinos, M.D., an Australian physician who found that half the
Aborigines given immunizations died within a few days of getting the shots.[7] Dr. Kalokerinos found that many of the Aborigines were deficient in vitamin C, but those who had taken vitamin
supplements were protected against the negative side effects of
the shots.

Faced with a growing grassroots challenge, physicians and
public health officials seriously worry about the declining use
of immunizations. There is a belief in what's sometimes called
the "herd effect"—that if a majority of people are immunized,

a small number of nonimmunized people will also be protected. When fewer and fewer children and adults are immunized, the risk of an epidemic increases. On average, about 25 percent of toddlers in the United States are not immunized.[8]

Children aren't the only ones affected. Gregory A. Poland, M.D., of the Mayo Clinic in Rochester, Minnesota, pointed out that, three hundred to five hundred children die each year from vaccine-preventable infections. But according to Dr. Poland as many as eighty thousand adults die each year in the United States from vaccine-preventable infections.[9]

So, should you or should you not vaccinate? Even with their limitations, immunizations have considerable value. But to enhance their benefits and minimize their risks, you need to lay a good nutritional foundation before getting immunized. As you learned in Chapter 6, your immune system depends on a large number of vitamins and minerals in order to function properly. If you are deficient in key micronutrients, your immune system will not be able to effectively respond to invading microorganisms. Nor will your immune system be able to respond appropriately to an immunization. Adequate intake of vitamins helps immunizations work the way they are meant to, and they minimize the undesirable side effects.

If you assume that most diets provide adequate nutrients, then the fact that bad reactions to immunizations occur is puzzling—and this is exactly how many physicians view bad reactions to vaccines. If, however, you assume that most diets are poor, then the bad reactions start to make sense. We're convinced that many immunizations go awry when the diet has gone awry. In this situation, the immune system doesn't have the nutritional building blocks required for a healthy response. It is also possible that many infants at two or four months of age are simply too fragile for immunization. Many physicians do not mind delaying these scheduled immunizations for a number of months. Our advice is to talk to your physician about scheduling immunizations for children.

You can often ease the feverish side effects of immunizations.

In our experience, we have found that simply increasing intake of vitamin C shortly before and after getting a vaccination reduces the side effects. While we can't guarantee that supplemental vitamin C will lower the risk of severe side effects, we believe that it will. Again, there are practical problems. It's easy enough for an adult to take extra vitamin C and B vitamins, but how do you get vitamins down the mouth of an infant or small child? Schiff, a brand of vitamins sold through health food stores, markets a superb liquid vitamin C that can be easily added to infant formula or juice—a half-teaspoon for an infant, and a full teaspoon for a toddler daily should be sufficient. Other companies market liquid multivitamins.

In our opinion, mass immunizations pose a risk that most people don't hear about but which is more important than the occasional side effects. That risk is complacency. So long as physicians and public health officials regard immunizations as the cornerstone of preventive medicine, they will downplay the role of other factors, such as nutrition. Nutrition is the fundamental key to a healthy immune system, and vaccine-induced complacency can actually foster neglect of the immune status of people.

An additional aspect of complacency is the prevalent belief that, once vaccinated, a person is safe from serious infection. A person is not, because the vaccines cover only a small number of germs. Many supergerms lie in wait for the marginally nourished, whose susceptibility is increased relative to their dietary deficiencies. Mass immunization fails completely to address this serious problem.

A Sensible Approach to Antibiotics

Antibiotics are among the most remarkable drugs of the twentieth century. They have saved hundreds of thousands, and perhaps millions, of lives. But the more that you, as an individual, use antibiotics, the less effective they will become. That means antibiotics may not work when you're sick and need them the most.

To appreciate the scale of the problem, multiply yourself by hundreds of millions of people. All of these antibiotics end up killing the weak bacteria and selecting for the survival of large numbers of antibiotic-resistant bacteria. As you learned in earlier chapters, frequent exposures to antibiotics can leave you more susceptible to infections. And if you desperately need an antibiotic to save your life, you may then have difficulty finding one that works.

There are, however, ways out of this biological and medical conundrum, but they do take time and effort. Just as antibiotics kill off weak bacteria and select for the survival of the strongest supergerms, *not* taking antibiotics selects against antibiotic-resistant bacteria. In general, if you avoid antibiotics, you will eliminate most antibiotic-resistant bacteria from your body in ten days to two weeks.[10] That's because there is a natural turnover in the body's bacteria.

Practically speaking, though, people may not deselect antibiotic-resistant bacteria that fast because antibiotic-resistant bacteria are becoming more, not less, common. For example, if you avoid medically prescribed antibiotics but your spouse or children use them, you will acquire their antibiotic-resistant bacteria. The bacteria are transferred by touching each other or common objects, such as kitchen sponges. These bacteria may not be dangerous in themselves, but they can and often do share their antibiotic-resistant genes with dangerous bacteria. Furthermore, eating food treated with antibiotics is another avenue for acquiring antibiotic-resistant bacteria. That's why eating antibiotic-free, organically produced foods—meat, fruits, vegetables, milk—is so important. (See Chapter 9.) Otherwise, you will be exposed and reexposed to antibiotics—and never truly be free of them.

Here's another way to lessen your dependence on antibiotics. When you get sick and call your doctor, don't insist that he prescribe antibiotics. Let your physician make the diagnosis—then, if you wish, discuss various treatments with him. If you have a viral infection, such as the common cold or influenza, antibiotics will be of absolutely no benefit. Getting a prescription might warm the cockles of your heart, but it won't do anything to relieve the burning infection in your lungs.

Be assertive, perhaps pushy, in another way, also. If your doctor prescribes an antibiotic, ask him what type of bacteria he is trying to control. If he has cultured your throat and identified a strep infection, an antibiotic is completely appropriate. If he is not sure of the specific organism, and this is often the case, he may opt for a broad-spectrum antibiotic. This is a shotgun approach that assumes he'll hit something. So if a culture has not been taken, and assuming you're not deathly ill, ask your doctor to take a culture and order the test to confirm his diagnosis. He may or may not go along with your suggestion for any number of reasons.

Why might your doctor be reluctant to spend $20 to $50 to have the microorganism cultured? It could be that your insurer just does not want to pay for such tests routinely. In other words, a broad-spectrum antibiotic is cheaper than a test and a narrow-spectrum antibiotic. This situation is often worst in Health Maintenance Organizations (HMOs) because doctors often get paid more for what they don't do, including the lab tests they don't order. With some HMOs, more than half of a doctor's pay is tied to incentives, bonuses, and penalties. This approach tends to go against a physician's better judgment, but there are advantages to it as well. An antibiotic that wipes out most bacteria will also eliminate the remote risk of a serious bacterial infection—and a malpractice lawsuit.

It's not uncommon for the health-care industry, physicians, insurers, and the government to be working at cross purposes, with you, the patients, getting squeezed in the middle. For example, some companies have been developing new tests to quickly identify bacterial infections, but insurance companies often don't want to spend the money on these tests. Through legislation, the federal government has been discouraging physicians from doing these rapid tests in their offices—thus deferring them to testing laboratories that insurers don't want to pay.

One solution, obviously, is preventing infections in the first place. But if you or your child has an infection, you have to deal with that before thinking more about prevention. If you have a small child with an ear infection, discuss simple pain relief, such as using a hot compress or acetaminophen, with your doctor. While it's hard to watch an infant or child in pain, remind yourself that each infection helps program and build long-term immunity. Even waiting a couple of days before administering an antibiotic will help program the immune system a little.

At the same time, though, remain vigilant. Very high fevers, a stiff neck, projectile vomiting, significant behavioral changes, extreme lethargy, and the appearance of purple spots on the skin can be signs of very dangerous infections. There aren't any firm guidelines to offer here—parents sort of learn as they go along. But be wary of physicians who are always fast to draw their pen and prescription pad. You would do better with a doctor who is slower to prescribe and more methodical in his diagnosis.

There will, of course, be times when you or someone close to you really does needs an antibiotic. The key, according to Dr. Levy, is to use them prudently. Different antibiotics require different lengths of time to work effectively. Most are prescribed for seven to ten days—the duration will vary with the type of antibiotic and the nature of the infection. A few antibiotics can cure certain types of infections in only three days; others, such as isoniazid (for tuberculosis) must be taken for up to eighteen months. *Always* take antibiotics for the prescribed time. If you accidentally skip a day, call your physician for guidance. He may ask you to stop, to continue the regimen, double your dose for a day, or begin a new antibiotic. Then follow his advice.

In general, injected antibiotics have little effect on the beneficial bacteria that inhabit the gastrointestinal tract. Conversely, oral antibiotics frequently wreak havoc on intestinal bacteria. Oral antibiotics are prescribed far more often, so you must be prepared to rebuild your colony of intestinal bacteria. These good bacteria discourage the growth of disease-causing bacteria, and they also stimulate the immune system. You want to do your utmost to keep your intestinal bacteria healthy, and after taking antibiotics you'll have to be especially conscientious. Eat extra amounts of cultured foods, such as "live-culture" yogurt, and consider taking probiotic capsules, which contain beneficial bacteria. In sum, whenever you take antibiotics, consume extra amounts of cultured-food products for at least a month afterward.

Staying Out of Harm's Way

From a practical standpoint, it's wise to enhance your immunity because it will improve your health in general—and because you never know when you will be exposed to a supergerm or other nasty infection. At the same time, it makes perfect sense to avoid exposures to supergerms. There's no sense in flirting with danger.

Here's a case in point. During the 1995 Ebola outbreak, Laurie Garrett, a seasoned *Newsday* reporter and author of *The Coming Plague* (Farrar, Straus and Giroux, New York, 1994), doffed her face mask shortly after arriving in Kikwit, Zaire, the center of the epidemic. The assumption was that Ebola was spread through blood and body fluids, not through the air. By the fall of 1995, Garrett's self-confidence had been shaken a little. During a lecture in Portland, Oregon, she related new research indicating that Ebola could be transmitted through aerosol mists comparable to those created in a sneeze.

Zaire, however, is half a world away. The average American risks encountering supergerms and other serious infections in one of two principal ways: (1) from other people, including family members, and (2) from food, either at home or in a restaurant. Depending on your sexual habits, you may also be at risk of contracting HIV or other venereal diseases. And if you camp in forests or travel in developing (third world) nations, you may increase your risk of contracting still other infections. In many developing nations, antibiotics are sold without a prescription—and antibiotic-resistant bacteria are common.

Most infections are transmitted through casual contact among family members, friends, and coworkers. The best example is how easily the flu spreads during the winter months, when people are crowded together in closed buildings. It's no surprise that the flu season reaches its peak around Christmas and New Year's Day. Schools, day care centers, airplanes (during the winter months), and hospitals are also high-risk environments for infection during the winter.

Consider how infections are spread through a day care center. One child with a cold or flu wipes his nose and then touches toys, other children, and adult caregivers. He sneezes, and virus-laden droplets atomize like a spray of perfume. Small children don't understand the importance of keeping their distance from a sick person or washing hands, but as an adult you should.

To protect yourself, try to maintain some physical distance between yourself and sick friends, coworkers, and family members. This may be nearly impossible if you are the parent of a sick child, so the next step is to wash your hands frequently with hot soapy water. Discipline yourself to wash your hands immediately after shaking hands with an infected adult or helping a toddler wipe his nose—before you casually touch your own nose, mouth, or ears, since these are the primary entry points of bacteria and viruses. If you have a runny nose, use and carefully dispose of tissues. Avoid handkerchiefs because they quickly become drenched with viruses and bacteria.

Food is another source of supergerms, and at home you can minimize the risk of food-borne infections through proper storage, handling, and cooking. While tainted meat has always been a problem, we think the situation has gotten worse in recent years. Many of the germs are antibiotic resistant, and some, such as *E. coli* 0157:H7, simply didn't exist years ago. We'll give you one brief example of how things have changed for the worse. Years ago, we enjoyed eating steak tartare—carefully ground and spiced *raw* beef. We haven't eaten it in years, because *E. coli* 0157:H7 have since become native to cattle.

Many packages of meat now contain instructions on their safe storage, and informative brochures are available from many supermarkets and local U.S. Department of Agriculture offices. Briefly, though, here are some tips:

- Try to use raw meats within a couple days of buying them. Keep meat refrigerated or frozen until you are prepared to cook it. Cooler temperatures slow bacterial growth, but they do not kill bacteria.
- Don't thaw frozen meat on a countertop for more than two hours. It's better to defrost it in the refrigerator, and then to cook it thoroughly. Heating does kill bacteria, such as *E. coli* and *Salmonella*, so cook meat thoroughly.
- Prepare raw meat on a separate wooden cutting board from the one you use to prepare vegetables, fruit, breads, and other foods. For some reason, bacteria transferred from meat are easier to wash out of wooden cutting boards, whereas they tend to breed in plastic cutting boards.
- Likewise, use separate plates and utensils for handling raw meat, cooked meat, and other foods. For example, *E. coli* can be spread by using the same knife to cut raw meat and then a cantaloupe.
- In terms of meat, hamburger poses the greatest risk of bacterial contamination, and cuts (such as steaks) offer a relatively low risk. If you want hamburger, ask your butcher to grind a round steak for you—right after he has cleaned and reassembled the grinding machine. In our personal experience, neighborhood German butchers tend to be very conscientious about their meat.

- Regularly clean kitchen sink sponges with hot water and replace them. Sponges are great media for growing colonies of bacteria.
- When dining out, it's best to patronize restaurants you know are conscientious about cleanliness. Look around. If you see waitresses taking puffs on a cigarette in between waiting on tables, you've got a big clue as to how seriously the manager or owner takes hygiene and sanitation. Also, read the newspaper for news of health departments downgrading restaurant ratings.
- Finally, whether you're at home or at a restaurant, always wash your hands after going to the bathroom. The densest colonies of bacteria live around the groin and anus, and they're spread by touch. Some unhygienic food handlers have spread infections, but we suspect some careless customers have done the same.

In terms of safe sex, there's little we can write that others have not already written. HIV is still a death sentence, and syphilis and gonorrhea are increasingly resistant to antibiotic treatment. Get to know your partner before you have sex—not a bad idea in general—and use condoms unless you're both committed to a long-term monogamous relationship and have tested negative for sexually transmitted diseases.

If you're camping and are bitten by a tick, have the bite examined by a physician. Lyme disease, which is transmitted through tick bites, typically starts with a ringlike rash and causes symptoms similar to the flu. In its early stages, the *Borrelia burgdorferi* parasite, which causes Lyme disease, can be treated effectively with antibiotics. If you wait a few months, the antibiotic becomes ineffective and the symptoms crippling.

When you're traveling outside of North America, eat only cooked food and drink only bottled liquids. Stick with more recognizable brands of bottled water. Recently, an acquaintance acquired a serious parasitic infection in France, but he had consumed only bottled water. One bottle happened to be a little-known brand, and the physician suggested that the bottled water may have come from a faucet rather than a spring.

Some Sample Vitamin Regimens

The best ongoing defense against supergerms is to maintain optimal immunity. If you are well you'll be less likely to have to resort to antibiotics. Although we have already described and provided dosages for many nutritional supplements, the following table provides several reference points for immune-boosting regimens. These dosages are guidelines and do *not* correspond to any specific products.

One way to approach supplementation is to begin with a high-potency multivitamin/multimineral formula, which should provide many of these nutrients. Then add individual supplements (such as vitamin C, A, and CoQ_{10}) to achieve the desired dosages. If you would like to add some of the supplements discussed in Chapter 16, such as flavonoids or bee propolis, follow label directions.

Recommending nutritional supplements for infants and small children is more difficult, and you must exercise some caution. Children's physiological ability to handle high-dose vitamins may be limited because a child's liver or kidneys may be immature. If you're a nursing mother, and your child is less than twelve months of age, take the vitamins yourself. Small, sufficient quantities will pass through your breast milk. You can also dab a little liquid vitamin C on your nipples as you begin breast-feeding. If you're bottle-feeding an infant, adding a very small amount of liquid vitamin C to the milk or formula might be helpful—again, follow label directions. If you're a parent and are able to get a toddler or small child to take a chewable children's vitamin each day, consider yourself ahead of many other parents.

But what if you have a difficult child, age four and up, who doesn't want to take vitamins? Here are several possible

✂

SAMPLE DAILY SUPPLEMENT DOSAGES FOR ADULTS

SUPPLEMENT	PREVENTIVE DOSE*	IMMUNE JUMP-STARTING**	VERY AGGRESSIVE***
Vitamin C	1,000–2,000 mg	2,000–10,000 mg	20,000+ mg
Vitamin A	5,000 IU	10,000 IU[a]	25,000+ IU[a]
Beta-carotene	25,000 IU	25,000 IU	50,000 IU
Selenium	50 mcg	100–200 mcg	400 mcg
CoQ_{10}	30 mg	60 mg	200 mg
Vitamin B_1[b]	10 mg	25 mg	50 mg
Vitamin B_2	10 mg	25 mg	50 mg
Vitamin B_3	100 mg	200 mg	300 mg
Vitamin B_6	10 mg	25 mg	50 mg
Vitamin B_{12}	10 mcg	25 mcg	100 mcg
Pantothenic acid	25 mg	100 mg	200 mg
Folic acid	400 mcg	400 mcg	800 mcg
Vitamin E	200 IU	400 IU	800 IU
Lysine	—	500–1,000 mg	2,000 mg
Carnitine	—	300 mg	1,000 mg
Glutathione	—	25 mg	50–100 mg
Zinc	10 mg	25 mg	50 mg
Copper	2 mg	4 mg	6 mg

*Preventive Dose: Consider taking every day.
**Immune Jump-Starting Dose: If you're prone to infections, or recover from them very slowly, consider taking for 1–3 months, then try to scale back to preventive dose levels.
***Very Aggressive: For the temporary treatment or amelioration of serious life-threatening infections. If your condition is long-term (e.g., tuberculosis, AIDS, etc.), consult your physician.
[a]If you are of childbearing age, take these dosages of vitamin A only under the supervision of a physician.
[b]Rather than take individual B vitamins, look for a B-complex supplement that provides levels of individual B vitamins similar to those listed here.

✂

approaches. Try to establish a daily routine in which your child takes one or two children's chewable multivitamin supplements. Flintstones® are a tasty brand of vitamins sold in drugstores and supermarkets, but health food stores sell many types of children's supplements. Many chewable vitamins will be sweetened with sugar, which is unfortunate, but it's often necessary to make bitter-tasting vitamins palatable for children.

If your child succumbs to one infection after another, try mixing some liquid vitamin C or a liquid multivitamin with apple or grape juice. If you do this consistently, your child may think that's the natural taste of the juice. Also, if your child has a respiratory infection (e.g., the flu), give him or her a little extra liquid vitamin C and, once or twice for a couple of days *only*, break open a capsule containing 10,000 IU of vitamin A and squeeze the contents into his juice. Because of the risk of overdose, do not give vitamin A to a child more often than one or two days a month.

As is always the case, it's best to work with a nutritionally oriented physician, and this is particularly important in preventing or treating infections in children. If you have trouble finding a doctor who appreciates vitamins, ask for a referral at your local health food store. Also, the Appendix of this book contains the names of organizations that can refer you to nutritionally oriented physicians.

AFTERWORD

❦

Epidemics and outbreaks of infectious diseases have appeared and often inexplicably disappeared throughout history. The Spanish flu of 1918, which likely occurred during the lifetime of your grandparents or great-grandparents, left millions of people dead in its wake. Today, the frightful emergence of AIDS and Ebola have instilled new fears in people.

Yet AIDS and Ebola are only two of the many supergerms people face. At a scientific meeting in December 1995, researchers warned that a new flu virus could mutate at any time and trigger a deadly worldwide pandemic. That's just how close the next supergerm might be.

When we began researching and writing this book, we knew supergerms and other infections were a major health problem. What struck us though was that we, as a society, have reached a crossroads. For the first time in history, we have the capability to truly optimize our immune systems. But it seems as though we are doing everything we can to weaken and injure immunity and to become more susceptible to disease.

Encroaching on, cutting, and burning the equatorial rain forests and dense deciduous and fir forests of North America have exposed people to countless new germs, from Lyme disease to AIDS and Ebola. The ongoing destruction of forests has also contributed to the greenhouse effect, one consequence of which is an increase in worldwide temperatures. Just slightly higher temperatures have enabled insects and animals that carry deadly bacteria and viruses to expand outward from their tropical habitats, spreading new contagions.

We have set the stage for new plagues in other ways as well. In the United States and many other countries, the reckless use of antibiotics has killed off many strains of bacteria while encouraging the survival of only the toughest and deadliest ones. Unbeknownst to most physicians, but well documented, is how some antibiotics and common pain-relieving drugs suppress the immune system and make us more susceptible to supergerms.

That's only part of an unparalleled assault on the immune system, our inborn defense against these microbial threats.

Much of our food supply has been intentionally contaminated with pesticides, which are toxic to the immune system. Intensive methods of farming have resulted in lower nutritional values in foods. Extensive food refining and manufacturing have created countless new products that titillate the taste buds but do not provide serious nutrition. The fewer the nutrients, particularly vitamins and minerals, the fewer building blocks of immunity we consume, and the more fragile our health becomes. Our bodies become the equivalent of homes without foundations.

All of us should be alarmed by attempts to gut the laws and regulations governing the use of pesticides, the quality of our water and air, and the safety of our food supply. The more our environment, food supply, and health degrade, the harder it will be to restore them. It doesn't matter whether you're a manufacturer or a consumer. We all have to live on the same Earth, and we're all susceptible to infections and other diseases.

The point is to look not at the past but to the future. As individuals and members of societies, we can curb the spread of supergerms by conscientiously washing our hands, by prudently prescribing or taking antibiotics, and by stopping the destruction of the environment. Those acts will lessen the outside forces influencing the emergence and spread of supergerms.

Whatever we do or don't do, though, we will still live in a sea of microorganisms. There is no escape from them, although some germs are clearly more dangerous than others.

Infections—whether chronic and low grade or the dangerous flash of a supergerm—add up to the third leading cause of death in the United States, a number that has somehow gotten lost in medical statistics. Furthermore, the immune system's response to infections sets in motion a cascade of biochemical events that then increases our risk of cardiovascular diseases and cancer, the first and second causes of death.

Even if we cannot control the germs around us—we are, after all, greatly outnumbered—we *can* enhance our bodies' response to them. Simply eating well and taking a few vitamin supplements reduces the physical damage associated with fighting infections.

Unfortunately, most people and their physicians have forgotten that a good diet provides the building blocks of immunity and overall health. When they do recognize the fundamental importance of diet, it's often in the form of lip service, and they wrongly assume that most diets are adequate. But the baseline against which we measure diets has shifted. Too many people are oblivious to the fact that good food is grown, not made.

As a society, we certainly do have the capability to eat well and to feed nearly everyone well. Organic foods are richer in vitamins and minerals and they are free of many hazardous chemicals. We also have at our fingertips, as Nobel laureate Linus Pauling observed, one of the most remarkable enabling technologies of the twentieth century: dietary supplements, which provide concentrated amounts of key nutrients, which optimize the function of the individual cells that make up our bodies.

One final thought. Late in 1995, researchers described an experiment in which a bacterium and its chromosomes were literally blown apart by a dose of radiation three thousand times more powerful than what would kill a person. It was sort of like being at ground zero during a nuclear explosion. In just a few hours, this bacterium had somehow reassembled its chromosomes exactly the way they had originally been. Humpty-Dumpty didn't have this unique talent, and neither do we. In a sense, that sort of tenacity is what we're up against in the microbial world. But we also have managed to coexist with such creatures for millions of years. If we're wise enough to preserve our immunity and overall health, we'll continue doing so.

Jack Challem
Richard P. Huemer, M.D.

APPENDIX

——————— ✂ ———————

There are many excellent sources for additional information on the roles of nutrition in health, as well as sources for nutritional supplements, organic foods, and other products. Your public library, a bookstore, or a health food store are good starting points. The following companies, publications, and organizations have impressed us.

Vitamins and Other Supplements

Many companies sell high-quality supplements. We prefer the brands sold in health food stores because they generally avoid the use of common allergens, artificial colors, and sugar. These are the names of some companies whose products we like and use. Most should be available through health and natural foods stores.

Allergy Research Group/Nutricology (vitamin supplements)
400 Preda Street
San Leandro, CA 94577
(510) 639-4572
1-800-545-9960

Ecological Formulas (vitamin supplements)
1061-B Shary Circle
Concord, CA 94518
1-800-888-4585

J. R. Carlson Laboratories, Inc. (vitamin supplements)
15 College Drive
Arlington Heights, IL 60004
(708) 255-1500
1-800-323-4141

Kyolic/Wakunaga of America (garlic capsules)
23501 Madero
Mission Viejo, CA 92691
(714) 855-2776
1-800-421-2998

Nature's Way (herb and vitamin supplements)
10 Mountain Springs Parkway
Springville, UT 84663
(801) 489-3639

Nature's Secret (vitamin supplements)
5485 Conestoga Court
Boulder, CO 80301
(303) 546-6306
1-800-525-9696

Twin Laboratories (vitamin supplements)
2120 Smithtown Avenue
Ronkonkoma, NY 11779
(516) 467-3140

VITALINE (vitamin supplements)
385 Williamson Way
Ashland, OR 97520
1-800-648-4755

Quigley Corporation (Cold-Eeze™ zinc lozenges)
Landmark Building
10 South Clinton Street
Doylestown, PA 18901
(215) 345-0919
1-800-505-COLD

George Eby Research (Fast Dry™ zinc lozenges)
2109 Paramount Avenue
Austin, Texas 78704
(512) 442-2933

Publication Resources

There are many good magazines, newsletters, journals, and books on nutrition and health. We recommend these.

Well-written and beautifully produced, *Natural Health* spans the field of natural health and alternative medicine. It's published six times a year.

Natural Health
Boston Common Press
PO Box 1200
Brookline Village, MA 01247
(617) 232-1500

The Nutrition Reporter™ newsletter summarizes recent medical journal articles on vitamin and nutrition research. It's suited for both physicians and consumers.

The Nutrition Reporter
PO Box 5505
Aloha, OR 97006
(503) 642-1372

The Townsend Letter for Doctors and Patients is really a magazine that provides a forum for the discussion of alternative medicine.

The Townsend Letter for Doctors and Patients
911 Tyler Street
Port Townsend, WA 98368-6541
(360) 385-6021

The Journal of Applied Nutrition
The International Academy of Nutrition and Preventive
   Medicine
PO Box 18433
Asheville, NC 28814
(704) 258-3243

The *Journal of Orthomolecular Medicine* contains articles on the therapeutic use of vitamins and other nutrients.

Journal of Orthomolecular Medicine
International Society for Orthomolecular Medicine
16 Florence Avenue
Toronto, Ontario Canada M2N 1E9
(416) 733-2117

The Third Line Press has published several books with comprehensive summaries on the role of vitamins and other nutrients in health. For example, the second edition of *Nutritional Influences on Illness*, by Mel Werbach, M.D., describes several thousand medical studies, all with references.

Third Line Press
4751 Viviana Drive
Tarzana, CA 91356
(818) 996-0076
1-800-916-0076

Organic Foods

Organic foods are increasingly popular, and nearly every city has a health or natural foods store with some selection. Larger cities often have one or more natural foods supermarkets, such as Whole Foods and Fresh Fields. Check your phone book.

Several companies also sell organic foods by mail. The largest is **Walnut Acres,** which sells canned foods, cereals, frozen meats, and (during part of the year) fresh produce. You can get a copy of Walnut Acres' forty-five page catalog by calling 1-800-433-3998, or by writing to the company at Walnut Acres Road, Penns Creek, PA 17862. Another mail order supplier of organic foods is **Diamond Organics** in Santa Cruz, CA. Call 1-800-922-2396 for a catalog.

ORGANIC AND HERITAGE SEED COMPANIES

If you're a home gardener and want to grow something besides the limited supermarket varieties of food, look into heirloom seeds. Two companies selling heirloom seeds are:

Abundant Life Seed Foundation
PO Box 772
Port Townsend, WA 98368
(360) 385-5660

Johnny's Selected Seeds
310 Foss Hill Road
Albion, ME 04910
(207) 437-4301

Organizations

The Alliance for the Prudent Use of Antibiotics (APUA) is directed by Stuart B. Levy, M.D., the foremost authority on antibiotic resistance. As the name suggests, APUA is an international organization that encourages the prudent use of antibiotics. Write to the organization at PO Box 1372, Boston, MA 02117-1372. Phone: (617) 636-6765.

The Northwest Coalition for Alternatives to Pesticides (NCAP) is a public advocacy group opposed to the use of pesticides. NCAP also maintains an extensive library of reference materials related to pesticides. Write to NCAP at PO Box 1392, Eugene, OR 97440. Phone: (541) 344-5044. Internet: ncap@igc.apc.org

The Environmental Research Foundation is a small environmental research and information organization that, over the years, has had significant impact on national policy. It publishes *Rachel's Environment & Health Weekly* newsletter, named after Rachel Carson the environmentalist. Write to the Environmental Research Foundation, PO Box 5036, Annapolis, MD 21403. Phone: (410) 263-1584. Internet: erf@rachel.clark.net

The National Pesticide Telecommunications Network (NPTN), a service of the Environmental Protection Agency, provides information about the toxicity of specific pesticides. Call EPA NPTN at 1-800-858-7378.

Vaccine Information & Awareness is a public advocacy group that believes people should have the freedom to choose whether they or their children get immunized. The organization is generally against the use of immunizations and has a wealth of information, pro and con, on the subject. Write to Vaccine Information & Awareness, PO Box 203482, Austin, TX 78720. Phone: 512-832-4176. Internet: via@eden.com.

Mothers and Others for a Livable Planet is dedicated to making environmental concerns, and a desire for organic foods, more practical. Membership in the organization includes an informative newsletter. Write to Mothers and Others, 40 West 20th Street, New York, NY 10011-4211. Phone: (212) 242-0010. Internet: MosNOthrs@aol.com.

Physician Referrals

If you have trouble locating a nutritionally oriented physician, contact one of the following groups for a referral. Send a long self-addressed envelope with postage for 2 ounces.

The American College for Advancement in Medicine
Post Office Box 3427
Laguna Hills, CA 92654

The American Preventive Medical Association
459 Walker Road
Great Falls, VA 22066
(703) 759-0662

The International Society for Orthomolecular Medicine
16 Florence Avenue
Toronto, Ontario Canada M2N 1E9
(416) 733-2117

The International Academy of Nutrition and Preventive Medicine
PO Box 18433
Asheville, NC 28814
(704) 258-3243

Price-Pottenger Nutrition Foundation
PO Box 2614
La Mesa, CA 92044-2614

NOTES

❦

CHAPTER 1

1. The *E. coli* narrative was derived from a variety of news sources, including the Tacoma *Morning News Tribune,* the *Oregonian,* and the Associated Press. For an excellent account of the Seattle-Tacoma *E. coli* outbreak, see "Race with the *E. Coli* Killer: In Search of a Scourge" and "Death Outruns *E. coli* Experts Groping in the Dark for Tiny Killer," by Elaine Porterfield and Sandi Doughton, Tacoma *Morning News Tribune,* April 19 and 20, 1993.

2. Porterfield, E., and Berliant, A., "Jack in the Box Ignored Safety Rules," *The News Tribune,* June 16, 1995.

3. The *Oregonian,* January 29, 1993.

4. USDA Food Safety and Inspection Service, "Talking Points on *E. coli* 0157:H7 Sampling Program," January 1995.

5. *Morbidity and Mortality Weekly Report,* Centers for Disease Control and Prevention, June 9, 1995;44:418–21.

6. Associated Press, July 13, 1995.

7. Associated Press, July 12, 1995.

8. Various sources, including the World Health Organization, Harvard School of Public Health (1990 figures), and Associated Press, December 6, 1994.

9. McGinnis, J. M., and Lee, P.R., "Healthy People 2000 at Mid Decade," *Journal of the American Medical Association,* April 12, 1995;273:1123–1129.

10. National Institute of Allergy and Infectious Diseases, *Report of the Task Force on Microbiology and Infectious Diseases,* Bethesda, MD, 1991.

11. Winker, M.A., et al., "Emerging and Reemerging Global Microbial Threats," *Journal of the American Medical Association,* January 18, 1995;273:241–242.

12. *Monthly Vital Statistics Report,* National Center for Health Statistics, Centers for Disease Control and Prevention, May 12, 1995;43:17.

13. Satcher, D., "Emerging Infections: Getting Ahead of the Curve," *Emerging Infectious Diseases Journal,* January–March 1995;1(1): distributed electronically via the Internet (http://www.cdc.gov/ncidod/EID/eid.htm) by the National Center for Infectious Diseases, Centers for Disease Control and Prevention. See also: Bennett, J. V., Holmberg, S. D., Rogers, M. E., Solomon, S. L. "Infectious and Parasitic Diseases," in *Closing the Gap: The Burden of Unnecessary Illness,* Amler, R. W., Dull, H. B., eds. New York: Oxford University Press, 1987.

14. Pinner, R. W., et al., "Trends in Infectious Diseases Mortality in the United States," *Journal of the American Medical Association*, January 17, 1996; 275:189–193.

15. McCaig, L. F., and Hughes, J. M., "Trends in Antimicrobial Drug Prescribing among Office-Based Physicians in the United States," *Journal of the American Medical Association*, January 18, 1995;273:214–219.

16. Mims, C. A., *The Pathogenesis of Infectious Disease*, 3d ed., Academic Press/Harcourt Brace Jovanovich, London, 1990.

17. Takala, A. K., et al., "Risk Factors for Primary Invasive Pneumococcal Disease among Children in Finland," *Journal of the American Medical Association*, March 15, 1995;273:859–864.

18. Associated Press, September 25, 1994.

19. Associated Press, June 15, 1994.

20. Jack Challem interview with Dan Dudley, April 12, 1995.

21. Troillet, N., et al., "Infections Invasives a Streptococcus pyogenes," *Schweizerische Medizinische Wochenschrift. Journal Suisse de Medecine*, June 18, 1994;124:1064–1069.

22. Jack Challem interview with Dan Dudley, April 12, 1995.

23. Associated Press, May 26, 1994.

24. *Newsweek*, June 20, 1994.

25. The *Oregonian*, January 12, 1995.

26. Associated Press, June 7, 1994.

27. Krause, R. M., "The Origin of Plagues: Old and New," *Science*, August 21, 1992;257:1073–1078.

28. *CD Summary*, Oregon Health Division, April 4, 1995.

29. Jack Challem telephone interview with Cathy Bakamus, April 7, 1995.

30. The *Oregonian*, March 19, 1995.

31. *CD Summary*, Oregon Health Division, April 4, 1995.

32. Gas heat and gas stoves, which cause indoor air pollution from the burning of hydrocarbons, have been implicated in many cases of allergy-like conditions, suggesting a direct impact on the immune system. See Randolph, T. G., *Human Ecology and Susceptibility to the Chemical Environment*, Charles C. Thomas Publisher, Springfield, IL, 1962, and Krohn, J., *The Whole Way to Allergy Relief & Prevention*, Hartley & Marks, 1991.

33. *CD Summary*, Oregon Health Division, Salem, Oregon, April 4, 1995.

CHAPTER 2

1. Associated Press, May 24, 1995.

2. Associated Press, March 20, 1995.

3. *Science News*, June 18, 1994.

4. *Newsday*, March 20, 1995.

5. Associated Press, July 26, 1994.

6. Jack Challem interview with Marc Lappé, Ph.D., September 12, 1994. Dr. Lappé said, "If one person has a cold, everyone on the flight will get it."

7. *Science News*, October 15, 1994.

8. Associated Press, March 2, 1995.

9. *Science News*, March 18, 1995.

10. Associated Press, March 2, 1995.

11. Bloom, B. R., and Murray, C. J. L., "Tuberculosis: Commentary on a Reemergent Killer," *Science*, 1992;257:1055–1064.

12. Associated Press, March 20, 1995.

13. Lappé, M., *Evolutionary Medicine: Rethinking the Origins of Disease*, Sierra Club Books, 1994.

14. Snider Jr., D. E., and Roper, W. L., "The New Tuberculosis," *New England Journal of Medicine*, March 5, 1992;325:703–705.

15. *Science News*, February 6, 1993.

16. Ezzell, C., "Captain of the Men of Death," *Science News*, February 6, 1993;143:90–92.

17. Small, P. M., et al., "The Epidemiology of Tuberculosis in San Francisco. A Population-Based Study Using Conventional and Molecular Methods," *New England Journal of Medicine*, June 16, 1994;330:1703–1709.

18. Alland, D., "Transmission of Tuberculosis in New York City. An Analysis by DNA Fingerprinting and Conventional Epidemiologic Methods," *New England Journal of Medicine*, June 16, 1994;330:1710–1716.

19. The *Oregonian*, July 27, 1995.

20. Tomasz, A., "Multiple-Antibiotic-Resistant Pathogenic Bacteria. A Report on the Rockefeller University Workshop," *New England Journal of Medicine*, April 28, 1994;330:1247–1251.

21. Naziri, W., "Pneumonia in the Surgical Intensive Care Unit. Immunologic Keys to the Silent Epidemic," *Annals of Surgery*, June 1994;219:632–640.

22. Ibid.

23. Hofmann, J., et al., "The Prevalence of Drug-Resistant *Streptococcus pneumoniae* in Atlanta," *New England Journal of Medicine*, August 24, 1995;333:481–486.

24. Breiman, R. F., "Emergence of Drug-Resistant Pneumococcal Infections in the United States," *Journal of the American Medical Association*, June 15, 1994;271:1831–1835.

25. *USA Today*, September 20, 1995.

26. Breiman, R. F., op. cit.

27. *Statistical Abstracts of the United States*, 1987 and 1991.

28. *Facts on File*, 1991.

29. Takala, A. K., "Risk Factors for Primary Invasive Pneumococcal Disease among Children in Finland," *Journal of the American Association*, March 15, 1995;273:859–864.

30. Ibid.

31. Nauts, H. C., *The Beneficial Effects of Bacterial Infections on Host Resistance to Cancer. End Results in 449 Cases*, Monograph No. 8, Second Edition, Cancer Research Institute, New York. 1980.

32. Anonymous, "Survey Shows Link between Antibiotics & Developmental Delays in Children," *Townsend Letter for Doctors and Patients*, October 1995:9.

33. Mandel, E. M., et al., "Efficacy of Amoxicillin with and without Decongestant-Antihistamine for Otitis Media with Effusion in Children. Re-

sults of a Double-Blind, Randomized Study," *New England Journal of Medicine*, February 19, 1987;316:432–437.

34. Findlay, S., "Easing the Agony of Childhood Earaches," *U.S. News & World Report*, January 27, 1992.

35. Cantekin, E. I., McGuire, T. W., and Griffith, T. L., "Antimicrobial Therapy for Otitis Media with Effusion," *Journal of the American Medical Association*, December 18, 1991;266:3309–3317.

36. Jaffe, D. M., et al., "Antibiotic Administration to Treat Possible Occult Bacteremia in Febrile Children," *New England Journal of Medicine*, November 5, 1982;317:1175–1180.

37. Williams, R. L., "Use of Antibiotics in Preventing Recurrent Acute Otitis Media and in Treating Otitis Media with Effusion. A Meta-analytic Attempt to Resolve the Brouhaha," *Journal of the American Medical Association*, September 15, 1993;270:1344–1351.

38. Reves, R. R., "Risk Factors for Fecal Colonization with Trimethoprim-Resistant and Multiresistant *Escherichia coli* among Children in Day-care Centers in Houston, Texas," *Antimicrobial Agents and Chemotherapy*, July 1990;34:1429–1434.

39. Fornasini, M., "Trimethoprim-Resistant *Escherichia coli* in Households of Children Attending Day-care Centers," *Journal of Infectious Diseases*, August 1992;166:326–330.

40. *U.S. News & World Report*, January 27, 1992, and the *New York Times*, April 27, 1994.

41. Kleinman, L. C., "The Medical Appropriateness of Tympanostomy Tubes Proposed for Children Younger than 16 Years in the United States," *Journal of the American Medical Association*, April 27, 1994;271:1250–1255.

42. Associated Press, July 14, 1994.

43. Nsouli, T. M., "Role of Food Allergy in Serous Otitis Media," *Annals of Allergy*, September 1994;73:215–219.

44. Duncan, B., "Exclusive Breast-feeding for at Least 4 Months Protects Against Otitis Media," *Pediatrics*, May 1993;91:867–872.

CHAPTER 3

1. Kunin, C., "Resistance to Antimicrobial Drugs—A Worldwide Calamity," *Annals of Internal Medicine*, April 1, 1993;118:557–561.

2. Levy, S. B., *The Antibiotic Paradox: How Miracle Drugs Are Destroying the Miracle* (New York: Plenum, 1992).

3. Challem, J., "Defend Yourself against Supergerms," *Natural Health*, March/April 1995.

4. Meeting of the American Association for the Advancement of Science, February 16–21, 1995, Atlanta, Georgia.

5. Radicella, J. P., Park, U. P., and Fox, M. S., "Adaptive Mutation in *Escherichia coli*: A Role for Conjugation," *Science*, April 21, 1995;268:418–420.

6. Galitski, T., and Roth, J. R., "Evidence That F Plasmid Transfer Replication Underlies Apparent Adaptive Mutation," *Science*, April 21, 1995;268:421–423.

7. Levy, S. B., op. cit.

8. Kunin, C., op. cit.

9. Neu, H. C., "The Crisis in Antibiotic Resistance," *Science*, August 21, 1992;257:1064–1073.

10. Levy, S. B., op. cit.

11. Adapted from Lappé, M., *Evolutionary Medicine*, Sierra Club Books, 1994, 76.

12. Lappé, M., *Germs That Won't Die: Medical Consequences of the Misuse of Antibiotics*, Anchor Press/Doubleday, New York, 1982.

13. Lappé, M., *Evolutionary Medicine*, Sierra Club Books, 1994.

14. Levy, S. B., et al., "High Frequency of Antimicrobial Resistance in Human Fecal Flora," *Antimicrobial Agents and Chemotherapy*, December 1988;32:1801–1806.

15. Summers, A. O., "Mercury Released from Dental 'Silver' Fillings Provokes an Increase in Mercury- and Antibiotic-Resistant Bacteria in Oral and Intestinal Floras of Primates," *Antimicrobial Agents and Chemotherapy*, April 1993;37:825–834.

16. Shearer, B. G., "Dental Amalgam and Multiple Antibiotic Resistance: An Untested Hypothesis," *Antimicrobial Agents and Chemotherapy*, August 1993;37:1730.

17. Summers, A. O., et al., "Author's Reply," *Antimicrobial Agents and Chemotherapy*, August 1993;37:1730–1731.

18. Tomasz, A., "Multiple-Antibiotic-Resistant Pathogenic Bacteria," *New England Journal of Medicine*, April 28, 1994;330:1247–1251.

19. *Morbidity and Mortality Weekly Report*, Centers for Disease Control and Prevention, August 6, 1993;42:597–599.

20. Shulkin, D. J., et al., "The Economics of Infections. An Analysis of Hospital Costs and Charges in Surgical Patients with Cancer," *Archives of Surgery*, April 1993;128:449–452.

21. Henderson, E., and Love, E. J., "Incidence of Hospital-Acquired Infections Associated with Caesarean Section," *Journal of Hospital Infection*, April 1995;29:245–255.

22. Stone, R., "Search for Sepsis Drugs Goes on Despite Past Failure," *Science*, April 15, 1994;264:365–367.

23. Tomasz, A., op. cit.

24. Emori, T. G., and Gaynes, R. P., "An Overview of Nosocomial Infections, Including the Role of the Microbiology Laboratory," *Clinical Microbiology Review*, 1993;6:428–442.

25. *Morbidity and Mortality Weekly Report*, Centers for Disease Control and Prevention, August 6, 1993;42:597–599.

26. Noble, W. C., Virani, Z., and Cree, R., "Cotransfer of Vancomycin and Other Resistance Genes from *Enterococcus faecalis* NCTC12201 to *Staphylococcus Aureus*," *FEMS Microbiology Letters*, 1992;93:195–198.

27. *New York Times*, December 26, 1995.

28. Finland wrote about the emergence of serious infectious diseases in the antibiotic era in *Journal of the American Medical Association*, 1959;170:2188–2197.

29. Kunin, C. M., op. cit.

30. Anononymous, "Brief Summary of MMWR Recommendations and Reports," Centers for Disease Control and Prevention, September 22, 1995.

31. Associated Press, September 28, 1995.

32. Chren, M. M., and Landefelt, C. S., "Physicians' Behavior and Their Interactions with Companies: A Controlled Study of Physicians Who Requested Additions to a Hospital Drug Formulary," *Journal of the American Medical Association,* 1994;271:684–689.

33. Orlowski, J. P., and Wateska, L., "The Effects of Pharmaceutical Firm Enticements on Prescribing Patterns: There's No Such Thing As a Free Lunch," *Chest,* 1992;102:270–273.

34. Shorr, R. I., and Greene, W. L., "A Food-Borne Outbreak of Expensive Antibiotic Use in a Community Teaching Hospital," *Journal of the American Medical Association,* June 28, 1995;273:1908.

35. Named after Mary Mallon who, in 1915, infected dozens of people with typhoid fever in New York.

36. Unpublished study presented at the 1994 meeting of the Infectious Disease Society, Orlando, Florida. Reported by the Associated Press, October 7, 1994.

37. Associated Press, June 19, 1995.

38. Mastro, T. D., "An Outbreak of Surgical-Wound Infections Due to Group A Streptococcus Carried on the Scalp," *New England Journal of Medicine,* October 4, 1990;323:968–972.

39. Livornese Jr., L. L., et al., "Hospital-Acquired Infection with Vancomycin-Resistant *Enterococcus faecium* Transmitted by Electronic Thermometers," *Annals of Internal Medicine,* July 15, 1992;117:112–116.

40. *Annals of Internal Medicine,* January 15, 1993;118:156–157.

41. Weernink, A., "Pillows, an Unexpected Source of Actinetobacter," *Journal of Hospital Infection,* March 1995;29:189–199.

42. Dryden, M. S., Keyworth, N., Gabb, R., et al., "Asymptomatic Foodhandlers As the Source of Nosocomial Salmonellosis," *Journal of Hospital Infection,* November 1994;28:195–208.

43. Joseph, C. A., and Palmer, S. R., "Outbreaks of Salmonella Infection in Hospitals in England and Wales, 1978–1987," *British Medical Journal,* 1989;298;1161–1164.

44. *Science News,* March 18, 1995, 175.

CHAPTER 4

1. *Business Week,* September 4, 1995.

2. *Newsweek,* March 28, 1994.

3. Holmberg, S. D., et al., "Drug-Resistant Salmonella from Animals Fed Antimicrobials," *New England Journal of Medicine,* September 6, 1984; 311:617–622.

4. Spika, J. S., "Chloramphenicol-Resistant Salmonella Newport Traced through Hamburger to Dairy Farms," *New England Journal of Medicine,* March 5, 1987;316:565–570.

5. Jack Challem interview with Stephen Sundlof, D. V. M., Ph.D., September 19, 1995.

6. *The Stockman's Handbook*, 7th ed., Interstate Publishers, Danville, IL,

7. *The Merck Veterinary Manual*, 6th ed., Merck & Company, Rahway, NJ, 1986.

8. "Antibiotics in Animal Agriculture," *Food Insight*, International Food Information Council Foundation, November/December 1994.

9. Marshall, B., Petrowski, D., and Levy, S. B., "Inter- and Intraspecies Spread of *Escherichia coli* in a Farm Environment in the Absence of Antibiotic Usage," *Proceedings of the National Academy of Sciences of the USA*, September 1990;87:6609–6613.

10. Mims, C. A., *The Pathogenesis of Infectious Disease*, 3d ed., Academic Press/Harcourt Brace Jovanovich, London, 1990.

11. Levy, S. B., et al., "Changes in Intestinal Flora of Farm Personnel after Introduction of a Tetracycline-Supplemented Feed on a Farm," *New England Journal of Medicine*, September 9, 1976;295:583–588.

12. Hansen, L., "Will Healthier Birds Mean Sicker People," *Business Week*, September 4, 1995.

13. Renwick, R. A., et al., "Evidence of Direct Transmission of *Escherichia coli* 0157:H7 Infection between Calves and a Human—Ontario," *Journal of Infectious Diseases*, 1993;168:792–793.

14. Lyons, R. W., "An Epidemic of Resistant Salmonella in a Nursery, Animal-to-Human Spread," *Journal of the American Medical Association*, February 8, 1980;243:546–547.

15. Bezanson, G. S., "Nosocomial Outbreak Caused by Antibiotic-Resistant Strain of *Salmonella typhimurium* Acquired from Dairy Cattle," *Canadian Medical Association Journal*, February 15, 1983;128:426–427.

16. Ryan, C. A., "Massive Outbreak of Antimicrobial-Resistant Salmonellosis Traced to Pasteurized Milk," *Journal of the American Medical Association*, December 11, 1987;258:3269–3274.

17. Lappé M., *Germs That Won't Die: Medical Consequences of the Misuse of Antibiotics*, Anchor Press/Doubleday, New York, 1982.

18. Howe, K., and Linton, A. H., "An Investigation of Calf Carcass Contamination by *Escherichia coli* from the Gut Contents at Slaughter," *Journal of Applied Bacteriology*, 1976;41:37–45.

19. Linton, A. H., and Howe, K., "Antibiotic Resistance among *Escherichia coli* O-serotypes from the Gut and Carcasses of Commercially Slaughtered Broiler Chickens: A Potential Public Health Hazard," *Journal of Applied Bacteriology*, 1977;42:365–378.

20. Linton, A. H., and Howe, K., "The Colonization of the Human Cut by Antibiotic-Resistant *Escherichia coli* from Chickens," *Journal of Applied Bacteriology*, 1977;43:465–469.

21. Holmberg, S. D., op. cit.

22. Spika, J. S., op. cit.

23. *New York Times*, March 21, 1996.

24. Brown D. R., et al., "Role of Microglia and Host Prion Protein in Neurotoxicity of a Prion Protein Fragment," *Nature*, March 28, 1996; 380:345–347.

25. *Newsweek*, March 28, 1994.

26. *FDA Veterinarian*, Food and Drug Administration, November/December, 1994.

27. Millstone, E., et al., "Plagiarism or Protecting Public Health," *Nature*, October 20, 1994;371:647–648.

28. Brunner, E. J., et al., "BST and Animal Health: The Effect of Recombinant Bovine Somatotrophin on Somatic Cell Counts," December 12, 1993. Unpublished.

29. White, J. R., Brunner, E. J., and Millstone, E. P., "An Improved Estimate of the Effect of BST on Clinical Mastitis." Unpublished.

30. *Natural Foods Merchandiser*, May 1995.

CHAPTER 5

1. Elswood, B. F., and Strichker, R. B., "Polio Vaccines and the Origin of AIDS," *Medical Hypotheses*, June 1994;42:347–354; see also Curtis, T., "The Origin of AIDS," *Rolling Stone*, March 19, 1992.

2. Lappé, M., *Evolutionary Medicine: Rethinking the Origins of Disease*, San Francisco, Sierra Club Books, 1994.

3. Nowak, M. A., May, R. M., and Anderson, R. M., "The Evolutionary Dynamics of HIV-1 Quasispecies and the Development of Immunodeficiency Disease," *AIDS*, November 1990;4:1095–1103.

4. Ellison, B. J., and Duesberg, P. H., *Why We Will Never Win the War on AIDS*, Inside Story Communications, El Cerrito, CA, 1994.

5. Anonymous, "Update: Management of Patients with Suspected Viral Hemorrhagic Fever—United States," *MMWR*, 1995;44:475–479.

6. Anonymous, "Update: Management of Patients with Suspected Viral Hemorrhagic Fever—United States," *Journal of the American Medical Association*, August 2, 1995;274–275.

7. Associated Press, September 1, 1995.

8. Groen, J., et al., "Hantavirus Infections in the Netherlands: Epidemiology and Disease," *Epidemiology and Infection*, April 1995;114:373–383.

9. Coimbra, T. L. M., et al., "New Arenavirus Isolated in Brazil," *Lancet*, February 12, 1994;343:391.

10. Anonymous, "Arenavirus Infection—Connecticut, 1994," *Morbidity and Mortality Weekly Report*, September 2, 1994;43:635–636.

11. *USA Today*, June 23, 1995.

12. Associated Press, July 12, 1995.

13. Nowak, R., "Cause of Fatal Outbreak in Horses and Humans Traced," *Science*, April 7, 1995;268:32; and Murray, K., et al., "A Morbillivirus That Caused Fatal Disease in Horses and Humans," *Science*, April 7, 1995;268:94–97.

14. Maurice, J., "Russian Chaos Breeds Diphtheria Outbreak," *Science*, March 10, 1995;267:1416–1417.

15. Associated Press, May 10, 1995.

16. Associated Press, May 23, 1995.

17. The *Oregonian* (New York Times News Service), June 16, 1995.

18. Associated Press, June 16, 1995.

19. Associated Press, May 16, 1995.

CHAPTER 6

1. Pauling, L., "Orthomolecular Psychiatry," *Science,* April 19, 1968;160:265–271.

2. Pauling, L., *Vitamin C and the Common Cold,* W. H. Freeman & Company, San Francisco, 1970.

3. Cameron, E., and Pauling, L., *Cancer and Vitamin C,* Linus Pauling Institute of Science and Medicine, Menlo Park, CA, 1979.

4. Committee on Diet, Nutrition and Cancer, Assembly of Life Sciences, National Research Council, *Diet, Nutrition and Cancer.* Washington, DC: National Academy Press, 1982.

5. Ames, B. N., "Dietary Carcinogens and Anticarcinogens," *Science,* September 23, 1983;221:1256–1264.

6. Pauling, L., *College Chemistry,* W. H. Freeman & Co., San Francisco, 1951, 260.

7. Harman, D., "The Aging Process," *Proceedings of the National Academy of Sciences of the USA,* November 1981;78:7124–7128.

8. Simopoulos, A. P., "Omega-3 Fatty Acids in Health and Disease and in Growth and Development," *American Journal of Clinical Nutrition,* September 1991;54:438–463.

9. Adlercreutz, H., "Plasma Concentrations of Phyto-Estrogens in Japanese Men," *Lancet,* November 13, 1993;342:120912–1210.

10. Kinlen, L. J., "Fat and Breast Cancer," *Cancer Surveys,* 1987;6:585–599.

11. Yonemoto, R. H., "Breast Cancer in Japan and United States: Epidemiology, Hormone Receptors, Pathology, and Survival," *Archives of Surgery,* September 1980;115:1056–1062.

12. Stampfer, M. J., et al., "Vitamin Consumption and the Risk of Coronary Heart Disease in Women," *New England Journal of Medicine,* May 20, 1993;328:1444–1449.

13. Rimm, E. B., "Vitamin E Consumption and the Risk of Coronary Heart Disease in Men," *New England Journal of Medicine,* May 20, 1993;328:1450–1456.

14. Hatton, D. C., and McCarron, D.A., "Dietary Calcium and Blood Pressure in Experimental Models of Hypertension," *Hypertension,* April 1994;23:513–530.

15. Appel, L., "Does Supplementation of Diet with 'Fish Oil' Reduce Blood Pressure? A Meta-analysis of Controlled Clinical," *Archives of Internal Medicine,* June 28, 1993;153:1429–1438.

16. Rose, D. P., "Effects of Dietary Omega-3 Fatty Acids on Human Breast Cancer Growth and Metastases in Nude Mice," *Journal of the National Cancer Institute,* November 3, 1993;85:1743–1747.

17. Lamm, D. L., et al., "Megadose Vitamins in Bladder Cancer: A Double-Blind Clinical Trial," *Journal of Urology,* January 1994;151:21–26.

18. Hoffer, A., and Pauling, L., "Hardin Jones Biostatistical Analysis of Mortality Data for a Second Set of Cohorts of Cancer Patients with a Large

Fraction Surviving at the Termination of the Study and a Comparison of Survival Times of Cancer Patients Receiving Large Regular Oral Doses of Vitamin C and Other Nutrients with Similar Patients Not Receiving These Doses," *Journal of Orthomolecular Medicine*, Third Quarter, 1993;8:157–167.

19. Flynn, M. A., et al., "The Effect of Folate and Cobalamin on Osteoarthritic Hands," *Journal of the American College of Nutrition*, August 1994; 13:351–356.

20. Reid, I. R., et al., "Effect of Calcium Supplementation on Bone Loss in Postmenopausal Women," *New England Journal of Medicine*, 328:460–464.

21. Chapuy, M. C., et al., "Vitamin D_3 and Calcium to Prevent Hip Fractures in Elderly Women," *New England Journal of Medicine*, December 3, 1992;327:1637–1642.

22. Heaney, R., "Thinking about Calcium," *New England Journal of Medicine*, February 18, 1993;328:503–505.

23. Taylor, A., "Cataract: Relationships between Nutrition and Oxidation," *Journal of the American College of Nutrition*, April 1993;12:138–146.

24. Delafuente, J. C., "Nutrients and Immune Responses," *Nutrition and Rheumatic Diseases*, May 1991;17:203–212.

25. See Beisel, W. R., "Single Nutrients and Immunity," *American Journal of Clinical Nutrition*, February 1982 (Supplement); 35:417–468. Despite the date, this comprehensive review article and its 386 references is not "dated."

26. Coodley, G. O., "Micronutrient Concentrations in the HIV Wasting Syndrome," *AIDS*, December 1993;7:1595–1600.

27. Tang, A. M., et al., "Dietary Micronutrient Intake and Risk of Progression to Acquired Immunodeficiency Syndrome (AIDS) in Human Immunodeficiency Virus Type 1 (HIV-1)-Infected Homosexual Men," *American Journal of Epidemiology*, December 1993;138:937–951.

28. Baum, M. K., Letter, *AIDS*, May 1994;8:715.

29. Baum, M. K., "Inadequate Dietary Intake and Altered Nutrition Status in Early HIV-1 Infection," *Nutrition*, 1994;10:16–20.

30. Beisel, W. R., "Herman Award Lecture, 1995: Infection-Induced Malnutrition—from Cholera to Cytokines," *American Journal of Clinical Nutrition*, October 1995;62:813–819.

31. Santos, J. I., "Nutrition, Infection, and Immunocompetence," *Infectious Disease Clinics of North America*, March 1994;8:243–267.

32. Benito Lopez, P., et al., "Influencia del estado de nutricion en la respuesta del organismo a las enfermedades infecciosas," *Revista Clinica Española*, October 1993; 193:255–260.

33. Ames, B. N., Shigenaga, M. K., and Hagan, T. M., "Oxidants, Antioxidants, and the Degenerative Diseases of Aging," *Proceedings of the National Academy of Sciences of the USA*, September 1993;90:7915–7922.

34. Anderson, B. O., "Mechanisms of Neutrophil-Mediated Tissue Injury," *Journal of Surgical Research*, August 1991;51:170–179.

35. Maeda, H., "Oxygen Free Radicals as Pathogenic Molecules in Viral Diseases," *Proceedings of the Society for Experimental Biology and Medicine*, 1991;198:721–727.

36. Beisel, W. R., et al., "Single-Nutrient Effects on Immunologic Functions," *Journal of the American Medical Association*, January 2, 1981;245:53–58.

37. Beisel, W. R., "Single Nutrients and Immunity," *American Journal of Clinical Nutrition,* February 1982 (Supplement); 35:417–468.

38. Rosenbaum, M., "Nutrients and the Immune System," in *The Roots of Orthomolecular Medicine: A Tribute to Linus Pauling,* Huemer, R. P., ed., W. H. Freeman and Company, 1986.

39. Ibid.

40. Lonsdale, D., "Recurrent Febrile Lymphadenopathy Treated with Large Doses of Vitamin B1: Report of Two Cases," *Developmental Pharmacology and Therapeutics,* 1980;1:254–264.

41. Beck, M. A., et al., "Rapid Genomic Evolution of a Non-virulent Coxsackievirus B3 in Selenium-Deficient Mice Results in Selection of Identical Virulent Isolates," *Nature Medicine,* May 1995;1:433–436.

42. Gauntt, C., and Tracey, S., "Deficient Diet Evokes Nasty Heart Virus," *Nature Medicine,* May 1995;1:405–406.

43. Beisel, W. R., op. cit., 1995.

44. Ibid.

CHAPTER 7

1. Liebman, B., "The Changing American Diet," *Nutrition Action Healthletter,* May 1990.

2. Willett, W. C., "Trans Fatty Acids: Are the Effects Only Marginal?" *American Journal of Public Health,* May 1994;84:722–724.

3. Meydani, M., "Vitamin E Requirement in Relation to Dietary Fish Oil and Oxidative Stress in Elderly," *EXS,* 1992;62:411–418.

4. Horwitt, M. K., "Interpretations of Requirements of Thiamine, Riboflavin, Niaci-triptophane, and Vitamin E Plus Comments on Balance Studies and Vitamin B-6," *American Journal of Clinical Nutrition,* 1986;44:973–985.

5. Rose, D. P., "Effects of Dietary Omega-3 Fatty Acids on Human Breast Cancer Growth and Metastases in Nude Mice," *Journal of the National Cancer Institute,* November 3, 1993;85:1743–1747.

6. Beisel, W. R., et al., "Single-Nutrient Effects on Immunologic Functions," *Journal of the American Medical Association,* January 2, 1981;245:53–58.

7. McHugh, M. I., et al., "Immunosuppression with Polyunsaturated Fatty Acids in Renal Transplantation," *Transplantation,* October 1977;24:263–267.

8. *Newsweek,* January 8, 1996.

9. Cheraskin, E., Ringsdorf Jr., W. M., and Clark, J. W., *Diet and Disease,* 2d ed., Keats Publishing, New Canaan, CT, 1995.

10. Cheraskin, E., Ringsdorf Jr., W. M., and Sisley, E. L., *The Vitamin C Connection,* Harper & Row, New York, 1983.

11. *Science News,* October 14, 1989.

12. Pantos, C. E., and Makakis, P., "A Research Note: Ascorbic Acid Content of Artificially Ripened Tomatoes," *Journal of Food Science,* March/April 1973;38:550.

13. Yadav, S. K., and Sehgal, S., "Effect of Home Processing on Ascorbic Acid and Beta-carotene Content of Spinach *(Spinacia oleracia)* and Amaranth *(Amaranthus tricolor)* Leaves," *Plant Foods for Human Nutrition,* February 1995;47:125–131.

14. Prochaska, L. J., and Piekutowski, W. V., "On the Synergistic Effects of Enzymes in Food with Enzymes in the Human Body. A Literature Survey and Analytical Report," *Medical Hypotheses*, 1994;42:355–362.

15. Ibid.

16. Kilshaw, P. J., Heppell, L. M., and Ford, J. E., "Effects of Heat Treatment of Cow's Milk and Whey on the Nutritional Quality and Antigenic Properties," *Archives of Disease in Childhood*, November 1982;57:842–847.

17. Patterson, B. H., "Fruit and Vegetables in the American Diet: Data from the NHANES II Survey," *American Journal of Public Health*, December 1990;80:1443–1449.

18. See Block, G., "The Data Support a Role for Antioxidants in Reducing Cancer Risk," *Nutrition Reviews*, June 1992;50:207–213.

19. *Recommended Dietary Allowances*, 9th ed., National Academy Press, 1980.

20. *Recommended Dietary Allowances*, 10th ed., National Academy Press, 1989.

21. Lachance, P., and Langseth, L., "The RDA Concept: Time for a Change?" *Nutrition Reviews*, August 1994;52:266–270.

22. Williams, R. J., *Biochemical Individuality: The Basis for the Genetotrophic Concept*, John Wiley & Sons, 1956.

23. Pauling, L., *How to Live Longer and Feel Better*, W. H. Freeman & Company, New York, 1986.

24. Hemilä, H., "Does Vitamin C Alleviate the Symptoms of the Common Cold? A Review of Current Evidence," *Scandinavian Journal of Infectious Diseases*, January 1994;26:1–6.

25. Stampfer, M. J., et al., "Vitamin Consumption and the Risk of Coronary Heart Disease in Women," *New England Journal of Medicine*, May 20, 1993;328:1444–1449.

26. Rimn, E. B., "Vitamin E Consumption and the Risk of Coronary Heart Disease in Men," *New England Journal of Medicine*, May 20, 1993;328:1450–1456.

27. Selhub, J., et al., "Vitamin Status and Intake as Primary Determinants of Homocysteinemia in an Elderly Population," *Journal of the American Medical Association*, December 8, 1993;270:2693–2698.

28. Ubbink, J. B., "Vitamin B-12, Vitamin B-6, and Folate Nutritional Status in Men with Hyperhomocysteinemia," *American Journal of Clinical Nutrition*, January 1993;57:47–53.

29. Naurath, H. J., et al., "Effects of Vitamin B12, Folate, and Vitamin B6 Supplements in Elderly People with Normal Serum Vitamin Concentrations," *Lancet*, July 8, 1995;346:85–89.

30. Santos, J. I., "Nutrition, Infection, and Immunocompetence," *Infectious Disease Clinics of North America*, March 1994;8:243–267.

31. Ibid.

32. Yudkin, J., *Sweet and Dangerous*, Peter H. Wyden Publishers, 1972.

33. Jack Challem interview with J. Yudkin, 1975.

34. DaCosta, J. C., and Beardsley, E., "The Resistance of Diabetes to Bacterial Infection," *American Journal of Medical Science*, 1908;136:361.

35. Richardson, R., "Measurements of Phagocytic Activity in Diabetes Mellitus," *American Journal of Medical Science*, 1942;204:229.

36. Kijak, E., Foust, G., and Steinman, R. R., "Relationship of Blood Sugar

Level and Leukocyte Phagocytosis," *Journal of the Southern California Dental Association*, September 1964;32:349–351.

37. Ibid.

38. Sanchez, A., et al., "Role of Sugars in Human Neutrophilic Phagocytosis," *American Journal of Clinical Nutrition*, November 1973;26:1180–1184.

39. Nalder, B. N., et al., "Sensitivity of the Immunological Response to the Nutritional Status of Rats," *Journal of Nutrition*, 1972;102:535–542.

40. Ringsdorf Jr., W. R., Cheraskin, E., and Ramsay Jr., R. R., "Sucrose, Neutrophilic Phagocytosis and Resistance to Disease," *Dental Survey*, December 1976;52:46–48.

41. Marhoffer, W., et al., "Monitoring of Polymorphonuclear Leukocyte Functions in Diabetes Mellitus—A Comparative Study of Conventional Radiometric Function Tests and Low-Light Imaging Systems," *Journal of Bioluminescence and Chemiluminescence*, May/June 1994;9:165–170.

CHAPTER 8

1. Munoz, J., et al., *Proceedings of the Society of Experimental and Biological Medicine*, 1950;75:367–379.

2. Forsgren, A., et al., "Effect of Tetracycline on the Phagocytic Function of Human Leukocytes," *Journal of Infectious Diseases*, October 1974;130:412–415.

3. Martin, R. R., et al., "Chemotaxis of Human Leukocytes: Responsiveness to *Mycoplasma pneumoniae*," *Journal of Laboratory and Clinical Medicine*, April 1973;81:520–529.

4. Martin, R. R., et al., "Effects of Tetracycline on Leukotaxis," *Journal of Infectious Diseases*, February 1974;129:110–116.

5. Forsgren, A., and Schmeling, D., "Effect of Antibiotics on Chemotaxis of Human Leukocytes," *Antimicrobial Agents and Chemotherapy*, April 1977;11:580–584.

6. Belsheim, J., Gnarpe, H., and Lofberg, J., "Granulocyte Function during Prophylaxis with Doxycycline," *Scandinavian Journal of Infectious Diseases*, 1979;11:287–290.

7. Belsheim, J. A., Gnarpe, G. H., and Persson, S., "Tetracyclines and Host Defense Mechanisms: Interference with Leukocyte Chemotaxis," *Scandinavian Journal of Infectious Diseases*, 1979;11:141–145.

8. Belsheim, J., et al., "Tetracycline Influence on Leukocyte Functions," *Acta Oto-Rhino-Laryngologica Belgica*, 1983;37:635–648.

9. Belsheim, J. A., and Gnarpe, G. H., "Antibiotics and Granulocytes. Direct and Indirect Effects on Granulocyte Chemotaxis," *Acta Pathologica et Microbiologica Scandinavica—Section C, Immunology*, August 1981;89:217–221.

10. Forsgren, A., and Gnarpe, H., "The Effect of Antibacterial Agents on the Association between Bacteria and Leukocytes," *Scandinavian Journal of Infectious Diseases—* Supplementum, 1982;33:115–120.

11. Voiculescu, C., et al., "Experimental Study of Antibiotic-Induced Immunosuppression in Mice. II. Th, Ts and NC Cell Involvement," *Comparative Immunology, Microbiology and Infectious Diseases*, 1983;6:301–312.

12. Sheng, F. C., Freischlag, J., Backstrom, B., et al., "The Effects of In Vivo Antibiotics on Neutrophil (PMN) Activity in Rabbits with Peritonitis," *Journal of Surgical Research*, September 1987;43:239–245.

13. Roszkowski, K., et al., "Intestinal Microflora of BALB/c-mice and Function of Local Immune Cells," *Zentralblatt Für Bakteriologie, Mikrobiologie, Und Hygiene—Series A, Medical Microbiology, Infectious Diseases, Virology, Parasitology,* November 1988;270:270–279.

14. Pulverer, G., et al., "Digestive Tract Microflora Liberates Low Molecular Weight Peptides with Immunotriggering Activity," *International Journal of Medical Microbiology,* March 1990;272:318–327.

15. Pulverer, G., et al., "Bacteria of Human Physiological Microflora Liberate Immunomodulating Peptides," *International Journal of Medical Microbiology,* April 1990;272:467–476.

16. Pulverer, G., Ko, H. L., and Beuth, J., "Effets immunomodulateurs des antibiotiques influencant les flores digestives," *Pathologie Biologie,* October 1993;41:753–758.

17. Nord, C. E., Kager, L., and Heimdahl, A., "Impact of Antimicrobial Agents on the Gastrointestinal Microflora and the Risk of Infections," *The American Journal of Medicine,* May 15, 1994;76:99–106.

18. Ibid.

19. Ibid.

20. Nord, C. E., Heimdahl, A., Kager, L., et al., "The Impact of Different Antimicrobial Agents on the Normal Gastrointestinal Microflora of Humans," *Reviews of Infectious Diseases,* March/April 1984, 6 Supplement 1:S270–275.

21. Belsheim, J. A., Gnarpe, G. H., and Persson, S., op. cit., 1979.

22. Florey, H. W., "Penicillin: A Survey," *British Medical Journal,* August 5, 1944;170:4361–4363.

23. *Science News,* October 7, 1995.

24. Stevens, D. L., "Could Nonsteroidal Antiinflammatory Drugs (NSAIDs) Enhance the Progression of Bacterial Infections to Toxic Shock Syndrome?" *Clinical Infectious Diseases,* October 1995;21:977–980.

25. Ibid.

26. Cohen, S. P., et al., "Salicylate Induction of Antibiotic Resistance in *Escherichia coli:* Activation of the Mar Operon and a Mar-Independent Pathway," *Journal of Bacteriology,* December 1993;175:7856–7862.

27. Truss, C. O., "The Role of *Candida albicans* in Human Illness," *Journal of Orthomolecular Psychiatry,* 1981;10:228–238.

28. Lecture by C. O. Truss, M.D., at Nutritional Medicine Today Conference, Toronto, Canada, April 30, 1993; also Challem, J., "What Doctors Said at a Breakthrough Vitamin Conference," *Let's Live,* September 1993:12–21.

29. Crook, W. G., *The Yeast Connection and the Woman,* Professional Books, Jackson, TN, 1995.

30. Nord, C. E., op. cit., 1984.

31. Iwata, K., and Uchida, K., "Cellular Immunity in Experimental Fungus Infections in Mice: The Influence of Infections and Treatment with a Candida Toxin on Spleen Lymphoid Cells," in *Medical Mycology,* 1978; Supplement 1:72–81.

32. Iwata, K., and Yamamoto, Y., "Glycoprotein Toxins Produced by *Candida albicans*," *Proceedings of the Fourth International Conference on the Mycoses*, June 1977, PAHP Scientific Publication #356.

33. Nelson, R. D., et al., "Candida Mannan: Chemistry, Suppression of Cell-Mediated Immunity, and Possible Mechanisms of Action," *Clinical Microbiology Reviews*, January 1991;4:1–19.

34. Pakhomova, E. N., and Bykov, V. L., "Macrophage Interaction with *Candida albicans* in Immunosuppression," *Zhurnal Mikrobiologii, Epidemiologii i Immunobiologii*, January/February 1994;(1):14–16.

35. Ferrari, F. A., et al., "Inhibition of Candidacidal Activity of Human Neutrophil Leukocytes by Aminoglycide Antibiotics," *Antimicrobial Agents and Chemotherapy*, January 1980;17:87–88.

36. Fisher-Hoch, S. P., and Hutwagner, L., "Opportunistic Candidiasis: An Epidemic of the 1980s," *Clinical Infectious Diseases*, October 1995;21:897–904.

37. Aspelin, A. L., *Pesticide Industry Sales and Usage: 1992 and 1993 Market Estimates*, U.S. Environmental Protection Agency, 1994.

38. *CD Summary*, Oregon Health Division, April 18, 1995.

39. Telephone interview with J.C., June 9, 1995.

40. Davis, J. R., et al., "Family Pesticide Use in the Home, Garden, Orchard and Yard," *Archives of Environmental Contamination and Toxicology*, 1992;22:260–266.

41. Wagner, S. L., and Orwick, D. L., "Chronic Organophosphate Exposure Associated with Transient Hypertonia in an Infant," *Pediatrics*, July 1994;94:94–97.

42. Wagner, S. L., and Gallant, J. D., "Organophosphate Intoxication from Over-the-Counter Insecticides," *Annals of Emergency Medicine*, July 1989;18:802.

43. Dandliker, W. B., et al., "Effects of Pesticides on the Immune Response," *Environmental Science and Technology*, 1980;14:204–210.

44. Esser, C., "Dioxins and the Immune System: Mechanisms of Interference. A Meeting Report," *International Archives of Allergy and Immunology*, 1994;104:126–130.

45. Kerkvliet, N. I., and Brauner, J. A., "Mechanisms of 1,2,3,4,6,7,8-heptachlorodibenzo-p-dioxin (HpCDD)-Induced Humoral Immune Suppression: Evidence of Primary Defect in T-cell Regulation," *Toxicology and Applied Pharmacology*, 1987;87:18–31.

46. Thigpen, J. E., et al., "Increased Susceptibility to Bacterial Infection as a Sequela of Exposure to 2,3,7,8-tetrachlorodibenzo-p-dioxin," *Infection and Immunity*, December 1975;12:1319–1324.

47. Yao, Y., et al., "Dioxin Activates HIV-1 Gene Expression by an Oxidative Stress Pathway Requiring a Functional Cytochrome P450 CYP1A1 Enzyme," *Environmental Health Perspectives*, March 1995;103:366–371.

48. *Science News*, July 15, 1995.

49. Davis, D. L., et al., "Medical Hypothesis: Xenoestrogens As Preventable Causes of Breast Cancer," *Environmental Health Perspectives*, October 1993;101:372–377.

50. Wolff, M. S., "Blood Levels of Organochlorine Residues and Risk of Breast Cancer," *Journal of the National Cancer Institute*, April 21, 1993;85:648–652.

51. Raloff, J., "Something's Fishy," *Science News*, July 2, 1994;146:8–9.

52. Montague, P., "A New Era in Environmental Toxicology," *Rachel's Hazardous Waste News #365*, November 25, 1993.

53. See Hileman, B., "Environmental Estrogens Linked to Reproductive Abnormalities, Cancer," *Chemical and Engineering News*, January 31, 1994;19–23.

54. Dandliker, W. B., op. cit.

55. Hermanowicz, A., and Kossman, S., "Neutrophil Function and Infectious Disease in Workers Occupationally Exposed to Phosphoorganic Pesticides: Role of Mononuclear-Derived Chemotactic Factor for Neutrophils," *Clinical Immunology and Immunopathology*, 1984;33:13–22.

56. Giurgea, R., et al., "Beitrag zum Einfluss einiger organochlorurierter Pestizide auf die immunologische Reaktivitat der weissen Ratte," *Achiv für Experimentelle Veterinarmedizin*, 1978;32:769–774.

57. Street, J. C., and Chadwick, R. W., "Ascorbic Acid Requirements and Metabolism in Relation to Organochlorine Pesticides," *Annals of the New York Academy of Sciences*, September 30, 1975;258:132–143.

58. Associated Press, June 15, 1995.

59. Porter, W. P., "Toxicant-Disease-Environment Interactions Associated with Suppression of Immune System, Growth, and Reproduction," *Science*, June 1, 1984;224:1014–1017.

60. Ibid.

61. Holdren, C., "Entomologists Wane as Insects Wax," *Science*, November 10, 1989;246:754–756.

62. Various sources, including Vos, J. G., and Krajnc, E.I., "Immunotoxicity of Pesticides," in *Developments in the Science and Practice of Toxicology*, Hayes, A. W., ed., Elsevier Science Publishers, 1983, 229–240; Thomas, P. T., et al., "Immunologic Effects of Pesticides," in *The Effects of Pesticides on Human Health*, Baker, S. R., and Wilkinson, C. F., eds., Princeton Scientific Publishing, 1990, 261–295.

63. Associated Press, October 18, 1994.

64. Associated Press, August 17, 1995.

65. Associated Press, February 16, 1995.

66. Green, M. A., "An Outbreak of Watermelon-Borne Pesticide Toxicity," *American Journal of Public Health*, November 1987;77:1431–1434.

67. Associated Press, June 4, 1995.

68. The *Oregonian*, October 25, 1995.

69. Hallengren, B. and Forsgren, A., "Effect of Alcohol on Chemotaxis, Adherence and Phagocytosis of Human Polymorphonuclear Leucocytes," *Acta Medica Scandinavia*, 1978;204:43–48.

70. See Pillai, R., Nair, B. S., and Watson, R. R., "AIDS, Drugs of Abuse and the Immune System: A Complex Immunotoxicological Network," *Archives of Toxicology*, 1991;65:609–617.

71. Ibid.

72. An excellent assessment of the stresses from overwork appeared in "Breaking Point," *Newsweek*, March 6, 1995.

73. Fuller, R., "Probiotics in Man and Animals," *Journal of Applied Bacteriology*, 1989;66:365–378.

74. Fuchs, B. A., and Sanders, V. M., "The Role of Brain-Immune Interactions in Immunotoxicology," *Critical Reviews in Toxicology*, 1994;24:151–176.

75. Flach, J., and Seachrist, L., "Mind-Body Meld May Boost Immunity," *Journal of the National Cancer Institute*, February 16, 1994;86:256–258.

76. Cohen, S., Tyrrell, D. A., and Smith, A. P., "Psychological Stress and Susceptibility to the Common Cold," *New England Journal of Medicine*, August 29, 1991;325:606–612.

77. Flach, J., and Seachrist, L., op. cit.

78. Berk, L. S., et al., "Eustress of Humor Associated Laughter Modulates Specific Immune System Components," *Annals of Behavioral Medicine*, 1993 (Supplement);15:S111.

79. Nieman, D. C., "Exercise, Upper Respiratory Tract Infection, and the Immune System," *Medicine and Science in Sports and Exercise*, February 1994;26:128–139.

80. Sparling, P. B., Nieman, D. C., and O'Connor, P. J., "Selected Scientific Aspects of Marathon Racing. An Update on Fluid Replacement, Immune Function, Psychological Factors and the Gender Difference," *Sports Medicine*, February 1993;15:116–132.

81. Peters, E. M., et al., "Vitamin C Supplementation Reduces the Incidence of Postrace Symptoms of Upper-Respiratory-Tract Infection in Ultramarathon Runners," *American Journal of Clinical Nutrition*, February 1993;57:170–174.

82. Shepard, R. J., and Shek, P. N., "Infectious Diseases in Athletes: New Interest for an Old Problem," *Journal of Sports Medicine and Physical Fitness*, March 1994;34:11–22.

83. Cooper, K. H., *Antioxidant Revolution*, Thomas Nelson Publishers, Nashville, 1994.

CHAPTER 9

1. *Newsweek*, March 27, 1989.

2. *Living Earth and the Food Magazine* (England), May 1994; based on Pither and Hall, *Technical Memorandum 597*, Campden Research Station, Ministry of Agriculture, Fisheries and Food project no. 4350, 1990 (unpublished).

3. Ibid.

4. Jack Challem interview with Robert L. Smith, November 29, 1994.

5. Smith, B. L., "Organic Foods vs. Supermarket Foods: Element Levels," *Journal of Applied Nutrition*, 1993;45:35–39.

6. Jack Challem telephone interview with Robert L. Smith, November 29, 1994.

7. Smith, B. L., op. cit.

8. *Abundant Life Seed and Book Catalog*, Abundant Life Seed Foundation, 1995.

9. For a philosophical discussion of the value of heirloom seeds, see Ausubel, K., *Seeds of Change*, HarperSanFrancisco Publishers, 1994.

10. Ingham, E., "Soil Microbial Biomass Service: Interpretation of Microbial Information." (Unpublished.)

11. *Science News*, October 14, 1995.

12. Ingham, E., op. cit.

13. Ibid.

14. The *Oregonian*, April 20, 1995.

15. Flattau, E., "Organic Farming Maturing As a Competitive Alternative," The *Oregonian*, May 27, 1993.

16. *Science News*, October 14, 1995.

17. Adler, T., "Bugs for Hire: Siccing Good Insects on Bad Ones," *Science News*, May 13, 1995.

18. Jayaraj, A., and Rabindra, R. J., "The Local View on the Role of Plant Protection in Sustainable Agriculture in India," *Ciba Foundation Symposium*, 1993;177:168–184.

19. *Science News*, June 17, 1995.

20. Raloff, J., "Garden-Variety Tonic for Stress: Vitamins May Invigorate Leafy Plants," *Science News*, February 8, 1992;141:94–95.

21. *Science News*, October 14, 1989.

22. Jack Challem interview with Mel Coleman Sr., December 12, 1994.

23. Jack Challem telephone interview with Kay Weedon, June 29, 1995.

24. Jack Challem interview with Mel Coleman Sr., June 30, 1995.

25. *Natural Foods Merchandiser*, June 1995.

26. Ibid.

27. "Shattering a Myth: Organic Packaged Food Can Be the Cheapest Buy," *The Green Guide for Everyday Life*, Mothers and Others for a Livable Planet, April 14, 1995.

28. Stanley, V. G., et al., "Magnesium Sulfate Effects on Coliform Bacteria Reduction in the Intestines, Ceca, and Carcasses of Broiler Chickens," *Poultry Science*, January 1992;71:76–80.

29. Tengerdy, R. P., "Effect of Beta-carotene on Disease Protection and Humoral Immunity in Chickens," *Avian Diseases*, October–December 1990;34:848–854.

30. Tengerdy, R. P., "Vitamin E, Immune Response, and Disease Resistance," *Annals of the New York Academy of Sciences*, 1989;570:335–344.

31. Hogan, J. S., et al., "Role of Vitamin E and Selenium in Host Defense against Mastitis," *Journal of Dairy Science*, September 1993;76:2795–2803.

32. *Federal Register*, February 3, 1995.

33. The *Oregonian*, February 1, 1995.

34. Hays, S. M., "Natural Microbes Curb Salmonella," Agricultural Research, November 1994.

35. *Food and Nutrition Research Briefs*, USDA, April 1995.

36. Rasmussen, M. A., et al., "Rumen Contents As a Reservoir of Enterohemorrhagic *Escherichia coli*," *FEMS Microbiology Letters*, 1993;114:79–84.

CHAPTER 10

1. Weber, G. H., correspondence, March 16, 1992.

2. Salminen, S., et al., "Lactic Acid Bacteria in Health and Disease," in *Lactic Acid Bacteria*, Salminen, S., and von Wright, A., eds., Marcel Dekker, Inc., New York, 1993.

3. Salminen, S., "The Role of Intestinal Microflora in Preserving Intestinal Integrity and Health with Special Reference to Lactic Acid Bacteria," *Annals of Medicine,* February 1990;22:35.

4. Ballongue, J., "Bifidobacteria and Probiotic Action," in *Lactic Acid Bacteria,* Salminen, S., and von Wright, A., eds., Marcel Dekker, Inc., New York, 1993.

5. Torres-Alipi, B. I., "Colonizacion bacteriana de la cavidad oral del recien nacido," *Boletín Médico del Hospital Infantil de México,* February 1990; 47:78–83.

6. Hall, M. A., et al., "Factors Influencing the Presence of Faecal Lactobacilli in Early Infancy," *Archives of Disease in Childhood,* February 1990;65:185–188.

7. Salminen, S., op. cit.

8. Selwyn, S., "Natural Antibiotics among Skin Bacteria As a Primary Defence Against Infection," *British Journal of Dermatology,* 1975;93:487–493.

9. Ibid.

10. Ballongue, J., op. cit.

11. Gorbach, S. L., and Goldin, B., U.S. patent application number 724114, 1985.

12. Gorbach, S. L., "Lactic Acid Bacteria and Human Health," *Annals of Medicine,* 1990;22:37–41.

13. Ballongue, J., op. cit.

14. Silva, M., et al., "Antimicrobial Substance from a Human *Lactobacillus* Strain," *Antimicrobial Agents and Chemotherapy,* August 1987;31:1231–1233.

15. Pulverer, G., et al., "Digestive Tract Microflora Liberates Low Molecular Weight Peptides with Immunotriggering Activity," *International Journal of Medical Microbiology,* March 1990;272:318–327.

16. Pulverer, G., et al., "Bacteria of Human Physiological Microflora Liberate Immunomodulating Peptides," *International Journal of Medical Microbiology,* April 1990;272:467–476.

17. Belsheim, J., et al., "Tetracycline Influence on Leukocyte Functions," *Acta Oto-Rhino-Laryngologica Belgica,* 1983;37:635–648.

18. Pulverer, G., Ko, H. L., and Beuth, J., "Effets immunomodulateurs des antibiotiques influencant les flores digestives," *Pathologie Biologie,* October 1993;41:753–758.

19. Perdigon, G., et al., "Effect of Preorally Administered Lactobacilli on Macrophage Activity in Mice," *Infection and Immunity,* August 1986;53:404–410.

20. Perdigon, G., et al., "Enhancement of Immune Response in Mice Fed with *Streptococcus thermophilus* and *Lactobacillus acidophilus,*" *Journal of Dairy Science,* May 1987;70:919–926.

21. Perdigon, G., et al., "System Augmentation of the Immune Response in Mice by Feeding Fermented Milks with *Lactobacillus casei* and *Lactobacillus acidophilus,*" *Immunology,* January 1988;63:117–123.

22. Halpern, G. M., "Influence of Long-Term Yoghurt Consumption in Young Adults," *International Journal of Immunotherapy,* 1991;7:205–210.

23. Carper, J., *Food — Your Miracle Medicine,* HarperCollins Publishers, New York, 1993.

24. Siitonen, S., Vapaatalo, H., et al., "Effect of *Lactobacillus* GG Yogurt in Prevention of Antibiotic Associated Diarrhoea," *Annals of Medicine,* February 1990;22:57–59.

25. Isolauri, E., "Mucosal Barrier and Lactic Acid Bacteria," *14th Annual Meeting of the Society of Intestinal Microecology*, Helsinki, Abstracts, 3–4; see also Isolauri, E., et al., "A Human *Lactobacillus* Strain (*Lactobacillus casei* sp strain GG) Promotes Recovery from Acute Diarrhea in Children," *Pediatrics*, July 1991;88:90–97.

26. Saavedra, J. M., et al., "Feeding of *Bifidobacterium bifidum and Streptococcus thermophilus* to Infants in Hospital for Prevention of Diarrhoea and Shedding of Rotavirus," *Lancet*, October 15, 1994;344:1046–1049.

27. Oksanen, P., et al., "Prevention of Travelers' Diarrhea by *Lactobacillus* GG, *Annals of Medicine*, February 1990;22:53–56.

28. Lappé, M., *Germs That Won't Die: Medical Consequences of the Misuse of Antibiotics*, Anchor Press/Doubleday, New York, 1982, 157.

29. Neri, A., et al., "Bacterial Vaginosis in Pregnancy Treated with Yoghurt," *Acta Obstetricia Gynecologica Scandinavaca*, January 1993; 72:17–19.

30. Hallen, A., et al., "Treatment of Bacterial Vaginosis with Lactobacilli," *Sexually Transmitted Diseases*, May/June 1992;19:146–148.

31. Reid, G., et al., "Implantation of *Lactobacillus casei* var *rhamnosus* into Vagina," *Lancet*, 1994;344:1229.

32. Hilton, E., et al., "Ingestion of Yogurt Containing *Lactobacillus acidophilus* as Prophylaxis for Candidal Vaginitis," *Annals of Internal Medicine*, March 1, 1992;116:353–357.

33. Collins, F. M., and Carter, P. B., "Growth of *Salmonellae* in Orally Infected Germfree Mice," *Infection and Immunity*, 1978;21:41–47.

34. Hitchins, A. D., "Amelioration of the Adverse Effect of a Gastrointestinal Challenge with *Salmonella enteritidis* on Weanling Rats by a Yogurt Diet," *American Journal of Clinical Nutrition*, January 1985;451:92–100.

35. Alm, L., "The Effect of *Lactobacillus acidophilus* Administration upon the Survival of *Salmonella* in Randomly Selected Human Carriers," *Progress in Food and Nutrition Science*, 1983;7:13–17.

36. Alm, L., "Survival Rate of *Salmonella* and *Shigella* in Fermented Milk Products with and without Added Human Gastric Juice: An *In Vitro* Study," *Progress in Food and Nutrition Science*, 1983;7:19–28.

37. Hesseltine, C. W., "Mixed-Culture Fermentations," in *Applications of Biotechnology to Traditional Fermented Foods*, report of an ad hoc panel of the board on science and technology for international development, Office of International Affairs, National Research Council, National Academy Press, 1992.

38. See *Applications of Biotechnology to Traditional Fermented Foods*, report of an ad hoc panel of the board on science and technology for international development, Office of International Affairs, National Research Council, National Academy Press, 1992.

39. Hughes, V. L., and Hillier, S. L., "Microbiologic Characteristics of *Lactobacillus* Products Used for Colonization of the Vagina," *Obstetrics & Gynecology*, 1990;75:244–248.

40. Roberfroid, M. B., et al., "Colonic Microflora: Nutrition and Health," *Nutrition Reviews*, May 1995;53:127–130.

41. Gibson, G. R., and Roberfroid, M. B., "Dietary Modulation of a Human

Colonic Microbiota: Introducing the Concept of Prebiotics," *Journal of Nutrition*, 1995;125:1401–1412.

42. Ibid.

CHAPTER 11

1. Abdullah, T. H., et al., "Garlic Revisited: Therapeutic for the Major Diseases of Our Times?" *Journal of the National Medical Association*, 1980;80:439–445.

2. Farbman, K. S., et al., "Antibacterial Activity of Garlic and Onions: A Historical Perspective," *Pediatric Infectious Disease Journal*, July 1993;12:613–614.

3. Block, E., "The Chemistry of Garlic and Onions," *Scientific American*, March 1985;252:114–119.

4. Cavallito, C. J., and Bailey, J. H., "Allicin, the Antibacterial Principle of *Allium sativum*. I. Isolation, Physical Properties of Antibacterial Action," *Journal of the American Chemical Society*, November 1944;66:1950–1951.

5. See Wills, E. D., "Enzyme Inhibition by Allicin, the Active Principle of Garlic," *Biochemical Journal*, 1956;63:514–520.

6. Spray, W., "The Importance of Taking Garlic," *Nursing Times*, February 16, 1978;295.

7. Rich, G. E., "Garlic an Antibiotic?" *Medical Journal of Australia*, January 23, 1995;1:60.

8. Lau, B. H. S., *Garlic Research Update*, Odyssey Publishing, Vancouver, B.C., Canada, 1991.

9. Itakura, Y., "The Composition of Garlic and Garlic Products: Some Newly Identified Ones," presented at the First World Congress on the Health Significance of Garlic and Garlic Constituents, Washington, DC, August 28–30, 1990.

10. Tonstad, S., "Kosttilskudd i behandling av hyperlipidemi," *Tidsskrift for Den Norske Laegeforening*, November 20, 1991;111:3398–4000.

11. Abdullah, T. H., op. cit.

12. Itakura, Y., op. cit.

13. Cavallito, C. J. and Bailey, J. H., op. cit.

14. Cavallito, C. J., and Bailey, J. H., "Allicin, the Antibacterial Principle of *Allium sativum*. II. Determination of the Chemical Structure," *Journal of the American Chemical Society*, November 1944;66:1952–1954.

15. Hirao, Y., et al., "Activation of Immunoresponder Cells by the Protein Fraction from Aged Garlic Extract," *Phytotherapy Research*, 1987;1:161–164.

16. Lau, B. H. S., "Detoxifying, Radioprotective and Phagocyte-Enhancing Effects of Garlic," *International Clinical Nutrition Review*, January 1989;9:27–31.

17. Lau, B. H. S., et al., "Garlic Compounds Modulate Macrophage and T-lymphocyte Functions," *Molecular Biotherapy*, June 1991;3:103–107.

18. Kandil, O. M., et al., "Garlic and the Immune System in Humans: Its Effect on Natural Killer Cells," *Federation Proceedings*, 1987;46:441.

19. Abdullah, T. H., "Enhancement of Natural Killer Cell Activity in AIDS with Garlics," *Deutsche Zeitschrift für Onkologie*, 1989;21:52–53.

20. Ibid.

21. See reference number 4, Chapter 11.

22. Chowdhury, A. K., et al., "Efficacy of Aqueous Extract of Garlic and

Allicin in Experimental Shigellosis in Rabbits," *Indian Journal of Medical Research,* January 1991;93:33–36.

23. Farbman, K. S., et al., op cit.

24. Rao, R. R., et al., "Inhibition of *Mycobacterium tuberculosis* by Garlic Extract," *Nature,* April 6, 1946;157:441.

25. Deshpande, R. G., et al., "Inhibition of *Mycobacterium avium* Complex Isolates from AIDS Patients by Garlic *(Allium sativum),*" *Journal of Antimicrobial Chemotherapy,* 1993;32:623–626.

26. Weber, N. D., et al., "In Vitro Virucidal Effects of *Allium sativum* (Garlic) Extract and Compounds," *Planta Medica,* October 1992;58:417–423.

27. Mirelman, D., et al., "Inhibition of Growth of *Entamoeba histolytica* by Allicin, the Active Principle of Garlic Extract *(Allium sativum),*" *Journal of Infectious Diseases,* July 1987;156:243–244.

28. Soffar, S. A., and Mokhtar, G. M., "Evaluation of the Antiparasitic Effect of Aqueous Garlic *(Allium sativum)* Extract in Hymenoepiasis nana and Giardiasis," *Journal of the Egyptian Society of Parasitology,* August 1991;21:497–502.

29. Lun, Z. R., et al., "Antiparasitic Activity of Diallyl Trisulfide (Dasuansu) on Human and Animal Pathogenic Protozoa (*Trypanosoma* sp., *Entamoeba histolytica* and *Giardia lamblia*) In Vitro," *Annales de la Societe Belge de Medecine Tropicale,* March 1994;74:51–59.

30. Perez, H. A., et al., "In Vivo Activity of Ajoene against Rodent Malaria," *Antimicrobial Agents and Chemotherapy,*" February 1994;38:337–339.

31. Lau, B. H. S., *Garlic Research Update,* Odyssey Publishing, Vancouver, B.C, Canada, 1991.

32. Tadi, P. P., et al., "Anticandidal and Anticarcinogenic Potentials of Garlic," *International Clinical Nutrition Review,* October 1990;10:423–429.

33. Anonymous, "Garlic in Cryptococcal Meningitis. A Preliminary Report of 21 Cases," *Chinese Medical Journal,* February 1980;93:123–126.

34. Ibid.

35. Davis, L. E., Shen, J. K., and Cai, Y., "Antifungal Activity in Human Cerebrospinal Fluid and Plasma after Intravenous Administration of *Allium sativum,*" *Antimicrobial Agents and Chemotherapy,*" April 1990;34:651–653.

36. Adetumbi, M. A., and Lau, B. H. S., "*Allium sativum* (Garlic)—a Natural Antibiotic," *Medical Hypotheses,* 1983;12:227–237.

37. Harman, D., "The Aging Process," *Proceedings of the National Academy of Sciences of the USA,* November 1981;78:7124–7128.

38. Ames, B. N., Shigenaga, M. K., and Hagan, T. M., "Oxidants, Antioxidants, and the Degenerative Diseases of Aging," *Proceedings of the National Academy of Sciences of the USA,* September 1993;90:7915–7922.

39. Lin, X. Y., Liu, J. Z., and Milner, J. A., "Dietary Garlic Suppresses DNA Adducts Caused by N-nitroso Compounds," *Carcinogenesis,* February 1994;15:349–352.

40. Liu, J., Lin, R. I., Milner, J. A., "Inhibition of 1,12-dimethylbenz-[a]anthracene-Induced Mammary Tumors and DNA Adducts by Garlic Powder," *Carcinogenesis,* October 1992;13:1847–1851.

41. Jain, A. K., et al., "Can Garlic Reduce Levels of Serum Lipids? A Controlled Clinical Study," *American Journal of Medicine,* June 1993;94:632–635.

42. Sendl, A., et al., "Inhibition of Cholesterol Synthesis In Vitro by Extracts and Isolated Compounds Prepared from Garlic and Wild Garlic," *Atherosclerosis*, May 1992;94:79–85.

43. Jain, A. K., et al., op. cit.

44. Block, E., op. cit.

45. Kiesewetter, H., et al., "Effects of Garlic Coated Tablets in Peripheral Arterial Occlusive Disease," *Clinical Investigator*, May 1993;71:383–386.

46. *New York Times*, July 27, 1995.

CHAPTER 12

1. Stone, I., "Hypoascorbemia, the Genetic Disease Causing the Human Requirement for Exogenous Ascorbic Acid," *Perspectives in Biology and Medicine*, 1966;10:133–134.

2. See Stone, I., *The Healing Factor: Vitamin C Against Disease*, Grosset & Dunlap, New York, 1972.

3. Sato, P. H., and Grahn, I. V., "Administration of Isolated Chicken L-gulonolactone Oxidase to Guinea Pigs Evokes Ascorbic Acid Synthetic Capacity," *Archives of Biochemistry and Biophysics*, September 1981;210:609–616.

4. Stone, I., 1972, op. cit.

5. Ibid.

6. Pauling, L., *Vitamin C and the Common Cold*, W. H. Freeman and Company, San Francisco, 1970.

7. Pauling, L., "The Significance of the Evidence about Ascorbic Acid and the Common Cold," *Proceedings of the National Academy of Sciences of the USA*, November 1971;68:2678–2681.

8. Chalmers, T. C., "Effects of Ascorbic Acid on the Common Cold. An Evaluation of the Evidence," *American Journal of Medicine*, April 1975;58:532–536.

9. Hemilä, H., and Herman, Z. S., "Vitamin C and the Common Cold: A Retrospective Analysis of Chalmers' Review," *Journal of the American College of Nutrition*, April 1995;14:116–123.

10. Hemilä, H., "Vitamin C and the Common Cold," *British Journal of Nutrition*, 1992;67:3–16.

11. Hemilä, H., "Does Vitamin C Alleviate the Symptoms of the Common Cold? A Review of Current Evidence," *Scandinavian Journal of Infectious Diseases*, January 1994;26:1–6.

12. Hemilä, H., and Herman, Z. S., op. cit.

13. Ibid.

14. See references in Stone, I., *The Healing Factor: Vitamin C Against Disease*, Grosset & Dunlap, New York, 1972.

15. See references in Smith, L. H., *Vitamin C As a Fundamental Medicine. Abstracts of Dr. Frederick R. Klenner M.D.'s Published and Unpublished Work*, Life Sciences Press, Tacoma, WA, 1988.

16. Ibid.

17. Ibid.

18. Challem, J. J., and Lewin, R., "Vitamin C Stops Infections," *Let's Live,* July, 1982.

19. Ibid.

20. Ibid.

21. Cathcart, R. F., "Vitamin C, Titrating to Bowel Tolerance, Anascorbemia, and Acute Induced Scurvy," *Medical Hypotheses,* 1981;7:1359–1376.

22. Cathcart, R. F., "The Third Face of Vitamin C," *Journal of Orthomolecular Medicine,* 1992;7:197–200.

23. Cathcart, R. F., "Vitamin C in the Treatment of Acquired Immune Deficiency Syndrome (AIDS)," *Medical Hypotheses,* 1984;14:423–433.

24. Challem, J. J., and Lewin, R. L., "Vitamin C: The Megavitamin That Battles AIDS," *Let's Live,* August 1986.

25. Cathcart, R. F., "Proposal to Study the Therapeutic Effects of Intravenously Administered Ascorbate for the Treatment of AIDS," (unpublished) November 1983.

26. Goldschmidt, M. C., "Reduced Bacterial Activity in Neutrophils from Scorbutic Animals and the Effect of Ascorbic Acid on These Target Bacteria In Vivo and In Vitro," *American Journal of Clinical Nutrition,* December 1991;54:1214S–1220S.

27. Ibid.

28. Levy, R., and Schlaeffer, F., "Successful Treatment of a Patient with Recurrent Furunculosis by Vitamin C: Improvement of Clinical Course and of Impaired Neutrophil Functions," *International Journal of Dermatology,* November 1993;32:832–834.

29. Anderson, R., et al., "The Effects of Increasing Weekly Doses of Ascorbate on Certain Cellular and Humoral Immune Functions in Normal Volunteers," *American Journal of Clinical Nutrition,* January 1980;33:71–76.

30. Johnston, C. S., "Vitamin C Elevates Red Blood Cell Glutathione in Healthy Adults," *American Journal of Clinical Nutrition,* 1993;58:103–105.

31. Anthony, L. E., et al., "Cell-Mediated Cytotoxicity and Humoral Immune Response in Ascorbic Acid-Deficient Guinea Pigs," *American Journal of Clinical Nutrition,* August 1979;32:1691–1699.

32. Goldschmidt, M. C., op. cit.

33. Washko, P., "Ascorbic Acid in Human Neutrophils," *American Journal of Clinical Nutrition,* December 1991;54:1221S–1227S.

34. Kennes, B., et al., "Effect of Vitamin C Supplements on Cell-Mediated Immunity in Old People," *Gerontology,* 1983;29:305–310.

35. Hume, R., and Weyers, E., "Changes in Leukocyte Ascorbic Acid during the Common Cold," *Scottish Medical Journal,* January 1973;18:3–7.

36. Pauling, L., "Ascorbic Acid and the Common Cold," *Scottish Medical Journal,* January 1973;18:1–2.

37. Hume, R., and Weyers, E., op. cit.

38. Pauling, L., 1973, op. cit.

39. Anderson, R., and Lukey, P. T., "A Biological Role for Ascorbate in the Selective Neutralization of Extracellular Phagocyte-Derived Oxidants," *Annals of the New York Academy of Sciences,* 1987;498:229–247.

40. Anderson, R., et al., "Ascorbate and Cysteine-Mediated Selective Neu-

tralisation of Extracellular Oxidants during N-formyl Peptide Activation of Human Phagocytes," *Agents and Actions,* February 1987;20:77–86.

41. Cathcart, R. F., "A Unique Function for Ascorbate," *Medical Hypotheses,* May 1991;35:32–37.

42. Harakeh, S., and Jariwalla, R. J., "Comparative Study of the Anti-HIV Activities of Ascorbate and Thiol-Containing Reducing Agents in Chronically HIV-Infected Cells," *American Journal of Clinical Nutrition,* December 1991;54:1231S–1235S.

43. Nakanishi, T., "A Report on a Clinical Experience of Which Has Successfully Made Several Antibiotics-Resistant Bacteria (MRSA etc.) Negative on a Bedsore," *Igaku Kenkyu—Acta Medica,* February 1992;62:31–37.

44. Jack Challem interview with Dr. R. F. Cathcart, August 15, 1995.

45. Cathcart, R. F., "The Vitamin C Treatment of Allergy and the Normally Unprimed State of Antibodies," *Medical Hypotheses,* November 1986;21:307–321.

46. Amabile-Cuevas, C. F., et al., "Decreased Resistance to Antibiotics and Plasmid Loss in Plasmid-Carrying Strains of *Staphylococcus aureus* Treated with Ascorbic Acid," *Mutation Research,* November 1991;264:119–125.

47. Hickman, P., et al., "Neutrophils May Contribute to the Morbidity and Mortality of Claudicants," *British Journal of Surgery,* 1994;81:790–798.

48. Ibid.

49. Woodhouse, P. R., Khaw, K. T., et al., "Seasonal Variations of Plasma Fibrinogen and Factor VII Activity in the Elderly: Winter Infections and Death from Cardiovascular Disease," *Lancet,* February 19, 1994;343:435–439.

50. Khaw, K.T., and Woodhouse, P. R., "Interrelation of Vitamin C, Infection, Haemostatic Factors, and Cardiovascular Disease," *British Medical Journal,* June 17, 1995;310:1559–1563.

51. Challem, J. J., "Views on Vitamin C and Cancer. An Interview with Linus Pauling, Ph.D.," *Let's Live,* January 1991.

52. Cameron, E., and Pauling, L., *Cancer and Vitamin C,* Linus Pauling Institute of Science and Medicine, 1979.

53. Challem, J. J., "When It Comes to Vitamin Therapy in Advanced Cancer, More May Be Better," *The Nutrition Reporter,* March 1994.

54. Hoffer, A., and Pauling L., "Hardin Jones Biostatistical Analysis of Mortality Data for a Second Set of Cohorts of Cancer Patients with a Large Fraction Surviving at the Termination of the Study and a Comparison of Survival Times of Cancer Patients Receiving Large Regular Oral Doses of Vitamin C and Other Nutrients with Similar Patients Not Receiving These Doses," *Journal of Orthomolecular Medicine,* Third Quarter 1993;8:157–167.

55. Enstrom, J. E., "Vitamin C Intake and Mortality among a Sample of the United States Population," *Epidemiology,* May 1992;3:194–202.

56. Gaby, A. R., "Ester-C," *Townsend Letter for Doctors,* August/September 1995, 115.

CHAPTER 13

1. *Recommended Dietary Allowances,* National Academy Press, 1989.

2. Block, G., "The Data Support a Role for Antioxidants in Reducing Cancer Risk," *Nutrition Reviews,* June 1992;50:207–213.

3. Huemer, R. P., "Vitamin A and Cirrhosis," *Western Journal of Medicine,* July 1978;129:78.

4. Bendich, A., "Vitamins and Immunity," *Journal of Nutrition,* 1992;122:601–603.

5. Dennert, G., "Retinoids and the Immune System: Immunostimulation by Vitamin A," in *The Retinoids,* Sporn, M. B., Roberts, A. B., and Goodman, D. S., eds. Orlando: Academic Press, 1984;2:373–390.

6. Green, H. N., and Mallanby, E., "Vitamin A as an Anti-infective Agent," *British Medical Journal,* October 20, 1928;2:691–696.

7. Stephensen, C. B., et al., "Vitamin A Is Excreted in the Urine during Acute Infection," *American Journal of Clinical Nutrition,* September 1994,60:388–391.

8. Anonymous, "Lives on the Line," in *The Progress of Nations 1995,* New York: UNICEF, 1995, 13.

9. Sommer, A., "Vitamin A, Infectious Disease and Childhood Mortality: A 2¢ Solution?," *Journal of Infectious Diseases,* May 1993;167:1003–1007.

10. Ibid.

11. Sommer, A., "A Bridge too Far," in *The Progress of Nations 1995,* New York: UNICEF, 1995, 11.

12. Sommer, A., et al., "Impact of Vitamin A Supplementation on Childhood Mortality: A Randomized, Controlled Community Trial," *Lancet,* 1986;1:1169–1173.

13. Foster, A., and Sommer, A., "Corneal Ulceration, Measles, and Childhood Blindness in Tanzania," *British Journal of Ophthalmology,* 1987;71:331–343.

14. Sommer, A., 1995, op. cit.

15. Anonymous, "League Table of Action on Vitamin A," in *The Progress of Nations 1995,* New York: UNICEF, 1995, 12–13.

16. Fawzi, W. W., "Dietary Vitamin A Intake and the Risk of Mortality among Children," *American Journal of Clinical Nutrition,* February 1994;59:401–408.

17. Committee on Infectious Diseases, American Academy of Pediatrics, "Vitamin A Treatment of Measles," *Pediatrics,* May 1993;91:1014–1015.

18. Chytil, F., "The Lungs and Vitamin A," *American Journal of Physiology,* May 1992;262:L517–527.

19. Neuzil, K. M., et al., "Serum Vitamin A Levels in Respiratory Syncytial Virus Infection," *Journal of Pediatrics,* March 1994;124:433–436.

20. Ibid.

21. Ozsoylu, S., et al., "Vitamin A for Varicella," *Journal of Pediatrics,* December 1994;125:1017–1018.

22. Coutsoudis, A., et al., "Vitamin A Supplementation Enhances Specific IgG Antibody Levels and Total Lymphocyte Numbers while Improving Morbidity in Measles," *Pediatric Infectious Diseases Journal,* 1992;11:203–209.

23. Coutsoudis, A., et al., "The Effects of Vitamin A Supplementation on the Morbidity of Children Born to HIV-Infected Women," *American Journal of Public Health,* August 1995;85:1076–1081.

24. See Bendich, A., 1992, op. cit.

25. Committee on Diet, Nutrition and Cancer, Assembly of Life Sciences, National Research Council, *Diet, Nutrition and Cancer.* Washington, DC: National Academy Press, 1982.

26. Block, G., "Micronutrients and Cancer: Time for Action?" *Journal of the National Cancer Institute,* June 2, 1993;85:846–847.

27. Kardinaal, A. F. M., et al., "Antioxidants in Adipose Tissue and Risk of Myocardial Infarction: the EURAMIC Study," *Lancet,* December 4, 1993;342:1379–1384.

28. Allard, J. P., et al., "Effects of Beta-carotene Supplementation on Lipid Peroxidation in Humans," *American Journal of Clinical Nutrition,* April 1994;59:884–890.

29. Mayne, S. T., et al., "Dietary Beta-carotene and Lung Cancer Risk in U.S. Nonsmokers," *Journal of the National Cancer Institute,* January 5, 1994;86:33–38.

30. Lambert, L. A., et al., "The Protective but Nonsynergistic Effect of Dietary Beta-carotene and Vitamin E on Skin Tumorigenesis in Skh Mice," *Nutrition and Cancer,* 1994;21:1–12.

31. See Bendich, A., "Carotenoids and the Immune Response," *Journal of Nutrition,* 1989;119;112–115.

32. Ibid.

33. Ibid.

34. Umegaki, K., et al., "Beta-carotene Prevents X-ray Induction of Micronuclei in Human Lymphocytes," *American Journal of Clinical Nutrition,* February 1994;59:409–412.

35. Lunec, J., et al., "Free Radical Oxidation (Peroxidation) Products in Serum and Synovial Fluid in Rheumatoid Arthritis," *Journal of Rheumatology,* 1981;8:233–245.

36. See Bendich, A., 1989, op. cit.

37. Ibid.

38. Fuller, C. J., et al., "Effect of Beta-carotene Supplementation on Photosupression of Delayed-Type Hypersensitivity in Normal Young Men," *American Journal of Clinical Nutrition,* 1992;56:684–690.

39. Mikhail, M. S., et al., "Decreased Beta-carotene Levels in Exfoliated Vaginal Epithelial Cells in Women with Vaginal Candidiasis," *American Joural of Reproductive Immunology,* 1994;32:221–225.

40. Murata, T., et al., "Effect of Long-term Administration of Beta-carotene on Lymphocytes Subsets in Humans," *American Journal of Clincial Nutrition,* October 1994;60:597–602.

41. Baum, M., et al., "Inadequate Dietary Intake and Altered Nutrition Status in Early HIV-1 Infection," *Nutrition,* 1994;10:16–20.

42. Coodley, G. O., et al., "Micronutrient Concentrations in the HIV Wasting Syndrome," *AIDS,* December 1993;7:1595–1600.

43. Ullrich, R., et al., "Serum Carotene Deficiency in HIV-Infected Patients," *AIDS,* May 1994;8:661–665.

44. Garewal, H. S., et al., "A Preliminary Trial of Beta-carotene in Subjects Infected with the Human Immunodeficiency Virus," *Journal of Nutrition*, March 1992;122 (3 Suppl):S728–732.

45. Coodley, G. O., et al., "Beta-carotene in HIV Infection," *Journal of Acquired Immune Deficiency Syndrome*, 1993;6:272–276.

46. Challem, J. J., "Beta-carotene Can Help AIDS and CFS Patients," *The Nutrition Reporter*, May 1993.

47. Baum, M., op. cit.

48. Chen, H., and Tappel, A. L., "Protection by Vitamin E, Selenium, Trolox C, Ascorbic Acid Palmitate, Acetylcysteine, Coenzyme Q, Beta-carotene, Canthaxanthin, and (+)-catechin against Oxidative Damage to Liver Slices Measured by Oxidized Heme Proteins," *Free Radical Biology and Medicine*, 1994;16:437–444.

49. Committee on Infectious Diseases, American Academy of Pediatrics, op. cit.

50. Rothman, K. J., et al., "Teratogenicity of High Vitamin A Intake," *New England Journal of Medicine*, 333:1369–1373.

51. Bendich, A., and Langseth, L., "Safety of Vitamin A," *American Journal of Clinical Nutrition*, February 1989;49:358–371.

52. de Pee, S., et al., "Lack of Improvement in Vitamin A Status with Increased Consumption of Dark-Green Leafy Vegetables," *Lancet*, July 8, 1995;346:75–81.

CHAPTER 14

1. Committee on Dietary Allowances, Food and Nutrition Board, National Research Council, *Recommended Dietary Allowances*, National Academy Press, 1980.

2. Lehr, D., "A Possible Beneficial Effect of Selenium Administration in Antiarrhythmic Therapy," *Journal of the American College of Nutrition*, October 1994;13:496–498.

3. Beck, M. A., et al., "Rapid Genomic Evolution of a Non-Virulent Coxsackievirus B3 in Selenium-Deficient Mice Results in Selection of Identical Virulent Isolates," *Nature Medicine*, May 1995;1:433–436.

4. Beck, M. A., et al., "Increased Virulence of a Human Enterovirus (Coxsackie B3) in Selenium-Deficient Mice," *Journal of Infectious Diseases*, 1994;170:351–357.

5. Beck, M. A., et al., "Benign Human Enterovirus Becomes Virulent in Selenium-Deficient Mice," *Journal of Medical Virology*, 1994;43:166–170.

6. Beck, M. A., et al., "Vitamin E Deficiency Intensifies the Myocardial Injury of Coxsackievirus B3 Infection of Mice," *Journal of Nutrition*, 1994;124:345–358.

7. Beck, M. A., et al., 1995, op. cit.

8. McBride, J., "Nutritional Deficiency Causes Nice Virus to Mutate to Nasty," press release issued by the USDA Agricultural Research Service, April 10, 1995.

9. Gauntt, C., and Tracy, S., "Deficient Diet Evokes Nasty Heart Virus," *Nature Medicine,* May 1995;1:405–406.

10. Taylor, E. W., et al., "A Basis for New Approaches to the Chemotherapy of AIDS: Novel Genes in HIV-1 Potentially Encode Selenoproteins Expressed by Robosomal Frameshifting and Termination Suppression," *Journal of Medicinal Chemistry,* August 19, 1994;37:2637–2654.

11. Dworkin, B. M., "Selenium Deficiency in HIV Infection and the Acquired Immunodeficiency Syndrome (AIDS)," *Chemico-Biological Interactions,* June 1994;91:181–186.

12. Roy, M., et al., "Supplementation with Selenium and Human Immune Cell Functions. I. Effect on Lymphocyte Proliferation and Interleukin 2 Receptor Expression," *Biological Trace Element Research,* 1994;41:103–114.

13. Kiremidjian-Schumacher, L., et al., "Supplementation with Selenium and Human Immune Cell Functions. II. Effect on Cytotoxic Lymphocytes and Natural Killer Cells," *Biological Trace Element Research,* 1994;41:115–127.

14. Dworkin, B. M., op. cit.

15. Taylor, E. W., "Selenium and Cellular Immunity: Evidence That Selenoproteins May Be Encoded In the +1 Reading Frame Overlapping the Human CD4, CD8 and HLA-DR Genes," *Biological Trace Element Research,* May 1995;49:85–95.

16. Taylor, E. W., et al., "Do Some Viruses Encode Selenoproteins? Assessment of the Theory in the Light of Current Theoretical, Experimental and Clinical Data," presented at the International Society for Antiviral Research, eighth international conference, Santa Fe, NM, April 23–28, 1995.

17. Sandstrom, P. A., et al., "Lipid Hydroperoxides Induce Apoptosis in T cells Displaying a HIV-Associated Glutathione Peroxidase Deficiency," *Journal of Biological Chemistry,* January 14, 1994;269:794–801.

18. Dworkin, B. M., 1994, op. cit.

19. Written communication with Ethan Will Taylor, December 21, 1994.

20. Sappey, C., et al., "Stimulation of Glutathione Peroxidase Activity Decreases HIV Type I Activation after Oxidative Stress," *AIDS Research and Human Retroviruses,* 1994;10:1451–1461.

21. Piret, B., et al., "NF-Kappa B Transcription Factor and Human Immunodeficiency Virus Type 1 (HIV-1) Activation by Methylene Blue Photosensitization," *European Journal of Biochemistry,* March 1, 1995;228:447–455.

22. Sappey, C., et al., op. cit.

23. Schrauzer, G. N., and Sacher, J., "Selenium in the Maintenance and Therapy of HIV-Infected Patients," *Chemico-Biological Interactions,* June 1994;91:199–205.

24. Sappey, C., et al., op. cit.

25. Schrauzer, G. N., and Sacher, J., op. cit.

26. Tang, A. M., et al., "Dietary Micronutrient Intake and Risk of Progression to Acquired Immunodeficiency Syndrome (AIDS) in Human Immunodeficiency Virus Type 1 (HIV-1)-Infected Homosexual Men," *American Journal of Epidemiology,* December 1993;138:937–951.

27. "Vitamin Megadoses May Slow Onset of AIDS, Researchers Find," *Nation's Health,* January 1994;24:27.

28. Taylor, E. W., and Ramanathan, C. S., "Theoretical Evidence That the Ebola Virus May Be Selenium-Dependent: A Factor in Pathogenesis and Viral Outbreaks?," *Journal of Orthomolecular Medicine,* 1995;10 (3–4): 131–138.

29. Ibid.

30. Ziegler, J. L., "Endemic Kaposi's Sarcoma in Africa and Local Volcanic Soils," *Lancet,* November 27, 1993;342:1348–1351.

31. Schillhorn van Veen, T. W., et al., "Mineral Deficiency in Ruminants in Subsaharan Africa: A Review," *Tropical Animal Health and Production,* 1990;22:197–205.

32. Vanderpas, J. B., et al., "Iodine and Selenium Deficiency Associated with Cretinism in Northern Zaire," *American Journal of Clinical Nutrition,* December 1990;52:1083–1086.

33. Golden, M. H. N., correspondence, *Protozoological Abstracts,* 1993, 017–00398.

34. Taylor, E. W., and Ramanathan, C. S., op. cit.

35. Ibid.

36. Hou, J. C., et al., "Inhibitory Effect of Selenium on Complement Activation and Its Clinical Significance," *Chinese Medical Journal,* November 1993;73:645–646.

37. Taylor, E. W., and Ramanathan, C. S., op. cit.

38. E-mails with Will Taylor, December 15 and 28, 1995.

39. Stampfer, M. J., et al., "The Epidemiology of Selenium and Cancer," *Cancer Surveys,* 1987;6:623–633.

40. Clark, L. C., "The Epidemiology of Selenium and Cancer," *Federation Proceedings,* June 1985;44:2584–2589.

41. Ibid.

CHAPTER 15

1. Folkers, K., "Heart Failure Is a Dominant Deficiency of Coenzyme Q_{10} and Challenges for Future Clinical Research on CoQ_{10}," *Clinical Investigator,* August 1993;71:51S–54S.

2. Mitchell, P., "Protonmotive Redox Mechanism of Cytochrome b-c_1 Complex in the Respiratory Chain: Protonmotive Ubiquinone Cycle," *FEBS Letters,* August 1975;56:1–6.

3. Mitchell, P., "The Protonmotive Q cycle: A General Formulation, *FEBS Letters,* November 1975;59:137–139.

4. Luft, R., "The Development of Mitochondrial Medicine," *Biochimica et Biophysica Acta,* May 24, 1995;1271:1–6.

5. Ames, B. N., et al., "Mitochondrial Decay in Aging," *Biochimica et Biophysica Acta,* May 24, 1995;1271:165–170.

6. Bliznakov, E. G., and Hunt, G. L., *The Miracle Nutrient: Coenzyme Q_{10},* Bantam: New York, 1986.

7. Langsjoen, P. H., et al., "Effective Treatment with Coenzyme Q_{10} of Patients with Chronic Myocardial Disease," *Drugs Under Experimental and Clinical Research,* 1985;11:577–579.

8. Challem, J., "The Heart Remedy Your Doctor Never Heard Of," *Natural Health,* March/April 1994;44–50.

9. Langsjoen, P. H., et al., "Effective and Safe Therapy with Coenzyme Q_{10} for Cardiomyopathy," *Klinische Wochenschrift,* 1988;66:583–590.

10. See the entire supplemental issue of *Clinical Investigator,* August 1993;71S:145–149.

11. Challem, J., op. cit.

12. Ibid.

13. Bliznakov, E. G., and Hunt, G. L., 1986, op. cit.

14. Folkers, K., et al., "Survival of Cancer Patients on Therapy with Coenzyme Q_{10}," *Biochemical and Biophysical Research Communications,* April 15, 1993;192:241–245.

15. Lockwood, K., and Folkers, K., "Partial and Complete Regression of Breast Cancer in Patients in Relation to Dosage of Coenzyme Q_{10}," *Biochemical and Biophysical Research Communications,* March 30, 1994;199:1504–1508.

16. Lockwood, K., et al., "Progress on Therapy of Breast Cancer with Vitamin Q_{10} and the Regression of Metastases," *Biochemical and Biophysical Research Communications,* July 6, 1995;212:172–177.

17. Bliznakov, E. G., "Coenzyme Q in Experimental Infections and Neoplasia," in *Biochemical and Clinical Aspects of Coenzyme Q,* Folkers, K., and Yamamura, Y., eds., Elsevier Scientific Publishing, Amsterdam, 1977, 73–83.

18. Bliznakov, E. G., and Hunt, G. L., 1986, op. cit.

19. Stone, R., "Search for Sepsis Drugs Goes on Despite Past Failure," *Science,* April 15, 1994;264:365–367.

20. Lelli, J. L., et al., "Effects of Coenzyme Q_{10} on the Mediator Cascade of Sepsis," *Circulatory Shock,* 1993;39:178–187.

21. Jenkins, R., and Mowbray, eds., *Post-Viral Fatigue Syndrome,* John Wiley & Sons Ltd.: West Sussex, England, 1991.

22. Barak, Y., et al., MELAS Syndrome, Peripheral Neuropathy and Cytochrome c-oxidase Deficiency: A Case Report and Review of the Literature, *Israel Journal of Medical Science,* April 1995;31:224–229.

23. Folkers, K., and Simonsen, R., "Two Successful Double-Blind Trials with Coenzyme Q_{10} (Vitamin Q_{10}) on Muscular Dystrophies and Neurogenic Atrophies," *Biochimica et Biophysica Acta,* May 24, 1995;1271:281–286.

24. Folkers, K., "Biochemical Deficiencies of Coenzyme Q_{10} in HIV-infection and Exploratory Treatment," *Biochemical and Biophysical Research Communications,* June 16, 1988;153:888–896.

25. U.S. patent number 5,011,858.

26. *Journal American,* Bellevue, Washington, November 11, 1993.

27. Interviews with J.C., April 22, 1994 and November 15, 1995.

28. Folkers, K., and Simonsen, R., op. cit.

29. Huemer, R. P., et al., "Mitochondrial Studies in Senescent Mice—II. Specific Activity, Buoyant Density, and Turnover of Mitochondrial DNA," *Experimental Gerontology;* 6:327–334.

30. Harding, A. E., "Growing Old: The Most Common Mitochondrial Disease of All?" *Nature Genetics,* December 1992;2:251–252.

31. Nutritional Medicine Today conference, Vancouver, Washington, April 30, 1994.

32. Challem, J. J., "CoQ$_{10}$ May Be the Miracle Nutrient of the 1990s," *Let's Live,* August 1995.

33. Folkers, K., et al., "Lovastatin Decreases Coenzyme Q Levels in Humans," *Proceedings of the National Academy of Sciences of the USA,* November 1990;87:8931–8934.

34. Lelli, J. L., op. cit.

35. Langsjoen, P. H., et al., 1988, op. cit.

CHAPTER 16

1. Griffith, R. S., et al., "A Multicentered Study of Lysine Therapy in Herpes Simplex Infection," *Dermatologica,* 1978;156:257–267.

2. Walsh, D. E., "Subjective Response to Lysine in the Therapy of Herpes Simplex," *Journal of Antimicrobial Chemistry,* November 1983;12:489–496.

3. Jirillo, E., et al., "Effects of Acetyl-L-carnitine Oral Administration on Lymphocyte Antibacterial Activity and TNF-alpha Levels in Patients with Active Pulmonary Tuberculosis. A Randomized Double Blind versus Placebo Study," *Immunopharmacology and Immunotoxicology,* 1991;13:135–146.

4. De Simone, C., et al., "High Dose L-carnitine Improves Immunologic and Metabolic Parameters in AIDS Patients," *Immunopharmacology and Immunotoxicology,* January 1993;15:1–12.

5. De Simone, C., et al., "Carnitine Depletion in Peripheral Blood Mononuclear Cells from Patients with AIDS: Effect of Oral L-carnitine," *AIDS,* May 1994;8:655–660.

6. Wu, D., et al., "In Vitro Glutathione Supplementation Enhances Interleukin-2 Production and Mitogenic Response of Peripheral Blood Mononuclear Cells from Young and Old Subjects," *Journal of Nutrition,* May 1994;124:655–663.

7. Sappey, C., et al., "Stimulation of Glutathione Peroxidase Activity Decreases HIV Type I Activation after Oxidative Stress," *AIDS Research and Human Retroviruses,* 1994;10:1451–1461.

8. Kalebic, T., et al., "Suppression of Human Immunodeficiency Virus Expression in Chronically Infected Monocytic Cells by Glutathione, Glutathione Ester, and N-acetylcysteine," *Proceedings of the National Academy of Sciences of the USA,* February 1, 1991;88:986–990.

9. *New York Times,* May 3, 1994.

10. Johnston, C. S., et al., "Vitamin C Elevates Red Blood Cell Glutathione in Healthy Adults," *American Journal of Clinical Nutrition,* July 1993;58:103–105.

11. Chandra, R. K., and Purl, S., "Vitamin B-6 Modulation of Immune Responses and Infection," in *Vitamin B-6: Its Role in Health and Disease,* Reynolds, R. D., and Leklem, J. E., eds., Alan R. Liss Inc., New York, 1985, 163–175.

12. Meydani, S. N., et al., "Vitamin B6 Deficiency Impairs Interleukin 2 Production and Lymphocyte Proliferation in Elderly Adults," *American Journal of Clinical Nutrition,* 1991;53:1275–1280.

13. Baum, M. K., et al., "Association of B6 Status with Parameters of Immune Function in Early HIV-1 Infection," *Journal of Acquired Immune Deficiency Syndromes,* 1991;4:1122–1132.

14. Reeve, V. E., et al., "Pyridoxine Supplementation Protects Mice from Suppression of Contact Hypersensitivy Induced by 1-acetyl-4-tetrahydroxybutylimidazole (THI), Ultraviolet B Radiation (280–320 nm), or cis-urocanic acid," *American Journal of Clinical Nutrition*, March 1995;61:571–576.

15. Bendich, A., et al., "Dietary Vitamin E Requirement for Optimum Immune Responses in the Rat," *Journal of Nutrition*, 1986;116:675–681.

16. Meydani, M., "Vitamin E," *Lancet*, January 21, 1995;345:170–175.

17. Meydani, S. N., et al., "Vitamin E Supplementation Enhances Cell-Mediated Immunity in Healthy Elderly Subjects," *American Journal of Clinical Nutrition*, 1990;52:557–563.

18. Meydani, M., et al., "Effect of Long-term Vitamin E Supplementation on Lipid Peroxidation and Immune Responses of Young and Old Subjects," *FASEB Journal*;1993;7:A415.

19. Wang, Y., and Watson, R. R., "Potential Therapeutics of Vitamin E (Tocopherol) in AIDS and HIV," *Drugs*, September 1994;48:327–338.

20. Kline, K., et al., "Growth Inhibitory Effects of Vitamin E Succinate on Retrovirus-Transformed Tumor Cells In Vitro," *Nutrition and Cancer*, 1990;14:27–41.

21. Passwater, R. A., "Lipoic Acid against AIDS: An Interview with Dr. Lester Packer, *Whole Foods*, December 1995;50–60.

22. Stoll, S., et al., "The Potent Free Radical Scavenger Alpha-lipoic Acid Improves Cognition in Rodents," *Annals of the New York Academy of Sciences*, June 30, 1994;717:122–128.

23. Suzuki, Y. J., et al., "Alpha-lipoic Acid Is a Potent Inhibitor of NF-kappa B Activation in Human T Cells," *Biochemical and Biophysical Research Communications*, December 30, 1992;189:1709–1715.

24. Godfrey, J. C., "Zinc Gluconate and the Common Cold: A Controlled Clinical Study," *Journal of International Medical Research*, June 1992;20:234–246.

25. Kelley, D. S., et al., "Effects of Low-Copper Diets on Human Immune Response," *American Journal of Clinical Nutrition*, August 1995;62:412–416.

26. Sobota, A. E., "Inhibition of Bacterial Adherence by Cranberry Juice: Potential Use for the Treatment of Urinary Tract Infections," *Journal of Urology*, May 1984;131:1013–1016.

27. Avorn, J., et al., "Reduction of Bacteriuria and Pyuria after Ingestion of Cranberry Juice," *Journal of the American Medical Association*, March 9, 1994;271:751–754.

28. Fleet, J. C., "New Support for a Folk Remedy: Cranberry Juice Reduces Bacteriuria and Pyuria in Elderly Women," *Nutrition Reviews*, May 1994;52:168–170.

29. Berg, P. A., and Daniel, P. T., "Effects of Flavonoid Compounds on the Immune Response," in *Plant Flavonoids in Biology and Medicine II: Biochemical, Cellular, and Medicinal Properties*, Cody, V., et al., eds., Alan R. Liss Inc., New York, 1988, 157–171.

30. Otake, S., et al., "Anticaries Effects of Polyphenolic Compounds from Japanese Green Tea," *Caries Research*, 1991;25:438–443.

31. *Science News*, April 18, 1993.

32. Nakayama, M., et al., "Inhibition of the Infectivity of Influenza Virus by Tea Polyphenols," *Antiviral Research*, August 1993;21:289–299.

33. Mukoyama, A., et al., "Inhibition of Rotavirus and Enterovirus Infections by Tea Extracts," *Japanese Journal of Medical Science and Biology*, August 1991;44:181–186.

34. Horiuchi, Y., et al., "Protective Activity of Tea and Catechins against *Bordetella pertussis*," *Kansenshogaku Zasshi—Journal of the Japanese Association for Infectious Diseases*, May 1992;66:599–605.

35. Chosa, H., et al., "Antimicrobial and Microbicidal Activities of Tea and Catechins against *Mycoplasma*," *Kansenshogaku Zasshi—Journal of the Japanese Association for Infectious Diseases*, May 1992;66:606–611.

36. Toda, M., et al., "Antibacterial and Bactericidal Activities of Tea Extracts and Catechins against Methicillin-Resistant *Staphylococcus aureus*," *Nippon Saikingaku Zasshi—Japanese Journal of Bacteriology*, September 1991;46:839–845.

37. Kono, K., et al., "Antibacterial Activity of Epigallocatechin Gallate against Methicillin-Resistant *Staphylococcus aureus*," *Kansenshogaku Zasshi—Journal of the Japanese Association for Infectious Diseases*, December 1994;68:1518–1522.

38. Stavric, B., "Quercetin in Our Diet: From Potent Mutagen to Probable Anticarcinogen," *Clinical Biochemistry*, 1994;27:245–248.

39. Kaul, T. N., "Antiviral Effect of Flavonoids on Human Viruses," *Journal of Medical Virology*, 1985;15:71–79.

40. Zumla, A., and Lulat, A., "Honey—A Remedy Rediscovered," *Journal of the Royal Society of Medicine*, July 1989;82:384–385.

41. Subrahmanyam, M., "Honey-Impregnated Gauze versus Amniotic Membrane in the Treatment of Burns," *Burns*, August 1994;20:331–333.

42. Efram, S. E., et al., "The Antimicrobial Spectrum of Honey and Its Clinical Significance," *Infection*, July–August 1992;20:227–229.

43. al Somal, N., et al., "Susceptibility of *Helicobacter pylori* to the Antibacterial Activity of Manuka Honey," *Journal of the Royal Society of Medicine*, January 1994;87:9–12.

44. Zumla, A., and Lulat, A., op. cit.

45. Qiao, Z., and Chen, R., "Isolation and Identification of Antibiotic Constituents of Propolis from Henan," *China Journal of Chinese Materia Medica*, August 1991;16:481–482.

46. Krol, W., et al., "Synergistic Effect of Ethanolic Extract of Propolis and Antibiotics on the Growth of *Staphylococcus aureus*," *Arzneimittel-Forschung*, May 1993;43:607–609.

47. Ikeno, K., et al., "Effects of Propolis on Dental Caries in Rats," *Caries Research*, 1991;25:347–351.

48. Takaisi-Kikuni, N. B., and Schilcher, H., "Electron Microscopic and Microcalorimetric Investigations of the Possible Mechanism of the Antibacterial Action of a Defined Propolis Provenance," *Planta Medica*, June 1994;60:222–227.

49. Lab sample #1803E1, October 27, 1995.

50. Focht, J., et al., "Bactericidal Effect of Propolis In Vitro against Agents Causing Upper Respiratory Tract Infections," *Arzneimittel-Forschung*, August 1993;43:921–923.

51. Rao, C. V., et al., "Inhibitory Effect of Caffeic Acid Esters on

Azoxymethane-Induced Biochemical Changes and Aberrant Crypt Foci Formation in Rat Colon," *Cancer Research*, September 15, 1993;53:1482–1488.

52. Reiter, R. J., and Robinson, J., *Melatonin: Your Body's Natural Wonder Drug*, Bantam, New York, 1995.

53. Nelson, R. J., and Blom, J. M., "Photoperiodic Effects on Tumor Development and Immune Function" *Journal of Biological Rhythms*, 1994;9:233–249.

54. Grad, B. R., and Rozencwaig, R., "The Role of Melatonin and Serotonin in Aging: Update," *Psychoneuroendocrinology*, 1993;18:283–295.

55. Lissoni, P., et al., "A Study of the Mechanisms Involved in the Immuno-stimulatory Action of the Pineal Hormone in Cancer Patients," *Oncology*, November/December, 1993;50:399–402.

56. Giordano, M., et al., "Seasonal Variation in Antibody-Dependent Cellular Cytotoxicity Regulation by Melatonin," *FASEB Journal*, August 1993;7:1052–1054.

57. Maestroni, G. J., "The Immunoneuroendocrine Role of Melatonin," *Journal of Pineal Research*, January 1993;14:1–10.

58. Ben-Nathan, D., "Protective Effects of Melatonin in Mice Infected with Encephalitis Viruses," *Archives of Virology*, 1995;140:223–230.

59. Reiter, R. J., and Robinson, J., *Melatonin: Your Body's Natural Wonder Drug*, Bantam, New York, 1995, 51.

60. Muroi, H., and Kubo, I., "Bactericidal Effects of Anacardic Acid and Totarol on Methicillin-Resistant *Staphylococcus aureus*," *Biosci Biotech Biochem*, 1994;58:1925–1926.

61. Braunig, B., et al., "*Echinacea purpurea* Radix for Strengthening the Immune Response in Flu-like Infections," *Z Phytother*, 1993;13:7–13.

CHAPTER 17

1. Moskowitz, R., "Immunizations: A Dissenting View," 133–166; in *Dissent in Medicine: Nine Doctors Speak Out*, Contemporary Books, Chicago, 1985.

2. Woodin, K. A., et al., "Physician and Parent Opinions. Are Children Becoming Pincushions from Immunizations?" *Archives of Pediatric and Adolescent Medicine*, August 1995;149:845–849.

3. See *Vaccination: 100 Years of Orthodox Research Shows That Vaccines Represent a Medical Assault on the Immune System*, Scheibner V, self-published, 1993.

4. Ibid.

5. Coulter, H. L., speaking at the Nutritional Medicine Today conference, Vancouver, B.C., Canada, April 30, 1994.

6. Kalokerinos, A., *Every Second Child*, Keats Publishing, New Canaan, CN, 1981.

7. Jack Challem interview with Lendon H. Smith, December 14, 1995.

8. Associated Press, August 24, 1995.

9. The *Oregonian*, October 24, 1995.

10. Jack Challem telephone interview with Dr. Levy, January 5, 1996.

INDEX

꙰

Italic page numbers indicate material in tables or illustrations.